The

BODY LANGUAGE

of

HEALTH

Hamish MacGregor

©First Edition 2008
Published & distributed by
Eclipse Naturalcare Ltd
1 Prime Parkway, Derby, DE1 3QB
United Kingdom
Tel: 0044 (0)1332 365318
Fax 0044 (0)1332 292003
Email: info@eclipsenaturalcare.com
Web: www.eclipsenaturalcare.com
ISBN 978-0-9557909-0-4

CONTENTS

The Body Language of Health

The Body Language of Health

The Body Language of Health

INTRODUCTION

When my wife Elsie developed a craving for lettuce, it didn't take me very long to realise how important that was. Her body somehow knew she needed lettuce because it contains chemicals called sulphorathanes.

She had breast cancer.

I am sure she had developed a craving for lettuce because sulphorathanes are nature's defence against cancers of all kinds. But how did her body know? As a forensic scientist I am used to looking for clues, and I discovered that most health problems seem to reveal themselves early in subtle signs and symptoms, provided you know how to read the signs. Some signs reveal themselves as cravings, others might be poor skin condition, the inability to remember your dreams, even sneezing in bright sunlight. These signs form a fascinating new language which is not difficult to learn.

I have called it Body Language. And it is very simple to understand. Notice these symptoms early, and you could well improve your chances of leading a long and fruitful life.

I have extended this new language into the most comprehensive health diagnostic questionnaire on the internet, with over 1400 Body Language questions that allow the diagnostic system to interpret your answers and give you targeted nutrition to ease and hopefully eradicate your ailments. It has taken years of painstaking work and nowhere else will you find such a comprehensive, complete diagnostic system.

Surprisingly, no-one seems to have studied and accumulated these signs and symptoms before, at least, not to any great extent. Doctors, of course use this system to a limited extent every day without you realising, and I am sure their methods are much more sophisticated. All I have done is explain why these signs are valid. Yet I am nevertheless surprised these signs are not so well known. We're all tuned into many other kinds of 'early warning signs' of problems in other aspects of our everyday life. Like that annoying rattle which alerts us to an imminent problem with our car. Or a sick plant that highlights a problem in our garden. Just like Body Language, these early symptoms are not important in themselves, but if left unobserved, they could become serious.

Take earlobe creases, for example. A diagonal crease on the fleshy part of your earlobe is claimed to be a reliable indicator of cardiovascular disease. You should use this early indicator to make improvements to your diet and lifestyle, and at the same time review your weight and get more exercise. Perhaps these actions could save you from a heart attack.

The Body Language of Health

Body Language is not a substitute for medicine. Body Language complements it, as part of an integrated medical approach to health. Acting on Body Language signs and symptoms won't be detrimental and it will almost certainly give you added benefits. With Body Language signs and symptoms, you have everything to gain and nothing to lose.

Body Language is a fascinating insight into numerous little signs and symptoms that allow us to tap into the body's early warning system. A system that tells us all may not be well. But don't take these too seriously. The main purpose of this book is to show you that your body is a complex machine, and that one problem can be indicative of another. In fact during the discovery of Body Language I have set out to explain some of the intricacies of the body in non-medical terminology.

Mostly, the conditions that Body Language highlights can be controlled with better diet as a means of boosting some deficiency or other. So wherever practicable I have listed foods that are rich in the missing mineral, element or vitamin. But I have resisted the page-filler route that many health books have taken of including lots of tempting recipes. The only recipe you'll find in this book is a recipe for good health.

Only a few of the Body Language signs are indicative of very serious medical problems; and even most of those are quite minor 'early warning symptoms'. However that doesn't mean you can ignore these because if the problem goes unchecked it could often lead to other, much more serious health problems. Like all matters of health, if you have any concerns whatsoever you should consult your doctor. No doctor ever complains about you wasting their time, on the contrary they will be delighted you are taking more interest in your personal health as long as your concern is genuine.

Learn Body Language and you will learn to listen to your body. It has an important message for you.

If you want to find out more about Body Language, I recommend you look at the on-line questionnaire at www.mybodylanguage.co.uk and find out what your body is really thinking.

I wrote this book because I was concerned that the EU was eroding the opportunities of the public to buy supplements. Did you know that most of our common herbs, and many of the essential ingredients to herbal and mineral remedies will no longer be available once the legislation kicks in? All because the greedy pharmaceutiucal giants want all the business for themselves. Time to kick them out, I say.

Before it is too late to save our vital supplements, herbs and minerals.

FOOD AND FOOD FADS

Do you crave lettuce?

Why all cravings should be taken very seriously

I expect you already know that pregnant women often crave particular foods. At one time, they were renowned for eating pieces of coal, before the days of central heating when the coal scuttle resided by the hearth. But I had never come across a craving for lettuce until it entered into my life in a sinister way.

After 25 years of happy marriage, my wife Elsie suddenly and inexplicably developed a new passion. But it wasn't a torrid affair with another man, it wasn't an obsession with buying shoes, it wasn't even a fetish for kinky underwear, unfortunately. No. Her new passion was lettuce.

Lettuce came to dominate her diet. She took to eating at least two or three lettuces every day. But not in a salad. She would take a lettuce out of the 'fridge, cut slices off it with the bread knife, and chomp away at it, eating maybe half a lettuce or even a whole lettuce at one sitting.

This straight away aroused my suspicions, because I had heard of a condition called 'pica' which is an obsession for eating any kind of food. The medical books say that 'pica' is usually a phobia, but my wife had no other symptoms we could identify, and she certainly was not prone to phobias, except for the usual women's fear of spiders and replacing the toilet roll. Apparently pica can be stress related but the only stress she had was the worry that she might run out of her lettuce supply before the shops opened again.

I did some investigating on the internet. There was nothing about lettuce craving and precious little about lettuce and nutrition. Lettuce seemed to be nearly all water. A craving for lettuce appeared to be unheard of previously. That's a big failing of the internet; you only get out what you put in. But, you could say, that was the tip of the Iceberg. (That's a popular variety of lettuce, by the way).

One day, about a month after this pica developed, Elsie was washing in the bathroom in front of the bathroom mirror, lit by a shaft of sunlight from the window, and she spotted a dimple on the side of her breast that she hadn't noticed before.

She went to the doctor. Meanwhile, I tried a different tactic for searching the Internet. I put *lettuce* and *cancer* into the search this time. Within seconds I found something that sent the hairs on my neck tingling. Lettuce is rich in chemicals called sulphorathanes. These naturally occurring chemicals can kill human cancers and they are currently being investigated as potential anti-cancer drugs. Instinctively I knew straight away she had a big problem.

A few days later, biopsy results confirmed that she had developed breast cancer.

So what was happening here? It seemed as though her brain had been telling her mouth that it had to have lettuce. It's a lot more complicated than that, of course, her immune system was telling her brain that it had to have sulphorathanes. But she didn't even know that Webbs Wonderful lettuce was anything more than a bit of decoration in a salad, so how could that be?

Elsie was admitted to hospital for an operation, followed by a course of radiography. The strangest thing was, as soon as she had the operation, her interest in lettuce disappeared totally.

As time progressed, the consultant seemed pleased with my wife's progress, but not once did she ask, 'Still not interested in eating lettuce, Mrs MacGregor?' But to us, it was as important a part of the check up list as any of the tests that the Health Service had devised.

It seemed that her body knew what it needed, and switched on her craving to help fight the cancer with the sulphorathanes in the lettuce. If so, Webbs really is wonderful!

But how did her body know?

As a forensic scientist, I know that every action leaves behind evidence that can be pieced back together. We are taught that every contact leaves evidence of that contact. And for every 'outcome' there is a set of circumstances that was the 'cause' because everything in life is a series of 'cause and effects'. I believe this is just as true for the cause of a pica craving as it is for the cause of a fatal road accident that I might be called upon to explain.

I usually find there is a good reason for everything, even if the real reason is a bit obscure and requires an inquisitive mind to get to the bottom of it. The milk in tea debate is a good example. There is a typically English debate about whether milk should go into a teacup before you pour the tea, or whether the milk should be added after you have poured the tea. Theoretically it shouldn't really make much difference to the flavour, but the English are passionate about tea and this story has perpetuated for hundreds of years. So, you would suspect there might be something more to this story.

And there is. It seems that there was a lot of snobbery associated with the tea drinking ritual in the past, when tea was so expensive that tea caddies had locks on them to stop the servants from helping themselves. I know a bit about fluid mechanics, and I know that the milk disperses better when the tea is added to the milk rather than vice-versa. It also helps to cool the tea, and the reduced thermal shock to the milk is less likely to develop sterilised-fat compounds; so putting the milk in first is scientifically the more sensible approach.

But the real reason for the debate is more complicated. Early, cheap ceramics were liable to crack if boiling hot tea was poured into them, so putting the milk in the cup first would also help to cool down the tea and produce less of a thermal shock to the cup, so it was less likely to shatter. That suited most people, because they could only afford cheap crockery. Only the very wealthiest could afford to buy the finest porcelain recently imported from the far east, known as Bone China.

And so people who could afford the best 'China' cups would deliberately put the tea in first to demonstrate to their guests the superiority of their crockery. Hence the real reason for the big debate, all designed to bring attention to the fact that your cups were superior. It is all down to crockery-snobbery that has perpetuated to this day.

Incidentally, if you haven't already thought of it and aren't one step ahead of me here, that's also why we warm the teapot before filling it with tea and boiling water. It has very little with ensuring the tea is as hot as possible to extract the maximum flavour.

Following the lettuce addiction I started to gather a number of other examples of the body's signs and symptoms of deficiencies, disease and imbalance. I have called these signs and symptoms 'Body Language'. Remarkably, after extensive research, the collection extends to over 1400 separate questions about your body or your habits, so I have gathered them into one stupendous medical diagnostic system that you can complete for yourself on the internet at www.mybodylanguage.co.uk

Now, you can read this book from start to finish, and I hope that you do because it highlights some bizarre stories that are hidden within various categories, but you can also dip in and read up on individual Body Language signs, or try and resolve that niggling health issue that seems to stop you from enjoying perfect health.

The Body Language signs and symptoms have been put into categories, so you can focus in on your favourite part of the body. You will probably guess which one is mine.

The Body Language of Health

Now some Body Language signs are straightforward, but some need a bit of further investigation. Many are 'old wives tales' that have fallen out of favour, but where modern science has been able to explain why they are fundamentally sound, I have included what currently seems to be the logical explanation. These answers are not infallible, though, and I hope the categories will enable you to explore your symptom further, or do some lateral thinking for yourself as to cause and effect.

The power of information, and more pica stories

Having collected a lot of information about Body Language, I launched a home-made website listing a wide range of Body Language signs. Within a few days the newspapers featured extracts from the site, and the site received an incredible three quarters of a million hits in the first week. That site is still there under www.mybodylanguage.co.uk and it has received so much traffic that the site is listed on the first page of most web search engines even if you search for the ubiquitous 'body language'.

One of the surfers on the site was very fortunate indeed. Her mother crunched ice cubes like they were sweets. Not the occasional ice cube, but trays of them at one sitting. This was a particular type of pica that was hiding a chilling secret.

Do you crunch ice cubes?

You're probably IRON deficient

Pica isn't just a title explaining lettuce addiction, it is a fancy name given to an unusual craving for specific foods, especially ice cubes, which seems to be the most common 'pica' of all. Until I began my research, it had not been widely realised that many iron-deficient people develop a craving for ice cubes, despite the fact that these are not even rich in iron.

Iron deficiency is the most common nutritional disorder in the world. The numbers are staggering; as many as four to five billion people, that's 66-80% of the world's population, may be iron deficient. It is also estimated that two billion people, or more than 30% of the world's population, are clinically anaemic. This is mainly through iron deficiency in the food, but it happens to be much more common in women due to monthly blood loss in menstruation. And that is why most ice cube crunchers seem to be women.

The Body Language of Health

That's still a heck of a lot of ice cube crunchers.

When the press wrote about the Body Language website, for some reason they chose the ice cube crunching as a headline. Maybe it was something they did themselves, suggesting they too were short of iron. Funny, I always thought journalists had to have a lot of mettle. The press coverage of the Body Language website travelled round the world, and there were articles about Body Language in Chinese, Russian, and Arabic, much to my amusement.

The press article in one particular British newspaper included a sizeable piece of editorial and it just so happened that a copy of this newspaper was sent out to an ex-patriot Brit living in Belgium. This in itself is not surprising since everyone who has moved abroad must derive comfort from reading home news, or even keeping in touch with the score from last night's home-town football match. Unless of course it is an England football or cricket international, we normally keep quiet about those, for obvious reasons.

As usual, the Body Language story was described in this newspaper by the headline 'Do you crunch ice cubes? Luckily the reader of the story in Belgium had one of those 'Eureka' moments, though she wasn't reading the paper in the bath at the time. She immediately recognised that this strange habit of crunching ice cubes described her mother perfectly. Apparently her mother was crunching her way through three or four trays of ice cubes a day. Unbelievable, but true.

'I've read that crunching ice cubes indicates you may be deficient in iron', she said to her mother on the telephone back in Blighty. 'I really think you should get checked out for anaemia by your doctor straight away'.

Well, fortunately this reader's mother must have been different to most mothers, she actually heeded her daughter's advice and went to see her doctor. He not only found she was chronically anaemic, he discovered the reason why as well. She had bowel polyps that were at an advanced stage of bleeding, and these could well have caused her demise if they had been allowed to continue undiscovered. She was so anaemic because she was literally bleeding to death.

This woman had a simple operation to treat the condition, and is now fit and well. That chance reading of my website content in the local paper by her daughter all those miles away probably saved this woman's life. Such is the power of information.

The Body Language of Health

So why suck ice cubes? Well, iron deficiency can result in a 'hot mouth' syndrome in which your mouth seems to be burning, so maybe this is the underlying reason for sucking on an ice cube. Or perhaps we are conditioned from the ice age to suck glacier ice which might have been rich in minerals.

Iron deficiency is very complicated. It is affected by gastric bleeding from taking aspirin and non steroidal anti-inflammatory drugs (NDAIDS). Individuals with coeliac disease (celiac in USA) find iron is difficult to absorb so these people develop anaemia. Vegetarians and people with peptic ulcers often become anaemic.

Iron is vital to us all. We all need iron to produce haemoglobin, an essential constituent of blood. As a forensic scientist, I have occasionally had to search premises where murders have been committed, looking for bloodstains. You might think that this would entail looking for red marks, but you'd be wrong. Blood oxidises as it dries, and the iron in the haemoglobin turns the stain into iron oxide, or rust. That's why blood goes a dark brown, rusty colour, and is so difficult to remove from clothing unless you can attack it with an enzyme-containing detergent. So unless you're at the premises immediately after the dastardly deed is done, you need to look for rusty marks, not blood.

I remember one particular property where foul play was suspected. The mother came back from a long weekend away only to find her husband missing. Her grown up son, who was at home from university, had totally redecorated the flat in her absence. They do that all the time don't they?

Anyway this son had redecorated everywhere with fresh emulsion paint and had also washed and rehung the curtains too. I could tell because they were now three inches too short and needed ironing badly. Actually, they had already been ironed badly, or maybe they hadn't been ironed at all.

A couple of weeks after the mother had returned, faint brown splashes started to appear all over the lounge walls. The policeman who visited to investigate her report of a missing person got suspicious of this, and called in the forensic team. These splashes were the rusty marks from the bloodstains that the son had failed to wash off the wallpaper before he applied the emulsion paint. The water in the paint had eventually oxidised the blood into rust which had started to show through the paint. Ironically, in the decorating trade this effect is known as 'bleeding' through, though the effect refers to pigments below the paint, not usually to blood.

Blood splashes produce a tadpole shape with a head and a tail, and by looking at the height of the mark and the shape of the tadpole, the marks told me exactly which

The Body Language of Health

direction the splash came from, what height, and whether they were from one event or from several by their direction of travel. In that flat I counted 15 blows at head height produced with a blunt instrument.

Of course when scientists refer to a blunt instrument, they don't mean a nicely rounded piano, that would be silly. How could you hit someone with a piano? They don't even mean a musical instrument. A blunt instrument is any kind of apparatus capable of doing the job in hand. By the same reasoning a pencil may be referred to as a writing instrument. Although I suppose if it needs sharpening it could qualify as a blunt instrument as well. As a forensic scientist, what I mean by a blunt instrument is something handy that is rounded and pointless (for example, a fat politician). In this particular case I thought it likely that the blows were performed with a hammer. Maybe on the strength of this we could reclassify a hammer as a surgical instrument.

The fact that blood turns dark brown makes intestinal bleeding difficult to see, because faeces are coloured brown with a bile called bilirubin. More about that later. You need to be looking for exceptionally dark stools, almost black. Everyone I know blows their nose and then looks at the rubbish on the handkerchief, well we should all get into the habit of looking in the toilet at our stools. If you notice any difference to what you usually expect, you should investigate it further. If you find very dark, almost black stools you must report it to your doctor immediately. There is a section on stool inspections later. If you're a teacher don't panic, I said stool inspections not school inspections.

Body Language is all about simple symptoms, many of which could lead to more serious ailments. You can use them in several ways. Initially, if you have identified a particular Body Language sign that fits your condition, try and add some of the foods that give you that nutritional boost. You could also try a supplement. Don't worry if you don't need it, because your body will excrete the excess. But always stick to the recommended dose.

Does the food seem appealing? Body Language has apparently programmed you to desire the foods your body needs. If so, chances are it will be doing you good. In fact you should give in to your cravings.

If you do decide to choose a supplement, try it for two or three weeks, anything less and you may not see the benefit. Supplements are not like drugs, they are a lot slower acting. If you haven't seen any benefit in a month, chances are that's not what you are lacking, so you can track down something else similar in this book and try that.

In this book you will find other symptoms of anaemia to check, like a pale tongue that will help you confirm anaemia. Deficiencies like anaemia can occasionally have quite serious implications, like the reader's mother with her bowel polyps, so you should always consult your doctor if you think you are seriously anaemic.

You can also use the book for some clever lateral thinking too. Sufferers of cystic fibrosis lose all their salt, so that is a Body Language sign for them. Recently it has been found that inhaling a salt mist brings them great relief. You will find later in the book that feet are super-absorbent, so for cystic fibrosis sufferers it seems sensible that a daily salt foot spa will be just the ticket. Try it, because it certainly won't do any harm.

In this book I will mostly be scratching the surface, and not just in the section on skin. Your body is immensely complicated. Each of our one hundred trillion cells demand a complex supply system, and we are all different. So I cannot hope to cover each topic fully. I just hope that my explanations about nutrients will whet your appetite for more.

Some Body Language symptoms overlap, so to avoid overloading your palette with too much information, I have spread it out over several Body Language signs where possible. This means to get a full picture of anaemia or any other ailment you can browse through the book using the index to pick out particular topics of interest.

Do you crave Butter?

You probably have a deficiency of SODIUM

Sodium is another vital metallic element and it is found at some level in nearly everything we eat. The body uses sodium to regulate blood pressure, blood volume, water balance and cell function. Without the two common salts based on sodium and potassium we lose our 'renal function' which means that our body's water balance goes wonky. The medical term 'renal' means anything associated with the kidneys and 'waterworks'

Sodium deficiency results in a number of symptoms such as severe muscle cramps, extreme weakness, nausea and fainting. It can even cause someone to go into a coma if they are exercising hard in hot, humid weather when they sweat a lot. It can also happen as a result of severe vomiting or diarrhoea because that is how a lot of salts are lost.

The Body Language of Health

The most important source of sodium is common salt, which has the chemical formula NaCl or sodium chloride. But in chemistry, 'salt' has come to mean any compound that is made up from a metal combined to a non-metal. So magnesium sulphate, copper chloride and silver nitrate are all salts, but there is only one 'common salt' and that is sodium chloride.

Actually most foods contain at least a trace of sodium, as sodium chloride. Sodium or 'soda' is also a component of many chemicals including baking powder (that's why it is also called 'baking soda'), soy sauce and many preservatives such as sodium citrate, sodium nitrate, sodium phosphate, sodium ascorbate and monosodium glutamate. Salt is a great preservative. And butter contains salt, of course, or it should do. That's why people crave it when they are sodium deficient.

A brief History of Salt

Salt was so important historically that the Romans gave it to their troops as 'Salary'. And by Jove they needed it. Despite the European Union's obsession with foreign units of measurement, the British unit of distance is still the mile. Ironically, this British bastion of the old 'imperial' systems of weights and measures is European anyway because it got its name during the Roman occupation of Britain. The Roman measure of distance was one thousand paces of a soldier's marching step. They were able to measure out the distances between towns this way, counting the steps as they marched.

But not in our logical Arabic system of course, it would be CMXCV, CMXCVI, CMXCVII, CMXCVIII, CMXCIX .... M..... TERMINUS in their day.

The Roman symbol for a thousand is 'm' and comes from 'mille'. Today in the metric system, mille (as in 'millennium') still stands for one thousand. But that doesn't mean that Cardiff's Millennium Stadium holds only a thousand supporters.

The British took the distance the Romans marched one thousand steps as' the mille' which became the mile, Britain's unit of distance.

These Romans must have been big, healthy men because the Anglo Saxon's measure for a man's step is one yard and there are 1,760 yards in a mile. So while we walked 1760 paces the Romans marched 1000 paces. Roman soldiers therefore must have got quite a sweat on, hence the need for Hadrian to provide them with their regular salt ration while they were on duty on his wall in Northumbria. Perhaps that's why when marathon runners run out of energy they call it 'the wall'.

The Body Language of Health

Over the years, those who controlled a nation's salt supplies also controlled the population. The British were so possessive of their control of taxable products in their colonies that they performed some unusual and heroic feats. By 1869 they had constructed a customs barrier 2,904 miles long from one end of India to the other, from the Himalayas to the Bay of Bengal. This included the planting and maintaining of an impenetrable bramble hedge twelve feet wide and 1200 miles long. Imagine trimming that!!. And the purpose? It was constructed, maintained and ruthlessly policed so as to totally cut off movement of salt except when salt taxes were paid, in this very hot, humid country where salt was vital to life. Salt has been, and still is a commodity worth fighting for. Even now a worthy worker is said to be 'worth his salt'.

Commodities like this bring power. This and other similar taxes, such as huge income from taxing opium in China, is what made Britain the wealthiest and most powerful country in the world. But was it worth fighting the Opium wars for? Many say these early acts are only on a par with modern day drug patenting which turns resources essential to life into overpriced commodities. Britain was no worse than the drug multinationals who took the South African government to court to stop AIDS sufferers having access to affordable medicine.

My pet goat, Sally who died of old age recently was often given a variety of human foods as treats, such as biscuits and bread, and she had a particular liking for corn flakes. But she went crazy over potato crisps. In fact I have experimented with different flavours and her favourite by far was salt and vinegar. She gobbled down plain unsalted crisps too, but was less likely to nibble your fingers off for these, so I think her passion must have been for the salt rather than for the potato. She also had a salt block in her stall, but goats are not renowned for their housekeeping skills so she usually ended up peeing on the block which must have reduced its appeal somewhat. Perhaps she thought that after a good soaking with urine it tasted more like salt and vinegar. Her favourite!!

Even the first true 'roads' in Britain were the prehistoric 'Salt Pathways' connecting the country with ancient salt mines, so we know that salt has been highly prized right from the early days of human settlement, about ten thousand years ago. These towns can easily be identified in Britain now, because they usually have the suffix 'wich' resulting in towns with names such as Northwich, Middlewich, Norwich and Sandwich etc. Maybe the Earl of Sandwich, who gave his name to the bread and filling snack, enjoyed a pinch of local salt with his roast boar 'sandwich' while out hunting. Actually, I am told the Sandwich was really developed so the Earl could spend more time at the gambling tables. More factually correct but not so romantic.

The Body Language of Health

Now, some people develop a craving for crisps. You might imagine that the salt in the crisps could be the driving factor here, but actually crisp cravings are usually something different altogether and we will talk about that in a different category.

You can check the likelihood of any sodium deficiency for yourself, because once again your body will tell you when you are deficient. There are apparently three levels of salt deficiency in humans. Those people who don't want salt on their food aren't deficient; those that taste the food first and then add salt are probably mildly deficient; and those that add salt first before tasting have a severe shortage and need salt at all costs. We have an uncanny knack of knowing just how much sodium we need, and should always add salt 'to taste'

These days though, there are many people who would love to add salt but have been brainwashed by Government advertising and health notices that salt is bad for you. Many scientists think that to have insufficient salt intake can be even more dangerous for most of us.

The problem is that the western diet is overloaded with calcium and sodium, and at the same time it is deficient in magnesium and potassium. Sodium retention increases during stress and is exhausted with adrenal burnout, so stressed out individuals need potassium and magnesium while burned out individuals need salt, saturated fat, potassium and magnesium amongst other things!

Stress, consumption of alcohol, use of diuretics, bouts of diarrhoea, and excess dietary sodium all favour adrenal imbalances affecting the sodium/potassium ratio.

Your adrenal glands are each only about half the size of your thumb, but they dictate much of what happens in your body. Perched on each of your kidneys, they produce hormones that help regulate your metabolism, immune system, blood pressure and other essential functions. One such hormone is aldosterone, which manages your body's balance of sodium and potassium. In primary aldosteronism, your body produces too much of this hormone, causing you to retain sodium and lose potassium.

Aldosteronism was once thought to be rare, but now that testing can be done, doctors have found that around one in eight cases of high blood pressure are caused by excess aldosterone. It also produces headache, muscle weakness and cramps, fatigue, temporary paralysis, numbness, pricking, tingling sensation, excessive thirst, and excessive urination. This hormone is also responsible for panic attacks.

The Body Language of Health

A rare type of primary aldosteronism called glucocorticoid-remediable aldosteronism (GRA) runs in families. This condition may cause high blood pressure in children and young adults. Genetic testing can identify people at risk.

Eating potassium rich foods will rarely correct an imbalance as it takes months of several supplemental grams of elemental potassium every day to rebalance electrolytes and tissue stores. This quantity is equivalent to four to six medium sized bananas a day at least or 10 grams of a good potassium salt per day – much more than most individuals would ever consume unless under the guidance of a doctor, or when driven by a banana-pica caused by potassium deficiency.

Believe it or not, in spite of the current anti-salt trend, scientists still debate over whether we need more or less salt. What is actually more important is the balance between sodium and potassium, because that is what drives the renal system. Let's put straight the issue of whether salt is good for you or bad for you once and for all. If nothing else, I can ensure that the majority of you once more enjoy good old-fashioned British fish and chips (which are now available in almost any capital city in the world if you know where to look) with plenty of salt and vinegar. I can feel my mouth watering already.

Actually, to appreciate the importance of salt, we have to go back to our origins.

When scientists first analysed human blood plasma, they were amazed to find that the proportions of all the elements in our blood were in precisely the same proportions as the various elements in sea water. It is as though the human body evolved in harmony with the minerals in the sea. To explain why this is significant we have to look at the property of liquids and cells that undergo something called osmosis.

It is said that nature abhors a vacuum. Well, nature abhors differences in density too. Different concentrations of salt solutions in different places try to balance themselves out by osmosis. The water from the weaker solution passes through the cell walls into the stronger solution, until it becomes the same concentration as the weaker solution. When this happens, there is equilibrium and the driving force for osmosis is switched off because the same amount is going in as is coming out, like Mr McCawber's perfect bank account. This balancing act is called osmosis when it involves cell walls and membranes, and diffusion when it doesn't.

This principle is put to good use when making pickled onions. You don't just peel the onions and put them in some vinegar. Then you'd have 'onions in vinegar', not pickled onions, and in all probability the onions would go bad after a while because the vinegar has to soak right into the onions to preserve them. The proper way to do it is to peel the onions and then soak them for twenty four hours in a strong solution of salty water, known as brine. The brine has a greater density of salt than the fluid in the pickled onion, so osmosis drives some of the water out of the onion and into the brine. Nature is trying to dilute the brine until it is the same density as the water in the onion, by robbing the water from the onion by osmosis. If the brine was too strong, or the onions were left in there for too long, then the onions would end up looking like onion-flavoured prunes. But you don't leave them soaking long enough for this to happen.

After twenty four hours, you take the onions out, rinse the salty water off them, and put them in a jar of vinegar. Now the reverse happens. The partially dehydrated onion absorbs vinegar, again driven by osmosis, because the density of vinegar is much less than that of the previous solution of brine. This absorption of vinegar swells the onion again and the vinegar preserves the onion. The result is a jar of pickled onions that are a perfect companion to those fish and chips you're still thinking about. These pickled onions will last for years, if you have enough will power to resist eating them for that long.

So where did all those minerals in our body come from? The answer is that we have evolved a system in our body to extract them from food, and if we are deficient, we crave them until our demand is satisfied. This is what drove Sally's craving for salt and vinegar crisps, and it is what encourages us to put salt on our food. Fortunately though, we have never adopted the habit of putting salt on our food and then peeing on it.

Our body sees to it that our blood gets its mineral balance from the food in our gut. But why do we need these salts? And why should they be in the same ratio as those in the oceans?

Scientists suggest that we have the same mineral mix in our body as that in the ocean because we have evolved from aquatic animals, and to live in the ocean it is necessary to have the same mineral balance as the ocean. If the mineral content of our plasma was weaker than the ocean, osmosis would rob the water in our bodies to try and dilute the ocean. We would shrivel up, and could end up looking like human-flavoured prunes. Incidentally, ladies, this isn't the same process that affects a man's reproductive organs when swimming in British seas, that's the effect of the icy water.

Conversely if our bodily fluid mineral content was less than that of the ocean we would absorb water instead and swell up as the cells in our body absorbed water, driven on by osmosis until they ruptured.

The Body Language of Health

Clearly, we don't do either of these things, because we have the right body chemistry. So, this is a convincing argument to show that the previous history of the human race included a period in the ocean. Personally I think that we probably took to living at the water/ice edge during the prolonged ice ages when the only reliable food source would be aquatic. That is probably why fish should be such an important part of the human diet now. This period of the human race living in harmony with water is also thought to be why we have a ridge of hair down our back - a remnant from streamlining in water.

And that's also reputedly why we have a ridge on our top lip, known as the naso-labial fold. It is thought this is a remnant of the air seal that is produced between our nose and our lip when we screw our face up in the water. It sounds far-fetched but this is entirely feasible when you look at the protruding jawbone of early man. At this point I would encourage you to screw up your face to see if you can form an air seal between your nose and upper lip. See how the crease in your lip coincides perfectly with the fleshy part of your cupid's bow and naso-labial fold?

I can't think of any other reason for this particular trait, unless it is a drainage channel for a runny nose but then I would expect there to be two channels, one for each nostril. And it is hard to see what advantage this could provide to mankind, for it to have developed into a dominant genetic trait throughout the human race. Every feature that has shaped our evolution has to provide an advantage in long life, and especially in finding, satisfying and keeping your sexual partner, for it to survive as a dominant feature. In reality, most females are likely to be less than happy mating with a male who has a streaming snotty nose, labial drainage channel or not. But having a sealable naso-labial fold that prevents you from drowning, now that could be quite advantageous in the fight for survival and reproduction.

Oh sorry. You can stop gurning now and start breathing again!

Of course, you don't need to know about osmosis to be able to make good pickled onions, but osmosis is vitally important to every cell in our body. Osmosis controls the transfer of minerals and nutrients in and out of the cell, but for this to occur it is essential that the fluid in the body has exactly the right mineral content. If it is too high, the cell will shrink as it gives up its water. If it is too low, the cell will absorb water and eventually rupture. We have an incredibly sophisticated mineral balancing mechanism within our body that keeps check on the balance and adjusts it if necessary, even when food and drink is sporadic. This balance is called the electrolyte stability, and it depends on supplies of sodium and potassium to maintain a balance suitable for cells to operate efficiently, controlled by aldosterone.

And that's why we need enough salt in our diet.

The Body Language of Health

Unfortunately, though, salt is made by industrial extraction processes that can deplete it of certain essential minerals. One scientist friend of mine says salt is 'made in a test tube and is no longer natural'. By that, I think he means it is devoid of all the other thousands of 'salts' that are in natural sea salt. If so, our bodies could still be craving for salt long after our desire is satisfied, simply because our body is still searching for those missing elements. Many nutritionists believe we are still looking for these missing nutrients in modern food, that is why we eat too much and become obese. This is a feature of modern food, which I will come back to later.

There is another unusual feature of the human body worth mentioning. Our feet are super absorbent. When we go paddling in the ocean, our feet are absorbing the minerals we need from the seawater. If we are already topped up with all the minerals we require, electrolyte balance ensures that we won't absorb any more. Osmosis guarantees that a paddle in the sea tops up our minerals until each element is balanced with its requirement. The only explanation I can think of for this phenomenon is that it was advantageous to us in the ice ages when food was scarce. Those people who were better at absorbing salts from the sea had a nutritional advantage over the others, and hence produced more offspring carrying this beneficial trait. Whenever you happen to be at the seaside, you should go for an invigorating paddle to top up your salt level. Although, in my opinion it's still not as much fun as a plate of fish and chips, with plenty of salt and a pickled onion.

When we have eaten too much salt, our body simply excretes the excess in urine. In theory it is not possible to build up an excess of salt because the body's electrolyte stabilising mechanism will excrete what it doesn't need. In fact our mouth is the main moderator of salt, since we will reject food that tastes salty when we already have enough in our body, that is where the concept of 'adding salt to taste' comes from, and this process drives all our food cravings.

Recently there have been several cases in the British courts concerning babies that appear to have died because their bodies contained high salt levels. And several parents have been convicted of killing their babies by allegedly deliberately feeding them excess salt, but legal appeals have now suggested that these babies were either given too much salt in hospital for their underdeveloped kidneys to cope with, or in some cases had adult breakfast cereal that was high in salt. It is also possible these babies had a problem with their bodily salt control system. We should all be aware that babies are especially sensitive to salt because we control their diet for them and they cannot make those decisions for themselves.

So, does this philosophy of 'salt to taste' apply to us all?

The Body Language of Health

Unfortunately, it doesn't look like it. Science and biology are never that simple. We are told that about 9 per cent of the population of Britain are sodium sensitive. These people have a salt control mechanism that doesn't work efficiently. This control mechanism is there to get rid of excess salt in the urine, so the balance is maintained, but in these people that does not happen efficiently. If you are in this 9% then you should actually take the government advice and limit your salt. For these people, intake of salt appears to be linked to the condition of high blood pressure; that is precisely why the government tell all of us to cut down on salt intake, because they can't tell who is and who isn't susceptible to this problem.

The other 91% probably actually need more sodium, and could risk serious deficiency especially if they sweat or exercise a lot. If you're in this group, put salt on your fish and chips and help yourself to the pickled onions. Not only do you deserve it, your body needs it.

It is impossible to know who is and who isn't sensitive to sodium until hypertension develops. Moreover, several studies have demonstrated that sodium sensitivity, just like glucose intolerance, increases with age. This could be due to a reduction in the efficiency of the electrolyte balancing mechanism. Therefore, while you may not be sodium sensitive now, you could become so in the future. It is also possible that the genetic resistance to sodium is weakened by chronically high sodium intake over a lifetime and by other factors such as stress.

So what do you do? This of course is the dilemma the Government and their medical advisers are in. Their advice, inevitably is eat less salt because they must issue one guideline for everybody.

But now you're better informed. Remember our diet is overloaded with calcium and sodium, but deficient in magnesium and potassium. Sodium retention increases during stress and is exhausted with adrenal burnout, so stressed out individuals need potassium and magnesium while burned out individuals need salt, saturated fat, potassium and magnesium.

You can probably decide which group you are in. You're probably best advised to 'add salt to taste' as your senses will be advising you just how much salt you need. Of course you should also listen to your Body Language. Do you crave butter? If so, add the salt. And be aware that what ius really important is your sodium/potassium ratio.

The best answer I can give you is that it's also a jolly good idea to get into the routine of testing your blood pressure occasionally especially now that there are many excellent home blood pressure machines available that cost very little.

Although the government is still advising on salt as the culprit for blood pressure, new research suggests that the real culprit in causing high blood pressure is a diet low in calcium, potassium and magnesium, and nothing to do with the level of sodium you take at all. Most people eating a healthy balanced diet will usually ingest sufficient sodium, potassium and magnesium to meet these requirements and will be OK, but most don't eat healthily. We cover this again elsewhere.

Of course, since a few people are salt sensitive, it's best to have low salt in everything and then add it to taste, and to deliberately increase our potassium and magnesium intake. That makes sure everyone's desires are satisfied.

This is all very complicated, simply because your body is such a sophisticated machine. Every one of its one hundred million million cells have chemical demands and control their own environment. It's like looking after the diet of every individual on earth a million times over. And so much of the processed food in our diet is laden with salt, and masked by flavourings. Life was so much simpler when we bought raw fruit and vegetables or grew our own, and cooked everything ourselves.

Do you have Cystic Fibrosis?

Now here is a fascinating fact that I have uncovered. It seems that cystic fibrosis patients tend to excrete much more sodium in their sweat than normal and are therefore even more at risk from sodium deficiency than the rest of us. But more importantly, they lack a protein that controls osmosis in the lungs driven by salt.

Salt loss could actually be the key to sufferers of cystic fibrosis, because it has recently been reported that Australian surfers found their cystic fibrosis was much better after exposure to salt spray. Sufferers who later had pulmonary flare ups reported they were milder and they recovered quicker.

Cystic fibrosis is one of the most common potentially fatal genetic diseases and one of the side effects is a thick mucous that clogs the lungs. This leads to chronic infections and lung damage. The medical team investigating this realised that there was too little liquid in the lining of the lungs, impairing the ability to water down and clear mucous from the bronchial tubes.

It seems their lungs were pretending to mimic those pickled onions we talked about earlier, because the mucous is kept moist by osmosis driven by the presence of salt. Because they have a problem controlling salt their lungs get too dry, producing thick mucous.

The Body Language of Health

Salty ocean sprays breathed in while surfing got their mucous moving normally by substituting a normal osmotic function to their lungs.

Do an internet search with cystic+fibrosis+salt and you will see this phenomenon is widely reported, even on trusted websites like the BBC site. This looks like such a simple and inexpensive treatment it is surprising we have not heard of it. Even the Cystic Fibrosis Institutions don't refer to it on their websites. Do you think it has anything to do with the fact that no-one can get rich supplying simple salt sprays that can't be patented? A simple sterile saline pack and a nebulizer should do it.

Based on these surfing stories, saline inhalers appear to make a big difference to cystic fibrosis sufferers. Regular paddling in the sea to top up their salt levels won't come amiss either. Those Australian surfers who discovered this inexpensive treatment for what is often a fatal condition have certainly proved to be 'well worth their salt'.

I could have studied the body language characteristics of cystic fibrosis sufferers, in their tendency to excrete salt excessively, and I might have pointed them in the right direction. Look out for further cases in this book where Body Language signs could point the way to a simple cure. There are lots of them. We should never be afraid to try out simple experiments with natural substances like salt, minerals, vitamins and micronutrients, to see if they improve our health. Try to think laterally.

For example, if you know anyone with cystic fibrosis try to encourage them to take daily foot baths with a sprinkling of sea-salt added to the water to see if it helps them. Body Language suggests it will, because of our porous feet. What is the perfect mixture? Well, actually, that which copies the salt level in the ocean.

Before we leave the issue of salt in the diet, lets have a look at an interesting fact about fingerprints. Humans have developed a remarkable capability to excrete much more salt from the sweat pores on our fingertips than from any other sweat pores on our body. Typically the fingertips excrete around ten times more salt that anywhere else on the body, making the fingers super gooey. As a forensic scientist I like this because it guarantees that a criminal leaves behind nice sticky fingerprints on anything they touch.

The reason for this evolutionary stroke of genius seems to be that sticky fingers are perfect for gripping anything smooth, giving us extra dexterity. For example, they are especially good for picking up a smooth beer glass. In fact if we put on our scientific irrationality hat we could argue that the smooth beer glass has been an evolutionary influence on our ability to develop especially sticky fingers. Could this mean we have evolved to be beer drinkers? Try using this excuse on your wife the next time you're heading off to the bar.

'I can't help it, Dear, it's part of my evolutionary duty to maintain the 'sticky finger gene", he said, as he put on his scientific irrationality hat and went off down the pub.

This evidence certainly suggests that man's love of beer has been vital in guaranteeing the evolutionary advantage of sticky fingers, to the dismay of criminals everywhere.

A bit of flawed logic there, I think. But if you know any cystic fibrosis sufferers you should certainly be discouraging them from turning to crime, their extra salty fingerprints would be their downfall.

Incidentally, if you don't believe this story about salty fingerprints, just lick your fingers. If they taste 'salty' you must have more salt on your fingers than the level of salt that is currently in the rest of your body. If your fingers have the same level as the salt in the saliva, they won't taste salty at all. The taste buds on the tongue can only taste 'difference' because your tongue is bathed in saliva with the natural level of salt that is in the body. By the same reasoning, when you eat something that tastes bland, it has less salt than your body's equilibrium value, and when it tastes salty it contains more than your equilibrium value. This is another factor that your body uses to decide whether you need more salt or not. A prehistoric cave man in natural surroundings would seek out a saltier diet, probably of sea fish. And of course we already know that salt sources were highly prized and worth guarding or fighting over. Even cats love to lick furniture we have handled; to them it must taste super-salty.

Maybe you like a lot of salt on your food and you also like butter? Do you also get heartburn after fatty food, especially at night? This could be another body language symptom. It seems to be well established now that indigestion and heartburn are more likely to be caused by low acid levels in the stomach rather than high acid levels. This makes the fatty food more difficult to digest no matter how much bile you excrete. Indigestion tablets might give you a short-term cure, but in the long term are more likely to make the problem worse because they neutralise the acid in your stomach.

The reason for your love of salt could be due to the fact that the chemical name for salt is sodium chloride, and the acid in your stomach is hydrochloric acid. The link between these is chlorine, the element that is used in making both these compounds. You can't drink hydrochloric acid, your body has to make it from chlorides it consumes. You get the chlorine from salt; sodium chloride.

The Body Language of Health

Unlike other salts, every known chloride is highly soluble. So even if you consume enough chloride in your food, you stand a good chance of losing a lot of it if you take diuretics, like drinking a lot of coffee or tea.

How can you tell if you are short of stomach acid? Easy, just use a bit of simple logic. Next time you get indigestion after fatty food, drink a little fresh lemon juice and reflect on what this little extra dose of weak acid does to your indigestion. Does your indigestion feel a bit better? If so you were short of stomach acid. Does it feel a bit worse? In that case your problem is either too much stomach acid or an inflamed or irritated stomach lining or sphincter. If the latter, you should discuss this with your doctor.

Low stomach acid can also be detected by looking at your stools, and we describe this in a later section. But what causes low stomach acid? Well, one little-known reason happens to concern whether you have a hearty breakfast or not. If you skip breakfast, your stomach has nothing to do for hours and learns to throttle back on the acid production. Eventually the acid system decides enough is enough and you get heartburn at night when the acid you need is absent. The best answer to fighting heartburn at night is therefore to start the day with a decent breakfast. It's pretty obvious when put in these simple terms, isn't it?

You might have noticed there is one little flaw in this whole argument about salt, and were wondering when I was going to address it. So far we have described a craving for butter being driven by the desire for more salt, however butter nowadays contains very little salt. The reason for this pica seems to be that in the past, before the evolution of the refrigerator, plenty of salt was added to butter to preserve it. Like the craving for ice cubes which don't have any iron in them now, it doesn't really matter if the butter is salted or not, the craving still exists. It is as if Body Language is conditioned in our brains from a time when food was not 'manufactured' but was produced in simpler ways. In those days, salt would be an essential ingredient in butter to help its keeping properties, just as ice would come from glaciers and mountain streams in winter, or else would be collected and stored snow from the winter, and was probably rich in iron.

Before you go and load up your food with salt, check out sodium and then potassium in the index. Then try and strike a happy balance that relates to your condition.

So to sum up, the answer for most of us is, take salt to taste, and stay well preserved.

Do you wheeze eating fruit & vegetables?

You might have a deficiency of MOLYBDENUM

Molybdenum deficiency can lead to wheeziness because of something called sulphite sensitivity.

Sulphites are sulphur-based chemical preservatives used a lot on light coloured fruit and vegetables to stop them going brown prematurely. Sulphites are also used to prevent black mould forming on seafood, and inhibiting the growth of micro organisms in fermented foods such as wine and dough. But sulphites give off the gas sulphur dioxide, which causes irritation in the lungs. This irritation makes the lining of the lungs produce mucous as a protective layer. And that is what makes you wheeze.

In Britain, many products are preserved by sulphites in this way, even bread. There are only a handful of bakeries supplying bread dough in the whole country. You might argue this point, if your local supermarket has an in-store bakery and emits mouth-watering baked bread smells that entice you to buy lovely fresh-baked bread whenever you enter the store. What could be healthier?

But the local bakeries almost certainly just buy pre-mixed dough from one of these main suppliers and then just bake it on their premises. So it is a pretty safe bet that you consumed some bread today that has been hanging around for quite a while protected by its antiseptic cloud of sulphites and other preservatives, until your supermarket bunged it in the oven.

The effects from these sulphites can sometimes be serious too. They can cause a severe attack of asthma in sufferers who are sensitive to sulphur compounds. The reaction that develops can vary from chest tightness, nausea, hives, or even anaphylactic shock. This can happen especially if your body is lacking molybdenum. It doesn't have to be sulphites, either. Some people develop wheeziness when eating onions, presumably because onions are a rich source of sulphur compounds.

Most people have probably never heard of molybdenum. It is a metal that has a particular affinity for sulphur, when it readily forms molybdenum disulphide; a compound that is more commonly known to motorists as 'MolySlip' or Slick 90, both of which are oil additives for your car engine. Molybdenum sulphide happens to form particularly slippery platelets, like the structure of graphite, so it is ideal for lubricating an engine. You probably remember the advertisement where a car had all its oil drained out of the engine and then could be driven for hundreds of miles before it seized up. That was all thanks to molybdenum disulphide.

We all need traces of molybdenum in our body, and we get it from the minerals in plants, and they get it from the soil. Molybdenum in the blood also has the ability to mop up sulphites and sulphur dioxide, producing molybdenum sulphide molecules in the body which is harmlessly broken down and excreted.

A deficiency of molybdenum prevents the body from neutralising the sulphites in our food, and this can accentuate wheeziness, so much so that several experts even quote molybdenum deficiency as a factor that can promote the development of asthma.

Now, wheeziness when eating fruit and vegetables you can live with, but molybdenum deficiency can be much more serious, because it has also been associated with the development of cancer in some parts of the world.

In China and Japan, people who are living in areas where the soil is molybdenum-deficient have been found to have an increased risk of stomach and oesophageal cancers. This may be because the plants in these regions are molybdenum-deficient and don't have the ability to metabolise and remove carcinogenic compounds known as nitrosamines as they grow. These remain in the plant when it is harvested and then consumed. When these compounds pass through the human digestive system unmetabolised they can be harmful.

There is a message for us all here, because the majority of our food is now imported from countries whose soil could be deficient in certain elements, and we could be leaving ourselves open to mineral deficiencies that have previously never been a problem in our country.

Serious molybdenum deficiency is rare and has only been seen in people who are on long-term tube or intravenous feeding or in those who have molybdenum co-factor deficiency, a rare genetic inability to fix and use molybdenum. Symptoms of serious deficiency include rapid heartbeat and breathing, headache, night blindness, anaemia, mental disturbance, nausea and vomiting. There may also be problems with sexual function and excessive dental decay in people deficient in molybdenum.

Molybdenum is only present in the body as a trace element, but is clearly vital to our well being. Deficiency of molybdenum has been strongly linked to attention deficiency hyperactive disorder (ADHD) and other behavioural problems, for example. Molybdenum also plays a vital role in supporting xanthine oxidase that is used to detoxify the body of purines that are consumed in great quantities in meat. This is just one of the many thousand 'metabolic pathways' in the body that are adversely affected by deficiencies of trace metals. Through one of these pathways a deficiency of molybdenum can lead to a poorly functioning immune system.

Wheezing after food can also often be a symptom of something called synthetic salicylate and phenol sensitivity. See 'Do you have nasal polyps'.

Legumes, such as beans, lentils, and peas, are the richest sources of molybdenum. Grain products and nuts are considered good sources, while animal products, fruits, and many vegetables are generally low in molybdenum. Because the molybdenum content of plants depends on the soil molybdenum content and environmental conditions, the molybdenum content of foods can vary considerably. We will talk about mineral deficiency in modern fruit and vegetables later, and why they could be responsible for the huge expansion of obesity in the western world.

Do you take diuretics?

You may have a CALCIUM, MAGNESIUM and POTASSIUM deficiency.

Diuretics are more commonly known as 'water tablets' because they make you urinate more frequently. They are routinely prescribed for people with high blood pressure, but they are also used to treat kidney or heart disorders where the reduced fluid level in your body eases the load on your organs.

That is fine, but in Britain it is thought that diuretics are over-prescribed. Some sources suggest that around 40% of people who are on diuretics should not be taking them. When you don't need them, they can be a problem to your health especially because water tablets will lead to mineral deficiency, which actually causes high blood pressure. Ironic, when they are prescribed to cure blood pressure problems!!

Taking diuretics will lead to deficiencies because some minerals are flushed out of your body with your urine. As we have seen in the section on craving butter, modern thinking is that blood pressure is affected by deficiencies in calcium, magnesium and potassium, so treating blood pressure by prescribing a diuretic will cause loss of calcium, magnesium, potassium and other elements from the body, and this can actually elevate blood pressure.

So far we have not discussed Potassium in any great detail, so let's have a look at this element. Gardeners will know potassium as 'potash', which simply means salts of potassium, such as potassium nitrate. Potash is important for fruit setting and ripening, so fertilisers like tomato plant feed will be rich in potash.

In our body, potassium is another essential element with a wide range of biochemical and physiological roles. Among other things, it is important in the transmission of nerve impulses, the contraction of cardiac, skeletal and smooth muscle, the production of energy, the synthesis of nucleic acids (DNA), the maintenance of cells and control of normal blood pressure. Pretty essential, actually.

As early as 1928, it was suggested that high potassium intake could have a balancing effect on blood pressure, something that these days we call an anti-hypertensive effect. Accumulating evidence suggests that diets high in potassium may be protective not only against high blood pressure, but also strokes and cardiovascular disease and possibly other degenerative diseases, as well. All you need to do to increase your potassium intake is switch from table salt to sea salt or potassium salt.

Magnesium is pretty important too, and you will find that a lot of Body Language symptoms lead to magnesium deficiency in this book.

In particular, bone health is supported by many factors, but the most important are calcium, magnesium, boron and vitamin D. There is a lot of evidence that magnesium deficiency is even more important in reducing postmenopausal osteoporosis than calcium is, and most osteoporosis is caused by magnesium deficiency, not calcium deficiency. This may be due to the fact that magnesium deficiency not only alters calcium metabolism but it also controls the hormones that regulate calcium.

These salts are all readily water soluble, and are excreted in urine, so you should definitely be very careful of water tablets if you are a woman old enough to have experienced the menopause, because diuretics may rob you of your skeleton.

Why should that be? Well, remember the effect of paddling in the oceans? When the body requires these elements, it absorbs them from the seawater, and when it doesn't need them, none are absorbed. That is because the chemical balance is driven by osmosis and diffusion. Your body is a closed system and you have a large reserve of magnesium, calcium and other minerals in your skeleton. Diffusion processes ensure your body uses its bones as a reserve of minerals. If the body is deficient, it borrows some magnesium and calcium from the bones, since the body has a controlling system to keep its osmotic pressure of minerals to provide for its cells. If it is a bit short in its diet, it borrows a bit to keep the balance right. Once the shortage is over, it makes a deposit back into its mineral bank, the skeleton. It's just one of the many defence systems the human race has to protect itself from times of famine.

The problem comes when these elements are not replaced in the diet. And if you are taking water tablets the minerals never get replaced, because they never become available, even when they are in your diet. Since 'Water Tablets' are usually prescribed for the rest of your life, you continually lose these minerals and your body never has a chance to make a deposit into your mineral bank. The result of this may be osteoporosis. You never get off them simply because these mineral deficiencies cause high blood pressure – in effect your osmosis system has lost control of its balance.

You should discuss this issue of putting magnesium into your skeleton bank with your doctor. If he doesn't give you a sensible explanation why you should keep on taking the water tablets, you should try to educate your doctor, as many are not very conversant with nutritional issues. Colleagues of mine have resorted to taking diuretics based entirely on how they feel, and have looked at controlling their blood pressure in other ways, with the approval of their doctors. This is just one of the reasons why a staggering 30% of all drugs given to patients in Britain are never taken. The quality of your bones is very important to your future and old age.

Another problem with diuretics is that the loss of minerals can cause sudden bouts of low blood pressure from the action of the diuretics, and that can be serious too. It is not uncommon for this to cause fainting fits. The most common problem is that you may collapse if you get up out of your chair quickly. Blacking out is especially dangerous because when diuretics have weakened your bones you run the risk of easily breaking bones when you fall, and those breaks may be more complicated and take longer to repair.

Magnesium

Several studies have suggested that magnesium supplementation may improve bone mineral density. In a study of older adults, a greater magnesium intake increased and maintained bone mineral density to a greater degree than a lower magnesium intake. And diets that provide recommended levels of magnesium have been found beneficial for bone health.

Magnesium is in the same chemical group as calcium and these two elements are often found together in nature. They work together. You should not just be taking calcium as a supplement, you should take it with magnesium and boron as well.

And don't be fooled by the marketing people into drinking milk in the misapprehension that the calcium is good for bones. It is true that cow's milk is rich in calcium. This is needed for the calf to grow rapidly and develop strong bones. But for human adults, the high level of protein in milk promotes high acidity levels and your body takes alkalines from other parts of the body, mostly from the bones. In fact there is good evidence that milk causes deterioration of your skeleton, despite what the marketing people would have you believe. Hard to swallow, I know, but true.

The Eskimos and Inuits have one of the highest protein diets in the world and also the highest incidence of osteoporosis in the world. Countries where dairy products and calcium supplements are consumed in the greatest quantity (USA, UK, Sweden, Finland) have high incidences of osteoporosis. Countries with the lowest incidence of osteoporosis are those where the least amount of dairy produce is consumed.

So how do you maintain your skeleton, especially when you are a woman at menopausal age, affected by hormonal changes? Well, you should read the section on osteoporosis for those answers (P295) and perform the annual home osteoporosis test.

Do you crave sugar, or have blood sugar swings?

If you do, you may be deficient in CHROMIUM. You may also suffer from INTOLERANCE TO CARBOHYDRATES or GUT FERMENTATION SYNDROME.

Like a growing number of people in our modern world, I happen to have hypoglycaemia, so this was an interesting Body Language symptom for me to research. At junior school in assembly I would occasionally lose my sense of hearing due to falling blood sugar. That was no hardship, if you have any memory of your own school assemblies. Hearing loss is one of the first signs of sugar starvation to the brain. But then my eyesight would develop black spots, and shortly afterwards my knees would buckle and sometimes I would collapse and pass out briefly. Nothing serious, just a gentle sinking to the floor. At other times an attack would simply cause me to go very pale and sweaty, and I would recover after a few minutes as long as I could sit down. It occasionally happened after strenuous exercise too.

These are classic symptoms of hypoglycaemia, and they are simply caused by lack of blood sugar. But like all body metabolism, there's a lot more to it than that.

I have rarely been able to face breakfast (another Body Language sign for hypoglycaemics). Funnily enough, it is different if I am staying at a hotel. Then I enjoy breakfast as long as I can take my time over it. As I got older, the problems of hypoglycaemia receded and it rarely gives me any trouble now. But when I don't have anything to eat, or after exercise, my blood sugar will drop and I feel I have to eat something or I may start to get a hot flush or begin to feel light headed. It is usually worse if I have been drinking alcohol, so I have learnt to avoid it except for the odd social drink. These are all typical Body Language signs for hypoglycaemics.

Mostly, sugar craving appears to be a response to a metabolic instability due to an imbalance of sugar and insulin because your glucose metabolism has gone wonky. Research suggests that this metabolism is driven by chromium and vanadium, and often hypoglycaemics are chronically deficient in chromium.

When most people think of chromium they will think of car bumpers, even though it is very rare to see a metallic bumper on a car these days because they are usually plastic. But chromium is everywhere around us, and chromium is responsible for many of the strongly coloured pigments especially in pottery, glass, and dyes. Even the name of this metal comes from the Latin 'cromos' meaning brightly coloured, and we get the word 'chromatography' and 'monochrome' and many others from this word.

But chromium is also an essential ingredient in our diet. However, it is deficient in our modern diet because refining most foods removes the chromium. So if you crave sugar you're probably deficient in chromium, and nutritionists advise that you will be heading for diabetes or insulin intolerance unless you can stabilise your metabolism with the right diet, rich in chromium. In this case I would suggest possibly taking chromium supplements, simply because so many modern foods are chromium deficient that I have struggled to identify a good natural source of nutritional chromium.

Another important step for hypoglycaemics is to remove refined sugar from your diet because this makes the body go into insulin hyperdrive and can eventually lead to type 2 diabetes and insulin intolerance. I have noticed that while I love to eat sweets (especially caramels) occasionally I find that a few minutes later I can start to feel light headed, then go into a sugar deficiency stage. It is as though the big hit from the sugar made my body flood the system with insulin, then it triggered a chain reaction. And what do I need to rectify that? Why, more caramels of course. This gets into a vicious cycle and only stops when I exercise my will power.

Diabetes affects 1.3 million people in the UK and there may be as many as a million other people who have the disease but don't know it yet. Nine out of ten people with diabetes have type 2 diabetes and over 80% of these people are overweight.

We should all be exercising more, and I don't just mean exercising our will power, either, or pedalling a vicious cycle. (I used to own one of those, it chewed up my trouser leg every few miles). However, exercise is not the full story. Many nutritionists believe that a large proportion of these people could be helped significantly if their chromium level was brought back to normal, and they could then probably manage their diabetes themselves without medication. This cheap, natural element that should be in our food but has been removed by processing could help to relieve diabetes that is costing the UK's Health Service £5 million every day.

I started taking chromium myself on and off some months ago, and I do think that my hypoglycaemia is hardly noticeable now. But there is another strange effect. No, it is not that my pee has turned poly-chrome (all the colours of the rainbow), either. It's to do with perspiration, and to find out, you'll have to sweat it out until a little later in the next topic.

Carbohydrate Intolerance

Research shows that as many as 40% of the population will be affected by food intolerance or sensitivity at some point in their lives.

Now, food intolerance has been a topic of controversy for many years, mainly because of the variability of tests that can be carried out to see if you are food intolerant. While some seem to work, others aren't so successful. Those that look at specific antibodies seem at least to be looking in the right area. Their variability occurs because food intolerance is not just one simple problem.

It is very difficult to identify individual foods that cause intolerance because food intolerance can be the cause of many different health problems, ranging in severity, and the effect can appear from two hours up to two days after eating particular foods.

Here is a list of the most common symptoms that are triggered by food intolerance:

- Irritable bowel syndrome (IBS) and other gastro-intestinal problems
- Migraines and headaches
- Acne
- Eczema and other skin conditions
- Rhinitis
- Arthritis
- Lethargy, tiredness, no energy

You will find food intolerance elsewhere in the book, so I am just going to look at carbohydrate intolerance here within this Body Language symptom.

Carbohydrate is basically starch. And in the body starch is converted into sugar. Virtually all the cultures on Earth have a basic source of carbohydrate, depending on their climate and agricultural abilities. In western Europe this source is potatoes. In Asia it is predominantly rice. Other countries use wheat to make pasta and bread, or millet or sorghum grains. Mexicans use maize flour.

Carbohydrate is metabolised in the body into sugars, and carbohydrate intolerance produces blood sugar swings that destabilise the body and aggravate the conditions listed above. Many of the food intolerance issues centre around sugar, either from consumption of refined sugar or excess of carbohydrate.

Many nutritionists argue that we didn't evolve to eat these foods. But looking back at our distant past, it seems likely that even though we were not able to grow these crops successfully, we foraged for them. In my opinion, what is different now is the way we prepare them. You can find out why in the section on irritable bowel syndrome.

Teenagers all over the developed world suffer from chronic acne as their hormone balance changes, and they spend a fortune on lotions and take antibiotics unnecessarily. But the best solution is usually to cut out sugar, and add lots of omega 3 oil – take three times the recommended dose and many acne problems will disappear. Zinc rich foods like seeds and nuts are also good. Taking measures to cut out sugar includes avoiding sweets, chocolate, fizzy drinks, and most prepared foods and junk food. Add lots of fresh fruit and vegetables, and drink lots of water. Berries are very good for your skin, and will supplement the omega 3 oil.

Acne appears to be principally due to one or more of five things. Sugar intolerance, milk intolerance, hormonal imbalance, lack of zinc and not enough Omega 3. No amount of lotion will cover these up. If you are over 25 and still have acne, you have almost certainly got to change your diet to add these things. You could make sure by adopting a food exclusion diet as described elsewhere in this book.

The Body Language of Health

Sugar addiction

The question of whether we could actually get addicted to food has always been controversial, but there are signs that irreversible changes to brain chemistry occur in animals that compulsively consume sugar, suggesting sugar might be addictive in some cases.

Bart Hoebel, a psychologist from Princeton University, believes we can be addicted to food - at least to sugar. He has shown that rats bingeing on sugar release dopamine in the same way as rats given high doses of addictive drugs, and doing so can cause lasting changes in the dopamine system, withdrawal symptoms and cross-sensitisation to other drugs, including amphetamines. Very sweet foods can induce a form of dependency, he believes.

I believe that too. Some people are just addicted to sugar, they can't do without cola, sweets, chocolate and cakes. They may be trying to treat their depression, because elevated blood sugar levels trigger the release of insulin, resulting in the production of a chemical called tryptophan. This is then converted in the brain to serotonin that lifts our mood. So sugar helps us to beat depression temporarily, though it is a short-lived fix, and once the effect subsides, these people want to repeat the experience. Production of serotonin is so pleasurable that it is known as the 'happiness hormone' and it may be why overweight people are usually thought of as jolly people.

The trouble with this addiction is that with continued consumption of excess sugar, receptors for insulin break down and become 'insulin tolerant'. If this pattern continues, the person will finish up with type 2 diabetes. It is no coincidence that type 2 diabetes has become one of the commonest ailments of the 21st century.

High sugar consumption is also responsible for obesity. Not only is sugar highly calorific, it triggers high insulin and stress hormones in the body. The resulting breakdown in insulin receptor function leads to all that unburnt sugar being stored as fat. That is why people with diabetes type 2 usually also have a problem controlling their weight. The only answer is to cut out all that sugar and increase your exercise levels. Sugar can also result in yeast infections in the gut that can lead to chronic fatigue syndrome.

Unfortunately our modern diet is loaded with sugar, simply because sugar is such an addictive substance. Manufacturers know this and want us addicted to their food, so we will buy more and more. Our stomachs and brains love sugar, but our mouths are programmed to control sugar intake, just like they are programmed for 'salt to taste'

But these days, many processed foods have so much sugar we would feel sick at the taste of it. Manufacturers actually get us to crave their sugar-loaded products by adding sweetness-masking chemicals to the food so our mouth won't reject it, leaving our reckless stomachs and brains to want more and more. Next time you buy food, take a look at the ingredients, and surprise yourself at the variety of sugar-based products you are consuming.

I just ate an apparently 'healthy' oat bar, which I thought tasted a bit sickly. On reflection I decided to have a look at the ingredients. Here they are in order of concentration:

- Toasted oats (60%)
- Glucose syrup (i.e. SUGAR)
- Golden Syrup (3%) (i.e. SUGAR)
- Partially inverted sugar syrup (i.e. SUGAR)
- Sugar (yes, your'e right, SUGAR)
- Vegetable oil Humectant (that is a fancy name for something that keeps it moist, probably lactic acid which is a metabolite of SUGAR)
- Molasses (yes, that's SUGAR)

So by my reckoning that 'Oat Goodness' oat bar I just consumed was almost 40% sugar. Eaten by a hypoglycaemic, this snack puts the body into hyperdrive for a half an hour flight, after which time the body crashes. I am a big fan of ice cream, which can contain an astonishing 30% of its weight as sugar. The best thing to do with sugar is not to consume it, we should be converting it into alcohol, then we can put it in our car's petrol tank...... and use it for driving down to the chip shop. Just joking on that last part.

Gut Fermentation Syndrome and Dysbiosis

Another possible reason for craving sugar is a problem called gut fermentation syndrome.

Your intestines are home to so many organisms that they easily outnumber the cells you have in your body. It is estimated there are around 100,000,000 (that's a hundred million) bacteria in your intestines. Around 500 species of bacteria, as well as many species of yeast and other organisms, live in your intestines and make up the "gut flora". In an average adult the live bacteria weigh about 1kg and about half of your faecal matter is dead bacteria. There are so many bacteria that scientists think of them as a 'population' all co-habiting with each other in an ethnic community that lives in harmony until things go wrong.

Gut fermentation syndrome usually refers to the unpleasant effect of mixing carbohydrate and protein at lunchtime. It's a common event in Britain as we are still hooked on the 'meat and two veg' diet and one of the vegetables usually is potatoes, a great source of starch. And starch is a carbohydrate; it breaks down to sugar.

Now the gut always gets started on digesting the protein first with hydrochloric acid and pepsin etc. in the stomach. So the carbohydrate you've eaten is forced to hang around waiting to be digested, and it become a perfect substrate for bacterial fermentation. And as the home-made beer and wine makers amongst you know, fermentation processes produce copious amounts of gas!

This proliferation of microorganisms in the gut can easily lead to imbalance in gut flora and overgrowth of pathogenic microbes. This is known as dysbiosis.

The gut flora perform many functions that keep us healthy. Major useful functions of friendly bacteria include:

- Producing short chain fatty acids
- Participating in the metabolism of hormones
- Producing valuable nutrients such as B vitamins and vitamin K
- Protecting you from infection by nasty bacteria
- Maintaining a healthy intestinal pH
- Helping your immune system
- Preventing yeast cells from taking over.

These bacteria live in harmony in your intestines and this symbiosis is essential to our good health. Once things get out of balance, that is when dysbiosis sets in.

So what can go wrong?

Nasty things start to occur in your gut when the population of friendly bacteria is reduced, then other undesirable organisms such as yeasts increase their numbers and take over the intestines. These yeasts then invade the whole body. And just like yeast in wine or beer, they ferment sugars as food. These yeasts consume sugars in your gut, leaving you with a feeling that you want more. Once these yeasts have invaded your body, they control your sugar intake, just like a tapeworm in your intestines devouring all the food. Your insatiable desire for sugar leads to all sorts of problems like chronic fatigue syndrome.

There are lots of factors that can disrupt the balance of organisms in the intestines and lead to overgrowth of these less desirable species. The most important factors are:

- Using antibiotics
- Using a birth control pill hormone
- Using hormones especially immunosuppressants such as steroids
- Diet rich in sugars and carbohydrates (potatoes, starch, white bread)
- Excessive consumption of alcohol
- Excessive stress

Probably the most important factor is the use of broad-spectrum antibiotics. These medications kill all bacteria, but they don't discriminate between friendly and nasty bacteria. This means that every time you take antibiotic drugs for an infection you are wiping out literally billions of friendly bacteria in your intestines that give protection from other, potentially harmful, intestinal residents like yeasts.

There has also been a lot of animal research showing that both antibiotics and steroids commonly cause substantial increases in Candida and pathogenic bacterial colonization, due to destruction of friendly bacteria, thereby reducing the immune defence system.

One of the common consequences of using popular antibiotics is *antibiotic induced diarrhoea*, which is caused mainly by a nasty pathogenic bacterium called Clostridium difficile that has now become resistant to many popular antibiotics. These cases are on the increase, with 3 million cases reported in 2005 in the United States. Clostridium difficile infection is appropriately named because it is difficult to treat and severe cases can even lead to death, especially in hospital patients who are already weakened by other kinds of infections. Treatment involves prescribing even more antibiotics, this time targeted at Clostridium difficile in particular.

In technical circles this Clostridium difficile is called CD which makes it sound quite friendly, really. So if you read or hear of someone who is struck down with a CD outbreak it won't be related to Max Bygrave's latest collection of old hits on compact disc. But it will mean a toilet roll shortage at their house, so if you visit, take your own.

A more common effect of antibiotics is the havoc it plays with your sense of taste. Until recently, antibiotic drugs were seen as a magic bullet without side effects. But we now know that not only is there a major problem with strains of bacteria becoming resistant to these antibiotics, they also create havoc with the body's natural defence bacteria, leading to systemic yeast infections or serious side effects like CD or the methicillin resistant staphylococcus aureus bacteria, more commonly (and easily) known as MRSA or the 'hospital superbug'.

Do you crave chocolate?

You could be deficient in PHENYLETHYLAMINE

Chocolate is the most psychoactive food on the shelves in the supermarket today. Theobroma, the Greek name for the cacao tree which yields cacao beans literally means 'food of the gods' and the Aztec economy was even based on these beans. Apparently 100 beans could buy a slave.

Placebo controlled trials have shown that chocolate may subtly enhance cognitive function – verbal and visual memory are enhanced by eating chocolate. This is because it is a veritable cocktail of brain chemicals. You'll need better cognitive function to be able to pronounce them – better start eating chocolate right now, then.

Chocolate contains a small amount of a chemical called anandamide, an endogenous cannabinoid found in the brain. There will never be enough to turn a bar of chocolate into a marijuana joint, but chocolate also contains two almost unpronounceable chemicals (n-oleolethanolamine and N-linoleoylethanolamine) that inhibit the metabolism of anandamide and so these prolong the effect of it in the brain. Nice.

Chocolate also contains caffeine, and theobromine, a chemical that is said to work even better than codeine at suppressing the coughing response. Great excuse to eat lots of dark chocolate if you have a cold, then (milk chocolate is no good because it has too much sugar, contains milk that causes mucous, and not enough theobromine). Most quality dark chocolate is dairy-free, not a lot of people know that.

It also has lots of tryptophan, an amino acid that controls the production of serotonin, the mood chemical. Nice again.

Acute monthly cravings for chocolate from pre-menstrual women probably occur because chocolate is rich in magnesium, and magnesium deficiency makes PMT worse.

Oddly, cravings are usually worse in the late afternoon and early evening, probably because progesterone makes your body store energy as fat during the day, leaving you with an energy gap that chocolate fills nicely in the early evening.

But despite all these chemicals, chocolate's key ingredient is probably phenylethylamine, or PEA. Phenylethylamine releases dopamine in the mesolimbic pleasure centres of the brain. That's the part that takes a key role in sexual orgasms.

Some scientists say that most of the PEA is metabolised before it gets to the brain by a reaction with the enzyme monoamine oxidase type b (MAOb), but we are very sensitive to even small amounts of PEA.

PEA can even produce characteristic behaviour found in amphetamine users. PEA helps mediate feelings of attraction, excitement, giddiness and euphoria. This is why chocolate is known universally as the sex substitute. In fact in one survey 50% of women said they preferred chocolate to sex.

Why are these chemical in the cacao bean? Well, plants have been around for a long time and since they cannot run away from their enemies they have developed an arsenal of chemicals to deter their predators. Bad luck for the cacao tree, then to have been discovered by a predator that gets PMT.

PEA might have a sinister side, because one of its metabolites is unusually high in people with paranoid schizophrenia. There is even a PEA theory of depression in a few people caused by MOAb and PEA reactions that go wrong. So, for these people, chocolate should perhaps be avoided.

Chocolate cravings are not unusual, especially in people who are especially switched on by brain chemistry, to stimulate the reward centre in particular. Chocolate contains high levels of sugar, copper, caffeine, theobromine and theophylline which are all dopamine "pleasure transmitter" agonists and hence are very addictive. Copper activates MAOa to breakdown all monamines like 5HT and NE apart from the all important dopamine and beta-phenethylamine.

So why should we crave these things? Well we all have addictive genes to some degree, and some people are more susceptible than others. The genes encoding MAO-A and MAO-B are located side-by-side on the short arm of the X chromosome, and variations from one person to another are associated with arousal and novelty seeking.

Cravings, even obsessions, are a part of modern culture. You only have to look at the following list to see that's true.

- 25% of members of Gamblers Anonymous UK have a problem with fruit machines
- $11.9 billion - global internet gambling revenue in 2005
- 2000 - the estimated number of internet gambling sites
- 23 million - number of online gamblers in 2005, 8 million of whom are in the US, and 4 million in UK
- 75% of adults in the US have gambled in the past year
- $82.2 billion - global gambling revenue in 2005, estimated to rise by over 50% by 2010
- 60 million - obese adults in the US with an eating problem
- 83% of 8 to 18-year-olds have a video game player
- 2 hours - time spent gaming each day in average US household
- 31 hours - average time spent online per month worldwide
- 9 kilograms - amount of chocolate consumed per person per year in UK. Do you eat your share? You can judge your 'addiction level' by it

Do you feel sleepy after eating?

You could have a CHROMIUM deficiency

It is quite common for people to feel contented and sleepy after a big meal like a Christmas dinner. Eating produces a rise in blood sugar and a surge in insulin production. This chemical activity sends tryptophan to the brain where it triggers serotonin, the 'mood chemical' that calms you and can send you to sleep. But you can be forgiven at Christmas, because that turkey you consumed is also a rich provider of tryptophan. The fact that you were up late playing Father Christmas, and awake before dawn watching your children open presents may also have something to do with it.

But some people feel really tired after most meals, irrespective of what they ate, and the most likely reason is that they are deficient in chromium. This will cause the pancreas to function erratically and overproduce insulin in response to a rise in blood sugar. Occasionally these people even get an adrenalin rush from caffeine (adrenergic hypoglycemia). What happens is that too much insulin uses up the available sugar quickly and you experience an 'energy gap' leaving you feeling weak and tired.

Hyperinsulinism and chromium deficiency-induced insulin resistance is commonly associated with post-prandial drowsiness. Never heard that term before? Neither had I. Although medical terms usually have a reasonably logical derivation, this is not the case with "prandial." It comes from the Latin "prandium" which meant "a late breakfast or lunch." "Prandium" was derived in turn from the Greek "pro-", before + "endios", midday. Now, however, "prandial" refers to any meal -- breakfast, lunch, supper or even a snack. I mention it because post-prandial drowsiness sounds a useful pseudo-medical term to bandy about if you are partial to an afternoon nap at work.

So if you feel post-prandial drowsiness you should take a chromium supplement with your meal, because chromium is essential in the reaction that converts glucose into energy through the action of insulin. Many cases of diabetes type 2 are believed to be due to chromium deficiency. Another reason for drowsiness can be fasting hypoglycaemia which occurs at the 4-6 hr range owing to deficient corticosteroids through not eating.

Zinc and vanadium are two more important minerals that are essential in the glucose cycle, and if you are eating too much sugar, this can also cause a vitamin B deficency which may also mimic hypoglycaemia.

Feeling sleepy after food has some slightly sinister overtones, too. Chromium deficiency often accompanies diabetes type 2, so your sleepy head is trying to tell you something. Rectify that chromium deficiency and you will be going a long way towards fending off insulin tolerance that signals diabetes type 2. Of course you need to top up your zinc and vanadium as well which means eating plenty of green vegetables and fresh fruit. Any vanadium supplementation neeeds to be done with care since an excess is associated with manic depression.

Recently a team of researchers at Manchester University have discovered that high blood glucose levels, similar to those after eating a big meal, can switch off the brain cells that normally keep all of us awake and alert to some extent.

'The findings make evolutionary sense since sleepiness could be the body's way of telling us to relax and conserve energy once we have found and eaten our food', says Denis Burdakov of the University of Manchester, UK, who led the research.

"It has been known for a while that people and animals can become sleepy and less active after a meal, but the brain signals responsible for this were poorly understood," he says.

Burdakov's team studied a group of brain cells called orexin neurons, which are found in the hypothalamus and produce proteins called orexins that are essential for maintaining normal wakefulness in humans. These neurons are less active at night and when they malfunction this can lead to narcolepsy, where sufferers cannot stay awake.

He believes this could also explain why it can be difficult to sleep when we are hungry, since the activity of the neurons would be higher when there is less glucose in the blood. And when they become faulty this could trigger obesity in later life.

Are you an alcoholic?

You could be deficient in B1, B3, B6, B12, Folate, Zinc, Magnesium and Lithium.

Everyone responds differently to alcohol. Are you the sort of person that becomes a poet after drinking? Perhaps you want to fight everyone! Are you the type of person that gets tipsy after one drink, or can you hold your liquor with the hardest drinker?

Your response to alcohol is determined by your *alcohol biotype*.

Identifying your alcohol biotype is important because that will help you control your drinking, and even allow you to derive the maximum enjoyment from alcohol. It might even save you from a life of alcoholism.

Several years ago I had the good fortune to meet Simon Galloway, a young neurological nutritionist with a mission to help members of society with drug or alcohol problems who were not getting suitable treatment from the Health Service. He reviewed the pathways by which people metabolise alcohol for me, and the following section is his review. To this day I have not seen anything similar or so succinctly written despite the vast sums that are needed to treat alcohol addiction. I have always found that the key to understanding a problem is to confront it head on.

This is biochemistry, and so it is a bit more complicated, but I have reproduced it here for those who want to begin to understand their drinking problem or use it as a stepping stone to read around the subject on the internet.

ALCOHOL METABOLISM. *The five alcoholic biotypes.*

When you drink alcohol it is rapidly absorbed from the stomach. Once in the bloodstream, it is broken down into a compound called acetaldehyde which is one of the substances that gives you a hangover. Acetaldehyde is then decomposed by an enzyme produced in the liver called alcohol dehydrogenase II (ADH2). In this book whenever you encounter a 'dehydrogenase' you can be sure it is an enzyme that breaks down whatever it is designed for. In the case of alcohol dehydrogenase, ADH2 uses one of the following routes.

- ADH2/1 is the enzyme that is predominant in white and black populations.

- ADH2/2 is a modification of the enzyme and it breaks down alcohol 40% faster in around 10% of Europeans and over 90% of Far Eastern Asian populations.

- ADH2/3 is another modification found in 15-25% of African Americans and American Indians.

Acetaldehyde is toxic and is the cause of alcoholic poisoning and hangovers, but it is slowly oxidized to harmless acetate by another enzyme, acetaldehyde dehydrogenase (ALDH) found in virtually everybody. One special case though, ALDH2/1, is an enzyme that is found in 45-50% of Orientals, but is rarely observed in Caucasians. These people develop a facial flushing response.

These different metabolic pathways have produced several *biotypes*.

Biotype 1. The THIQ Biotype.

This biotype suffers from the unpleasant effects of acetaldehyde poisoning, so this biotype can quite easily develop problem drinking over time.

As his tolerance to alcohol increases and his consumption rises to meet the demand his brain is eventually forced to adapt to the acetaldehyde by-product generated by the liver. But instead of acting as a drinking deterrent, acetaldehyde mixes with neurotransmitters in the brain to form addictive morphine-like substances called THIQ'S (tetrahydroisoquinolines) and anxiety-causing substances called THBC's (tetrahydro-beta-carbolines). They only become pronounceable once you're pissed. These cause an addiction to alcohol.

The drinker becomes dependent on these alcohol by-product effects to feel normal. To make matters worse, a substance called mTHBC (1-methyl-tetrahydro-beta-carboline) forms which is thought to be responsible for anxiety neuroses seen in this biotype when they stop drinking.

His high alcohol consumption ensures he receives a constant supply of the "biologically rewarding" and mood-enhancing THIQ's which keep him hooked and whilst he needs several drinks to get the feeling he seeks, there is little accompanying intoxication and usually no hangover by this time. His sobriety usually wont last long however because without the THIQ's he doesn't feel normal and the intensely anxiogenic THBC's in his system keep him running back to alcohol for relief.

This category is made up of Type-A personalities, compulsive with a strong sex drive, requiring little sleep to function properly. Alcohol gives them energy and improves their performance. These are the big drinkers who can consume alcohol all day and who stay on a high with little sign of inebriation or negative effects. They have a high tolerance for alcohol and after many years of drinking are more prone to develop liver problems than psychiatric symptoms.

Biotype 2. The Allergic-Addicted biotype:

He is allergic to grapes, grains, amyl alcohols, phenols or "congeners" in alcohol and addicted to the opioid-like substances they liberate in the brain resulting in a short term high followed by bad physical withdrawal.

Once opioids (opium-like chemicals) are exhausted the pleasant "biological reward" effects are interrupted and he will experience a rebound depression, aggression, or crying spells and allergic, "toxic" withdrawals the morning after. This biotype may also develop cravings for alcohol after exposure to stimulant chemicals like gasoline, formaldehyde, printers ink and hydrocarbons which activate the same processes in the brain as the alcohol congeners.

Often arising from Northern European or American Indian ancestors, this category is made up of the typical "bad-starters" who learn how to drink. They are often moody, changeable and unpredictable alcoholics who experience very bad hangovers and who may become socially disruptive, engaging in fights and arguments, dangerous driving, irrational or bizarre behaviour and even criminal acts after drinking.

Biotype 3. The PGE1 Deficient biotype:

He suffers with a lifelong depression resulting from a genetically low level of the neurotransmitter prostaglandin E1 (PGE1). Alcoholic drinks stimulate the release of PGE1 which temporarily lifts his low mood until brain stores are depleted and his depression returns. The rebound depression that follows is often worse than before because alcohol frustrates his body's naturally slow production of fresh PGE1 which has to be made by the body from omega 6 essential fatty acids.

Consequently, this person may crave crisps, or other fatty acid sources (fish and chips or battered Mars bars?). Often arising from Scottish, Welsh, Irish, and Scandinavian ancestors this category is made up of lifelong sombre, introverted and depressed individuals who visibly cheer up after drinking. They drink to banish their depression and may become suicidal once a tolerance builds up to the effects of the drug.

Biotype 4. The Hypoglycaemic biotype:

He is addicted to the sugars in alcohol because his body ordinarily produces too much insulin in response to sugar in the drink, which starves his brain of the glucose it needs. He feels a rapid lift after drinking, from the sugar, followed shortly thereafter by an exaggeration in his original hypoglycaemic symptoms like light-headedness, spaciness, confusion, weakness, sleepiness and lack of co-ordination. Consequently he gets very hungry after drinking. He has a low tolerance for alcohol and can easily be mistaken for an out of control drinker.

He usually experiences hangovers because alcohol triggers insulin shock which causes fatigue, lethargy, confusion, "brainfog", depression and irritability. This category is made up of individuals who cannot handle too much alcohol and who despite feeling a temporary increase in well-being after a drink or two, quickly show signs of neuroglycopenia (brain glucose starvation) resembling intoxication. (that's definitely me!)

Biotype 5. The Dopamine deficient biotype.

He inherits a genetic defect in the Dopamine D2 inhibitory auto-receptor and possibly other receptors in the brain. This has been dubbed "Reward Deficiency Syndrome" and results in an increased likelihood of addictive behaviours that temporarily raise dopamine, such as drinking, and risk taking. This group contains many of the seriously committed alcoholics, often incorporated with traits from other groups.

The Body Language of Health

This group's behaviour depends on their genetic tendencies to one of four Dopamine receptor genes, called the A1, A2, A3 and A4 alleles. The A3 and A4 variants are rare, whereas the A2 variant is found in nearly 75 percent of the general population and the A1 variant in about 25 percent of the population.

In any group of liver-damaged alcoholics, 69% have the A1 variant and 31% have the A2 variant, whereas in non-alcoholics 20% have the A1 variant and 80% have the A2 variant. Fortunately the craving seen by A1 carriers is not that great.

Biotype 5 is made up of the risk takers, gamblers, sexually promiscuous, compulsive overeaters, drug takers, and alcoholics who may show a lifelong tendency to antisocial behaviour, conduct disorders, violent behaviour, and criminal tendencies.

Many prisoners and re-offenders will fall into this category.

Which biotype are you?

You've probably been able to identify your biotype from the summary in each section; maybe you can place a few friends or celebrities into their category too. Most people fit into one or other even if they are not 100% one category, and have some overlap into others.

Your biotype is determined by your genetic background, you have your parents, or more likely, your grandparents to thank for your alcohol problem. And alcohol predisposition can be used to identify your other traits, such as risk taking, too.

So does this bring us any nearer a cure? Not at the moment. But knowing your biotype certainly helps you to understand your addiction and so it should help you to come to terms with it and modify your behaviour. That is why I am surprised this information is not more widely appreciated.

You will only give up alcohol, and other drugs for that matter if you really want to. Until that time, check out your biotype, come to terms with it and try to reduce your drinking pattern. Knowing how these addictions work, I have been instrumental in developed a range of psycho-nutritional products to alleviate each biotype's addiction, plus a product to help repair the liver damage from alcohol. But we would need financing to market these, so if you have a mission to fulfill and perhaps want to help others with addictions, I am sure this would become a worthy project. If you want more information you can contact me via the www.bodylanguage.co.uk website

The Body Language of Health

How much alcohol takes me to the safe driving limit?

During my career as a forensic scientist I have often been asked that question and my answer has always been the same. My answer is --- none.

I have attended scenes of a few serious vehicle accidents myself in the past. Most road accidents at night are due to alcohol. And 80% of hospital admissions after 10pm are also due to the effects of alcohol. There is no 'safe' level of alcohol intoxication if you are a driver, and no, alcohol doesn't make you a better driver either.

The amount of alcohol needed to take you over the limit is actually different for each individual, so there is no hard and fast rule about how much you can drink and then drive. Each person will also have a slightly different level from one day to another, as well, even if they replicate the drinking process again exactly, so it is very dangerous to 'calculate' your alcohol level when you are out drinking and considering driving. In fact any alcohol has been proven to adversely affect your driving skill, reaction time and judgement. Because it impairs your judgement, you just think it is making you drive better. This is because alcohol is not a stimulant, it is a depressant. But it works that way because the first thing it does is to depress your inhibitions.

Taking food, or exercising will have no significant effect on the rate of breakdown of the alcohol. This is a popular misconception. What food does is to make you feel a little better because it supplies you with blood sugars, which the alcohol will have starved you of as it passes into your body. That's why you often feel hungry after drinking alcohol.

But I fear there are a few drivers whom we will never fully convince to leave their car at home when they go out for a drink. And now, you probably know why? The answer is in the alcohol biotypes information. Some determined consumers of alcohol are risk takers, with a lifelong tendency to antisocial behaviour, conduct disorders, violent behaviour, and criminal tendencies. They don't care. The risk of getting stopped by a police patrol car is all part of the fun for these people, in some cases even when they have already had their licence confiscated.

And, don't forget, if the alcohol level reaches much above 250 to 300 mg (some three or four times over the limit, but not uncommon with binge drinking) you will get alcoholic poisoning. This is often fatal. The highest level I have ever encountered when testing blood from drink drivers in the forensic lab was 427 mg, (from a driver!!) and we all reckoned he was very lucky to still be alive.

He was a doctor, so he should have known better.

The Body Language of Health

Recently I got involved with a team of clever scientists in Germany who had perfected a system of analysing hair for the alcohol history of the donor. This can be very important for a number of reasons. Alcoholics usually deny their drinking habits or else they grossly underestimate the amount they drink, often quite innocently. So having a correct estimate of their drinking pattern is valuable in offering them the right sort of moral and medical support. The biggest value of hair analysis is that their history is locked into their hair strands as the hair grows, and most people will be able to donate around six months of history locked in their locks. So the alcohol history is available for experts to use as evidence of that person's drinking history.

The courts also find hair analysis valuable when they are faced with the problem of placing children with parents who are divorcing if there is a history of alcohol abuse in the family. Here, knowledge of the alcohol history of a parent is very helpful to the court team whom I find are genuinely concerned about taking the right action for the child and the parents as well.

The consumption of 60 grams of alcohol per day used to qualify someone with an alcohol 'problem' is quite significant. In the U.K. alcohol is based on 'units' to allow drinkers to establish their alcohol consumption. One unit is 8 grams (10 millilitres) of pure alcohol. However the amount of drink that equates to 60 grams depends on how strong the drink is. On average, one pub measure of wine, one half pint of average strength beer, and one 'short' of spirit are all one unit. So seven of these units provides $7 \times 8 = 56$ grams of alcohol. A 750ml bottle wine with 13% alcohol by volume would contain 750ml x 0.13% ABV ÷ 1000 = 9.75 units.

Alcoholism is now considered to be a disease, and we have seen that it is certainly strongly influenced by genetic tendencies. But not many people realise that alcoholism is also affected by vitamin and mineral deficiencies that predispose someone towards alcohol and result in alcoholism. Deficiencies of vitamins B1, B3, B6, B12 and folate produce this tendency, and so do deficiencies of zinc, magnesium and lithium.

So maybe you can tell by now that I am pretty well switched on by alcohol, without even touching a drop. Of course, alcohol is the most abused drug, and rates highly in the 'does the most harm' scale which incidentally is topped by nicotine. Yes, experts rate tobacco above crack cocaine in the harm stakes simply because tobacco is so invasive in society today.

Recently I used my knowledge of alcohol biotypes to invent a skin patch that reduced the effect of a hangover.

The Body Language of Health

Lots of products can be transmitted through a topical transdermal patch, because it is possible through careful use of skin dilatants to open up the pores to allow even large molecules through the skin. Patches are perfect for compounds which would normally be destroyed by the digestive system.

Apparently my patches, which are now sold widely across America and Europe, have been used extensively and users claim they work brilliantly. Of course, reducing the effects of a hangover should never be a reason to consume alcohol to excess, these patches are designed for those people in the non-addictive group who struggle to break down acetaldehyde.

The metabolic pathways described above rely on a suitable supply of precursor chemicals for them to work efficiently. In practice this means a suitable supply in the diet of vitamins B1, B3, B6, B12, and folate plus the minerals Zinc, Magnesium and Lithium. The most important is probably zinc. The problem here is that many alcoholics and social drinkers have a poor diet.

There is also good evidence that deficiency in these substances fuels the craving for alcohol. So one of the things that counsellors need to do in tackling alcohol abuse is to balance out the diet with supplements. One simple way to check for zinc deficiency is the Zinc Taste Test. Remember that you can tell if you have the 'sticky finger gene by licking your fingers? If your fingers have more salt than the salt content of your saliva, the fingers will taste salty. But if they are the same you won't taste anything? We are conditioned to look for differences like this, it is what drives our craving for minerals.

The zinc taste test gauges relative zinc deficiency based on whether the zinc tastes strong or not. It is the easiest and most accurate way to determine a zinc deficiency. Laboratory tests for zinc deficiency are not very accurate because most of the zinc is locked up in cells.

You can make your own Zinc Taste Test solution by mixing a 0.1% solution of zinc sulphate. You do that by adding 1 gram of zinc sulphate heptahydrate (ZnSo4 7 H20) in 1 litre of distilled water and mixing well. If you can't manage that you can buy a 0.1% solution by mail on www.eclipsenaturalcare.com. This solution is used as a treatment for anorexia and is sterile, but the solution you make is not sterile so it won't keep more than a day.

Don't eat, drink, or smoke for at least an hour before the test. Then take the equivalent of a liqueur glass of the fluid and rinse your mouth with the fluid for 5-10 seconds, after which you can either swallow or spit it out. Four different flavours now appear:

- No flavour or "like water" = typical chronic zinc deficiency.
- No flavour to begin with, but later a reaction occurs described as either "dry", "fluffy", "mineral", "like baking powder" or "sweet" = moderate zinc deficiency.
- A strong but not necessarily unpleasant flavour is registered immediately and builds up little by little = slight or no zinc deficiency.
- An unpleasant flavour is registered immediately. You might make a wry face and want to rinse you mouth with water = no zinc deficiency, good zinc status.

You can take this liquid as your zinc supplement. After three weeks you should be able to taste the zinc and exhibit the 'no zinc deficiency' category. If you don't you should see your doctor for a gastric acid examination.

The taste test can be used in all sorts of other ways using different minerals. Just apply the same rules as above to other salts.

Are you a Vegan?

You may be deficient in VITAMIN B12, ZINC and IRON

First, let's get the definition of a vegan and a vegetarian sorted out.

A vegetarian does not eat red meat (e.g. lamb, bacon, pork, beef), white meat or poultry (e.g. duck, chicken, turkey), fish or other sea creatures (e.g. tuna, cod, prawns, lobster) or slaughterhouse by-products (e.g. animal fat or lard, and gelatine, as it is made from crushed bones, horns etc).

A vegetarian may or may not eat eggs and dairy products (e.g. cow's milk, cheese, butter, yoghurt). Vegetarians who choose to eat dairy products and eggs are called Lacto-ovo-vegetarians.

Those who do not eat eggs, but choose to eat dairy products are called Lacto-vegetarians, and those who eat eggs but not dairy are called Ovo-vegetarians.

Those people who avoid all animal and bird products, including all dairy products, eggs and honey are called Vegans.

The Body Language of Health

So right from the start, a vegan has a restricted diet. You might think this would be a problem. But if a vegan can get hold of a good, organic source of fruit and vegetables, and eat a properly balanced diet, it should be possible to avoid deficiencies of minerals. The problem is that the soil used for agriculture has now become so depleted that it is lacking in many of the minerals and elements that the plants need for healthy growth. When we eat these plants we too become deficient.

So you may be surprised to find that many scientific studies comparing vegetarians with eaters of a typical Western diet have found that vegetarians are considerably healthier and less likely to suffer from a wide range of illnesses than meat eaters, and they tend to live longer.

What's more, there are apparently no illnesses which seem to affect vegetarians more than meat eaters. Since 1898, nutritionists have been telling us that a poor diet is the single most important factor in causing cancer than anything else. Many studies point to gluttonous consumption of meat as especially harmful.

In fact vegetarian diets are associated with reduced risk for a number of chronic diseases, including obesity, coronary artery disease, hypertension, diabetes, colorectal cancer, lung cancer, and kidney disease. In many developing countries of the world where few animal products are eaten, such diseases are virtually unknown.

But vegans can suffer from deficiency of vitamin B12, zinc and iron, because they do not eat meat.

Vitamin B12 is very important and lack of it in the body has been known to cause a range of problems including numbness down one side of the body. All manner of unusual effects can manifest themselves through eating a diet that lacks something or other. For vegans, vitamin B12 supplements are a good idea, along with a supply of iron supplements.

By now, you will have started to get the message that our body needs certain essential nutrients, and the modern diet is not providing the right nutrition. Refined sugar is alien to our diet, and is thought to be the major cause of so many ailments in modern society. Milk is designed for baby cows, and anecdotally has been associated with many allergies and even cancers. And, whatever your taste is in food, I have strong evidence that we were not designed to eat meat, and that meat can cause big problems to the human race.

Scientists have been telling us for years that we are omnivorous, we eat fruit, vegetables and meat. So why should I go against the trend and suggest humans are not meat eaters?

Well, humans have evolved along a certain path which has shaped our digestive system, our immune system, and our body's control mechanisms. We work best under those same conditions. Let's examine them in greater detail.

To understand why diet is so important, we need to look closely at our evolution.

Our Prehistoric Beginnings.

Why we know we are basically vegetarian in origin

Scientists still disagree over whether we are vegetarian, carnivores or omnivores but I believe the evidence is stacked in the favour of the vegetarians. Here's why.

We know that human evolution has been under way for between three and four million years. Modern humans, that is, people who are anatomically indistinguishable from us, date back at least 130,000 years and probably longer. During that time our fashion sense may have deteriorated, but our bodies and internal organs have changed relatively little.

Although there are no written records as old as that, we have still been able to piece together the history of the earth during those times. The deepest ice cores taken from Greenland go back as far as a quarter of a million years, and although there is no evidence of man, they tell us a remarkable story. Trapped in the ice are two isotopes of oxygen; one is prevalent in hotter climates, the other is prevalent in colder climates. By measuring the concentration of these isotopes, scientists have mapped out the global climate that man had to contend with during his evolution, and this relates to world-wide conditions, not just to local conditions in Greenland.

These oxygen isotope figures gave us two startling facts. The first is that the last 10,000 years, the period that geologists call the Holocene, have been unusually warm. To find any comparable time when the temperature was as warm for any period, we have to go back over 120,000 years. The second fact is that the Holocene has been a period of remarkable climatic stability. Prior to that the climate see-sawed from very very cold, to brief intervals when the climate was far hotter than it is today. The

The Body Language of Health

Holocene is therefore a very unusual period, and it seems that it has been crucial to the development of human civilisation. There has been nothing like it in the last 100,000 years, which is most of the period of time that 'modern' humans have been around.

This means that for 120,000 years 'modern man' eked out an existence in a hostile world with major temperature changes that make climate change today totally trivial. At times the climate would be unbearably hot. At other times, there were ice ages so severe that ice built up miles thick over much of today's populated continents. Remember, there was no central heating, no weapons, no power stations, no supermarkets, in fact nothing that we take for granted today. Then in the last ten thousand years, the climate stabilised and humans prospered and proliferated.

So it is no coincidence that the last ten thousand years also represents the dawn of our civilisations. Before the Holocene period, humans had developed as nomadic groups by necessity because we had to forage for food, and our diet then probably consisted of mainly nuts, berries and roots. The stable climate of the Holocene suddenly gave man the opportunity to settle, farm, collect seeds and cultivate them the following year; before the Holocene, the climate would have been too unpredictable for farming to succeed.

But ten thousand years, in evolutionary time, is nothing. And the age of 'enlightenment' of the human race brought about by science and medicine over the last 350 years is merely a fleeting moment in our evolutionary history. We have changed hardly at all physiologically. Our digestive system still functions like that of a cave man. So our digestive system still functions best with the diet consumed in prehistoric times.

For maximum health and longevity our diet should conform as nearly as possible to that in the Stone Age.

You've probably noticed that most wild animals stay sleek and healthy and don't become obese, even when food is plentiful. But you probably haven't noticed that this is true even for animals kept in zoos, and domestic animals, particularly dogs and cats, even when food is widely available. They only become obese when they are fed the wrong diet, such as introducing cereals and other carbohydrates to their meat diet. Goats weren't designed to eat potato crisps, after all. But as long as the diet is restricted to the animal's natural food, the animal stays healthy. And again, natural food means the diet the animal would have found in the wild, feathers and all. Cats and dogs only get fat when fed cream, cereals, chocolate and other foods they were not designed to eat.

The Body Language of Health

As a youth, I used to live in a small town in the Peak District of Derbyshire. The local shops had a range of products, and our diet was probably chosen from about one hundred different foods. If we visited the local Maypole grocers, (there was no such thing as a 'supermarket' then) we could perhaps choose from a couple of hundred products, because they introduced a few additional delicacies from the British colonies. Nowadays a very average supermarket gives us a choice of over twenty five thousand items.

But most of these are really processed products based on those few hundred basic ingredients. And we were not designed to eat most of these processed foods.

So how do we know what diet our body is designed for?

Anthropologists tell us that humans are omnivorous, they have evolved to eat anything. And the burger-meisters of America tell us we most definitely are carnivores with a propensity to 'fingerlickin'.

However by doing a little research of my own, I can tell you that there are compelling reasons to suggest that meat was not a significant part of prehistoric man's diet.

Our dental pattern most closely resembles that of the apes, like chimpanzees and gorillas. Their diet is mainly fruits and leaves, occasional insects and small animals, but rarely meat from larger animals. Our dental pattern is most unlike any of the meat-eating mammals.

But there is even more overwhelming evidence that our digestive system points towards a mainly herbivorous diet, with little meat. This is because our saliva contains an enzyme called ptyalin, which is needed for the pre-digestion of starchy plant material. This enzyme is not produced by any of the carnivores. They don't need it, because they don't eat starchy plants. But we do (or did).

The concentration of stomach acid in man is also lower than in carnivores and our intestines are much longer, because they are designed for the digestion of plant materials. Moreover, humans do not have the ability to convert uric acid, which is derived from dietary meat protein, to the more soluble product called allantoin which can be excreted. Our inability to do this causes high levels of uric acid in humans when they eat too much meat protein. And uric acid builds up in those people who have a 'rich' diet and precipitates out in the extremities in the very painful arthritic condition known as gout. Even the name 'rich' diet implies an unusually extravagant choice of meat which is much more expensive and labour intensive to produce compared with fruit and vegetables. You have to be wealthy to eat quality meat, even now (sorry but most burgers don't count as quality meat).

So it seems true that meat would have been an occasional treat in primitive man's diet, and it should be in ours. We have evolved very little in physiological terms from early primitive man.

The anatomy of humans still resembles that of the great apes. Our pair of eyes focus forwards on the same object, giving us stereoscopic vision which is better suited for delicate hand and eye coordination. This is essential for picking fruit off trees. Even our colour vision is ideally adapted with the optimum reception and colour balance in the red/green range of the spectrum, which helped us to find the ripest and most nutritious fruit on the trees. Our response to the blue end of the spectrum is poor but then there are not that many blue fruits requiring our skill in spotting them hiding behind leaves on the trees. And blue fruits only turn black as they ripen.

We should mention cooking. Man is unique in the animal kingdom in eating cooked food; these days we find uncooked meat and fish unpalatable, apart from a few exceptions like sushi which even now is not to everyone's liking. However, Man would not have had regular access to fire prior to 7,000 BC. This is the merest twinkling of an eye in evolutionary terms. So cooking meat to make it palatable is a very recent innovation, and it probably started as a means of drying the meat or cooking it so that it didn't go bad so quickly.

But the most convincing argument that humans evolved on a vegetarian diet happens to be another unique aspect of human physiology. It is our lack of ability to synthesis ascorbic acid, better known as Vitamin C.

Man, together with only one or two other mammalian species, (most particularly, the Guinea Pig) is unique in not being able to manufacture vitamin C in the body, even though this is one of the most important vitamins necessary for a healthy body. Because we cannot manufacture it ourselves we have to keep ourselves supplied with a regular source of Vitamin C in our food or else we are in big trouble. This is undoubtedly because historically we existed on a diet of fruit and vegetables, high in vitamin C, and therefore didn't need to develop the ability to manufacture it. Now, vitamin C is one of the main supplements taken in Western societies.

So I am confident that the human race is designed for vegetarianism with occasional treats of meat.

The Body Language of Health

This always offends many people, who for some irrational reason feel they should defend their meat-eating. Most people who are not vegetarians tend to argue that a vegetarian diet is not sufficient to produce a strong and healthy body, and that a high meat diet is required for strong muscles. They argue that we need meat for protein and iron. But we shouldn't forget that the biggest, strongest animals, like elephants and oxen, are herbivorous, and they have just as much need for iron in their blood. In fact our own growth rate is greatest in the first five months of life; yet human breast milk is only 10% protein.

Nowadays, our commercial success has become our downfall. In the western world, modern man is now accustomed to a cheap and readily available supply of food, high in fats and protein, most of it over-processed, with many of the nutrients destroyed.

But we are poorly equipped to cope with this excess. The evolutionary necessity to gorge on food when plentiful to safeguard against times of famine is still present, but now we have excess we can eat constantly, not for purposes of nutrition, but for entertainment and as a distraction. Consequently, our unsuitable diet contributes directly to the increasing incidence of the main human diseases:

- Cardiovascular disease caused by high refined sugar diets. This produces insulin secretion, increasing cholesterol biosynthesis and switching immune system from PGE1 and PGE3 to an inflammatory, prothrombotic and plaque-forming PGE2 series instead,
- Cancer caused by carcinogenic food additives which interrupt mitochondrial aerobic respiration and cause antioxidant/bioflavinoid deficiency (viz proton excess and over-acid intracellular energetics forced to switch from Krebs to Glycolysis and organic acid (lactate) production leading to metastasis),
- Diabetes (NIDDM) and obesity (syndrome X) caused by high refined sugar diets (insulin receptor desensitization, bacterial endotoxin dysbiosis-induced pancreatitis and immune cross reaction-induced destruction of pancreatic beta cells), refined sugar-induced essential nutrient deficiencies and chronic cortisolemia-induced subclinical potassium deficiency leading to hyperinsulinism),
- Not enough exercise.

The Romans took their excessive eating and made it into a fine art. They found that the shape of the stomach can be extended when lying on your left side propped up with an elbow or some cushions. They invented the Roman dining couch which looked rather like a chaise-long expressly for food orgies so the recumbent diner could eat to excess by utilising their extended stomach.

The current concerns about global warming suggest that the 10,000 year-long temperature stability of the Holocene might be coming to an end. We have no ideas why this stability occurred after millennia of wildly fluctuating temperatures, and we have no idea how to maintain its stability. The current panic about global warming might be a political tactic, but one thing is certain. We are all the product of the earth's previous excursions into arctic and tropical climates. It appears to be one of the factors that shaped our digestive system.

But times are changing, because in addition to this climatic uncertainty, we no longer know what we are eating.

Mineral Depletion of the Soil

...why a 'healthy diet' isn't so healthy any more.

We are now confident that human civilisation as we know it only appeared ten thousand years ago because of the Holocene, providing us with predictable seasons and rainfall. This stability allowed humans to save seed and plant crops annually, so the hunter-gatherer lifestyle developed into a stable and structured civilisation.

But farming was quite unsophisticated until very recently when some element of mechanisation was introduced into farming. Jethro Tull invented the first seed drill that started the agricultural revolution in 1701, around three hundred years ago. The Babylonians actually invented a similar device two thousand years ago in Iraq, one of the most important regions in the development of human civilisation, but we tend to ignore these things when it suits us. The gardens of Babylon, you may remember, were one of the seven wonders of the ancient world (Babylon is 50 miles south of Baghdad).

Reliable harvests led to stable food supplies, and the agricultural revolution led to cheaper food, and as food became plentiful, so the population grew. And grew. And grew.

As a consequence we have now been farming the same land for hundreds of years. This was fine in the beginning as long as the agricultural cycle was complete. Crops grew, we harvested them, we ate them, and we put our manure back on the soil. In biological terms this is a closed cycle. Minerals used by the plants are taken away in the crop, but they are replaced when we use sewage as fertiliser.

The Body Language of Health

But with the recent introduction of intensive farming, this cycle has been broken. We send the crop away to be consumed elsewhere, and our sewage ends up in landfill or else is flushed down the toilet and ultimately ends up in the ocean. Each time we pick an apple we are in effect extracting essential nutrients out of the soil in which the tree is growing, and removing it from that piece of land. If we eat it locally and fertilise the ground under the tree with our sewage, that's fine, the minerals are released for the plant to use again, but these days we ship commodities like apples round the world but we don't ship the shit back again. And even with the common agricultural policy (CAP) I doubt the French would be willing to receive supplies of English sewage in exchange for their apples. (we'll call that policy CRAP).

Instead of using manure, we use artificial fertiliser rich in nitrogen and phosphorus, but the essential minerals are still missing. Repeated use of the same land has been progressively depleting the soil of the minerals we need in our food.

Plants need these mineral for their own healthy growth, and we need them for our own health when we eat plants. It is what has shaped our evolution and our bodily needs. Our need for minerals is part of our evolutionary development.

Many plants nowadays have been chosen for their vigour, which includes their ability to thrive in soil that is depleted in essential minerals. Soil in which their plant ancestors would most probably have died. Gardeners know that soil used to grow roses year after year becomes so 'rose sick' that planting a new bush in that soil is a waste of time. The healthy newcomer will never amount to anything and most probably will be troubled by one ailment after another. The same thing would happen to fruit and vegetable plants, but we have carefully picked out the plants that nature has conveniently genetically modified for us to thrive in depleted soil.

It seems obvious to me that the same thing happens to humans. The fruit, vegetables and cereals which form the bulk of our diet have been found to be deficient in a range of minerals and trace elements compared to those 50 years ago. Similar findings were found in animal-derived foodstuffs, including meat and dairy produce.

But we have no way of knowing that our food is nutritionally deficient.

When we were foragers, we instinctively knew that scabby apples, deformed vegetables, and skinny beans were going to be poor in nutrition, and we would seek out the best specimens. I remember my Grandfather always told me not to eat deformed vegetables 'If there is something deformed about it that's not fit food for a human' he used to say, and I am sure he was right.

But modern agriculture / herbicide control / hydroponics / plant science / genetic modification / artificial ripening deceives our eyes. Blemish-free produce has very little to do with nutrition but we now have no visual signs of poor quality within. The nutrition and key mineral elements are missing. Ridiculously, the supermarkets' demands for perfect fruit and vegetables are so powerful that farmers have to throw away a third of everything they grow. Anything with a slight blemish gets ploughed back into the soil. And those that are sold have chemical added to maintain their blemish free appearance. All fruit is dipped into a sterilising solution or it is irradiated before it is packaged and stored until the price is ripe for selling it, often months after picking.

A detailed, well-controlled experiment measured a range of minerals and trace elements in a variety of vegetables, fruit meat and dairy products has been documented by an acquaintance of mine, renowned geologist David Thomas. He has shown that certain critical ratios of the minerals which are important to human physiology have changed drastically in recent years.

He has collected data from sources that began in 1940 and finished in 1991, so representing a 50-year experiment. The differences in mineral content in the soil over this time have been alarming.

As I have already suggested, intensive farming, and the use of inorganic fertilisers, has gone on since the 1920's, but these fertilisers consist mainly of nitrogen, phosphorus and potassium. Calcium, in the form of lime is used to maintain alkalinity. Iron is sometimes added, but the essential trace elements are never deliberately replaced.

Vegetables are probably the best indicators of change to mineral content, because of their rapid growth and short life cycles.

Severe depletion in the mineral content of vegetables.

Perhaps the most concerning results relate to the mineral loss in two of the West's main vegetables, carrots and potatoes. They lost 75% of their magnesium content, 48% of their calcium, 46% of their iron and 75% of their copper. We would need to eat up to four times as much just to maintain the same mineral intake, but we would then get fat with all those excess calories from carbohydrate.

Calculation of critical ratios: Calcium:Potassium, Sodium:Potassium, Magnesium:Calcium and Iron:Copper found a significant change in all these ratios, which will have a major influence on our body's biochemistry. Because of plant selection, and the ability for plants to thrive on minerally deficient soil, beautiful, colourful, healthy fruit and vegetables deceive us into thinking they are good for us. But because they are minerally deficient, we don't know what a 'healthy diet' consists of any more.

In David Thomas' experiments mineral losses in fruit were somewhat less, because only a small part of the plant is harvested, and tree root systems are deeper and more extensive than those of vegetables. Nevertheless there were still significant overall losses in mineral content. Meats and Dairy products also showed a general depletion because of course the animals were fed depleted plants.

The following Table summarises average changes in mineral content of different types of vegetables (27 varieties), fruit (17 types) and meat (10 cuts) measured between 1940 and 1991.

Mineral	Vegetable	Fruit	Meat
Sodium (Na)	-49%	-29%	-30%
Potassium (K)	-16%	-19%	-16%
Phosphorous (P)	+9%	+2%	-28%
Magnesium (Mg)	-24%	-16%	-10%
Calcium (Ca)	-46%	-16%	-41%
Iron (Fe)	-27%	-24%	-54%
Copper (Cu)	-76%	-20%	-24%

This is very important in itself, because we are supplying ourselves less and less key nutrients, but deficiency in our diet is made even worse by recent radical changes to our eating habits.

There has been a massive increase in manufactured convenience foods, often referred to as 'junk food'. These are high in saturated fats, sugars and processed carbohydrates.

And over the last 30 years new manufactured products have filled the shelves of supermarkets (one superstore has 134 types of yoghurt) and there is a generation of children who have eaten little else and regard it as an appropriate diet.

Consequently, we have created a society which is *overfed but malnourished of micronutrients*. These factors have contributed to the rise in certain diseases, such as diabetes, obesity, cardiovascular disease and osteoporosis, and many of the symptoms described in this book.

The Body Language of Health

There have been various half-hearted attempts to rectify this. Jamie Oliver, a well known television chef, tried to improve school meals with fresh food, and manufacturers use fortified additives to replenish one or other missing ingredient. But they all miss the fundamental point that even the freshest food lacks essential nutrients because the soil is worn out.

Many of the minerals and trace elements missing from our food are essential for healthy living. For example magnesium is required for 300 enzyme reactions and zinc is also required for over 200 of them. It is no surprise to me that these two metallic elements crop up in Body language signs over and over again as deficiencies.

Chemical substances derived from the diet also affect human behaviour. A recent study demonstrated that taking the recommended daily allowance (RDA) of micronutrients assisted in the correction of ant-social behaviour of juveniles.

In the West we over indulge in poor quality food with a low intake of essential micronutrients. There is plenty of evidence to suggest that we overeat because our need for certain minerals is never satisfied. Our body never says 'enough' because we still don't have our quota of essential nutrients.

But we can't replace the soil. So what do we do?

Actually, there are some quite simple things we can do, and they happen to be environmentally friendly too. But they need some radical changes to how we handle our waist, by controlling our waste.

Some years ago I was asked to investigate the corrosion of a handrail at an industrial plant in Milton Keynes. I arrived to find that the industrial plant was in fact a huge silo used to contain human sewage. Two hundred and fifty thousand gallons of (sh) it. Most of the silo had been emptied awaiting my arrival, but the spherical base still had a five feet deep lake of concentrated solids flushed from all the toilets in Milton Keynes.

The handrail was positioned round a metal plinth about six feet from the base of the silo.

On the *inside* of the silo.

The contractors had opened a manhole on the side of the silo, and had very considerately inserted a duct through an access hole in the roof, through which blew fresh air. There was also gas monitoring equipment present to make sure we wouldn't be blown up or suffocated by the remains of the methane in the silo. Can you imagine putting your head down the toilet bowl after it has been used for two weeks without flushing? That is how it smelt, only multiplied by the number of inhabitants of Milton Keynes.

That's 350,000 bottoms, making it 350,000 times stronger than a toilet bowl, or so it seemed. Milton, yes, but keen? No not really.

I remember precariously edging my way round the plinth, squelching the sewage solids under my feet, and my only hand hold was the slimy, turd-infested handrail which you will remember was corroded and likely to come off in my hand at any moment. I felt like the woodcutter sawing the very branch on which his ladder was resting. Anyway, I survived the ordeal to tell the tale. Phew.

But let me get to the point of the story. This sewage plant was ingenious. The silo filled with sewage sludge, and was then kept warm by hot water from a boiler in an adjacent building. Bacteria digested the sewage and produced huge quantities of methane, which bubbled to the top and was collected to fuel the boiler that kept the silo warm.

Once the silo was full, the sewage flow was diverted to another silo, while the one already full sat for a few days as the bacteria converted the sewage into fertilizer. After the process had finished, the contents were strained, the water was pressed out, and the compacted cake was fired in the boiler, again using the methane from the silos, until it turned to ash. This was then sold as fertilizer to the local farmers. The industrial plant was self contained, used no fuel, and excess methane was used locally as a source of energy. The boiler even provided local heating for businesses on industrial estates. More importantly, the process was a closed system, in that minerals were returned to the soil. This process could be repeated everywhere there is the need for sewage processing. And the sewage works itself emitted no smell, or so I was told. I was unable to verify this personally as I lost my sense of smell for the next six weeks.

Actually I shouldn't refer to it as 'my sense of smell' it was more a case of 'my sense of stench'

I don't make a habit of frequenting sewage works, but I had another job that happened to involve a gas holder filled with sewage gas. This gas holder was collecting the methane from a sewage sludge tank, in very much the same manner as that at Milton Keynes, but this one was at Hailsham, just a few miles from Brighton.

The Body Language of Health

We had several work experience school pupils with us at work at the time. One was my son, James, and the other was a local lad called Chris Phillips. The three of us set off from work, early in the morning, to survey this gas holder which was reported to be corroded and leaking.

This sewage works was fairly small, evidently Hailsham has a lot less bottoms than Milton Keynes. There was a small gasholder, along the lines of the old fashioned gasometer that used to be a familiar sight in most towns before the introduction of north sea gas. It had two flights of stairs spiralling round the outside, and a domed roof that was rather precarious to walk on because the handrail was incomplete on the edge of the roof. There was a boiler in an adjacent building, and the cesspits were to one side of the boiler room. The panoramic view from the gasholder roof was quite spectacular, lagoons of shit as far as the eye could see or the nose could detect.

Each of us put on a pair of overalls and a pair of gloves, not being sure what we might end up putting our hands in. Then we started our survey of the gasholder.

Gasholders are little more than upturned tumblers resting in a pit filled with water. As they fill with gas, the gas pressure lifts them up out of the water, and as the gas is used they sink down into the water again. That is fine for a few years but all that fart gas and water is no good for steel. However it's great for rust.

This gasholder was clearly so corroded it would have been melted down into tin cans years ago if it had been a car. It had a concrete path round it, then a gap of about a foot where the water could be seen, then the side of the gasholder towered up in front of us.

It turned out that the gas holder had corroded just below the water line, and had developed holes through the wall of the dome; consequently gas could escape. All three of us were leaning down into the gap between the concrete path and the gasholder, measuring the thickness of the metal, when there was an almighty gurgling sound, like someone was going to be sick. Suddenly the water in front of us heaved and a huge bubble of gas broke the surface, just like the surging of air and water that you see on films when a submarine comes to the surface.

I'm not sure whether it is grammatically more correct to say that the gas broke the surface, or to say that the contents of the gasholder broke wind, but the effect was staggering.

By that, I mean we did the staggering.

The Body Language of Health

The smell couldn't have been more concentrated if we'd had our head inside the gas holder. Or inside someone's bottom, come to that. The three of us leapt to our feet and staggered away from the gasholder, and down towards the boiler house, trying to avoid making sparks. The only position we could find that didn't stink of a million farts was holding our heads over the concrete wall surrounding the sewer outlet pipe to the sewage works, in comparison the stink of raw sewage was much less pungent than the stench of concentrated fart gas from the holes in the gas holder.

We stood there for quite a few minutes, getting our breath back, becoming ever more fascinated by the contents of the outlet pipe spewing onto the conveyor. Cotton buds by the hundred. Condoms by the dozen. Toilet paper in the colours of the rainbow by the thousand. Turds by the million. A comb!!!

'Let's stay here a bit longer and see if we see any false teeth,' Chris said.

I often wondered afterwards what Chris put into his school report for his work experience.

I have explained this in detail because the material from this boiler was also grey ash that contained all the minerals derived from the sewage, which in turn was derived from the food we eat and excrete down the toilet. And what did they do with it? They sold it to farmers at a cheap price and the farmers put it back on their soil. The cycle was completed.

Using sewage in this way is a perfect environmental exercise but it will not turn the clock back. Our sewage is already depleted in many of the essential minerals. These have now ended up in the oceans.

For millions of years the rain has been washing minerals off the land and depositing them in the sea. Something else we could do is isolate lagoons of seawater, let the water evaporate, collect the salt, extract the sodium chloride which we don't need, and put the rest back into the soil. This will be a mineral rich deposit containing all the minerals on earth. This is simply turning the evolutionary clock back.

The soil has been purged with rain for millennia, washing salts into the sea, but ordinarily that is no problem because soil itself consists of particles of rock which contains minerals and elements. Slowly, the acidity in rain and the digestive systems of insects and worms frees those minerals and releases them into the soil for plants to absorb. But when crops are grown intensively, the rate of release must be too slow

The Body Language of Health

to cope with mineral loss, because the figures produced by David Thomas demonstrate this.

A number of nutritionists now think that the future health of humans lies with nutritional supplementation, not drugs. And supporters of natural farming methods, like Prince Charles, believe that we should get back to natural food production in traditionally fertilised soil.

When the 2004 Tsunami swept seawater onto much of the coastal agricultural land in Indonesia and Thailand, it was assumed the soil would be ruined. So imagine everyone's surprise when the next crops thrived and yielded twice the quantity of first class quality produce. We know the reason, of course. The minerals from the seawater had replenished the soil, replacing all those essential elements that had been extracted from the soil over many years of intensive farming. Several far-sighted scientists have been recommending fertiliser made from sea salt to the deaf ears of agricultural ministers for many years.

This type of natural replenishment of the soil is however quite rare. Tidal waves, called Tsunami's in the far east, are usually due to earthquakes under water. The mass displacement can also be due to landslips, or volcanos. The 2004 Tsunami due to an earthquake in the Indian Ocean, was a particularly impressive one and affected Indonesia, Thailand, northwest Malaysia, Bangladesh, India, Sri Lanka, Somalia, Kenya, Tanzania and Eastern Africa.

We know that the minerals from the sea are great for agriculture, because we have been eating Jersey new potatoes in Britain for many years. The Jersey farmers use seaweed as a fertiliser. This provides the soil, and the crop, with iodine and all the ocean's minerals, and imparts a particularly good flavour to the potatoes.

All forms of life rely on photosynthesis for energy. First, sun-harvesting microbes, then algae, then higher plant life invented this cunning plan to turn sunlight into energy while they were swanning around one day with nothing to do. Actually, it has taken about three billion years to perfect the process. Now, photosynthesis produces an estimated yearly yield of three hundred billion tons of sugar, that is utilised as energy for plants, insects, reptiles, mammals, and humans.

In order to explain how they do this I would need to write another book, but in brief, they do this by structuring an energy cell called a protein pocket. Atoms vibrate with sunlight energy just like a spider in a web wafting in the breeze, and this energy is used to excite electrons that enable the plant to turn carbon dioxide (CO_2) and water (H_2O) into a sugar like glucose ($C_6H_{12}O_6$). The energy cell needs a collector, and the plant makes one by unfurling an antenna that photons of light energy just cannot resist. Each cell spreads out an array of chlorophyll molecules, about two hundred to each pocket. Each antenna positions itself like the plates on a space station solar cell, maximising the number of light photons that will hit it.

But one photon at a time isn't enough energy to get the cell primed and running. You need several photons at once to provide enough energy. Even the number two hundred has been fine tuned over millions of years of evolution. Too few and the efficiency is poor, too many and energy collecting space is wasted. If you hold up an array of two hundred pigment collectors instead of one, you are forty thousand times more likely to have photons hitting the cell when you want them. This is perfect to collect the right amount of photons. Once the cell is receiving, electrons are displaced and as they fall back to their rest state they give off a packet of energy. This energy is used in a cascade of other chemicals to wrestle carbon, hydrogen and oxygen atoms from their molecules, and reassemble them in sugar molecules. Why sugar? It is just a stable energy supply, rather like a battery. Cells can break down sugar and use the energy to fuel their own chemical reactions. And the waste products? Water and oxygen, there was no oxygen on earth until plants evolved. Now we consume oxygen and emit carbon dioxide, which is just as vital. And so the cycle continues.

There is currently a lot of controversy about humans emitting carbon dioxide and we will all have to catch the bus and leave our cars at home if the government gets its way. But an increase of carbon dioxide is a consequence of climate change, not a cause of it. Convenient propaganda, though, when the government has forgotten to build any new power stations, while the old ones are about to fail. The climate has always been changing. Scientists have calculated that when the giant reptiles as big as a house and insects as big as a pig were around, the oxygen level was 30%, not 20.947% as it is today.

In the beginning, there was just heaven and earth. Photolysis of water vapour and carbon dioxide from sunlight and ligntning produced traces of oxygen that kick started the origins of life. Eukaryotic metabolism could only have begun once the level of oxygen had built up to about 0.2%, or ~1% of its present abundance. Don't worry, a eukaryote is a technical name for a creature with one or more cells, like bacteria, amoeba or plankton. This must have occurred by ~2 billion years ago, according to the fossil record. We can plot the history of oxygen on earth from the 'red beds' of iron that mopped up a lot of that early oxygen to form rusty deposits in the ocean floor. The rest, as they say, is history.

Carbon dioxide currently comes in at around 0.038% - precious little for all those plants, who must be on their last gasp. That's another reason why trees wear their lungs (the leaves) on the outside. Carbon dioxide is readily soluble in water (that's what you put in your Scotch and all those fizzy drinks) and is simply absorbed by the vast oceans, so the balance is all down to thermodynamic kinetics, not car exhausts, animal's backsides, or politician's pontifications of hot air.

So, we have a lot to thank plants for. Our oxygen, and our food. That's why plants provide the fuel for all higher animals, insects and reptiles. Without them we would starve, because we have not evolved the process required to turn solar energy into stored chemical energy. It is also why plants that get shaded by others, or get buried underneath something struggle to survive, and will eventually die. They literally starve to death. As sunlight diminishes in Autumn, deciduous trees switch off chlorophyll production, because there isn't enough light to make sugars, that's when the natural yellow and red of their leaf structure shows through, giving us their autumn spectacle of colour.

Are plants smarter than humans?

Yes, in many respects they are. Plants don't often go on Mastermind, but they have other skills we can only dream of. While compiling the information for this book I came across some fascinating information about plants, and thought that since we have evolved in harmony with them I should share some of these facts with you. These facts explain why so many plants are essential to our well being.

Plants cannot get up and run away from their enemies, so they have developed some incredibly complex chemicals and responses to their predators, just like the cacao bean tree we discussed earlier. Plants can detect the saliva of the caterpillar that is eating the leaves, and even identify the species of moth or butterfly by analysing it. Then they can manufacture and emit a specific perfume that attracts the exact wasp which is a predator to the caterpillar that is eating their leaves. The wasp lays its eggs in the caterpillar, which then dies to feed the wasp larvae.

Not only that, but the plant sends a chemical signal to its neighbours of the same species, which triggers production of toxins that make them less palatable to future invasions of the same caterpillars.

How can stupid plants do that? Well, compared to plants, humans are mere beginners. If you go along with the current evolutionary views, humans have evolved over about 2 million years. But plants have evolved over three BILLION years. That's three THOUSAND MILLION, by the way, and 1500 times longer than the whole of the human race's lifespan. Plants are virtually the all time survivors on this planet. So they are much more advanced in so many ways we are only just starting to appreciate. Because they can't run away from their predators, they have developed a veritable army of chemicals and detection systems that can sense heat, light, and all manner of chemicals. So it's no wonder that plants contain so many chemicals that we can harness for our own use. We have evolved to live in harmony with them. That's why our modern processed diet that is removed from nature is so unnatural.

I've recently become worried that genetic modification totally ignores these vital skills that plants have, just focussing on making them bigger or more productive for human needs. How can a scientist choose parent genetic material when he doesn't even know what traits he is selecting, just focussing on size? It's like breeding a human crossed with an elephant and expecting the offspring to fit perfectly into society.

What is the future of healthcare? Not pharmaceuticals is what most switched-on scientists are saying. Instead, they say it will be targeted nutrition. Will plant-derived products take over? Well, they should, but not if the western world's focus on patents, profit and monopoly continues. This makes it unprofitable to develop plant-based products unless they can be patented (like genetic modified organisms).

But the global economy is changing. I am told that in 20 years or so the commercial centre will be China, and their medical business is centred very much on traditional botany. So the future may well be botanic, not pharmaceutical, if China has greater influence. I think it will.

There is also a new movement away from intensive agriculture and towards perennial crops that don't disturb the soil. These mimic natural savannahs, meadows and forests, which have evolved naturally to take nothing out of the soil. At the moment our intensive systems use annuals, which have to be set every year, but sustainable perennial mixes are best for the soil. Setting thousands of acres with the same variety attracts rampant disease, drives out predating wildlife, and leaves crops susceptible to storm damage or total crop failure. Mixing species allows different crop heights that can better weather the storm, makes disease more difficult to spread because of the biodiversity, and attracts natural predators that keep pests at bay. Crop yields are less, but there are so many other benefits that this system has a lot of merit.

Of course, the answer is less people. At 6.6 billion, and expected to rise to 9 billion by 2050, we are a species out of control. In Britain alone, about 750 million animals and 650 thousand tons of fish are slaughtered each year to feed us. But two things are certain. The future will be very interesting. And we shouldn't underestimate plants.

SLEEP

Do you remember your dreams?

If you don't, you may be deficient in VITAMIN B6

Usually I have very unusual, vivid dreams. In fact sometimes I can't wait to get back to sleep to see if I continue where I left off. Certain subjects seem to crop up time and time again in my dreams, or maybe they are just the more memorable parts.

It seems that if you cannot remember your dreams you may be deficient in Vitamin B6.

This is because Vitamin B6 is the master vitamin for processing amino acids—the building blocks of all proteins and a few hormones too. In particular, Vitamin B6 helps to make vital neurotransmitters such as serotonin, melatonin, and dopamine, which are essential for brain processing power. Their production affects the functioning of your brain, and they also affect your mood, and your powers of dreaming too. So if you can't remember your dreams, you may be B6 deficient.

Have you heard the old wives' tale that you will have vivid dreams after eating cheese? This is because cheese is a good source of Vitamin B6. It also contains amphetamine and morphine-like compounds such as phenylethylamine, (pronounced fee –nile- ee-thile- a –mean) and tyramine which trigger a reaction in the brain that mimics ecstasy and speed in a milder form.

A lot of brain chemistry is based on amines, actually. Tyramine is an indirectly acting sympathomimetic amine which is thought to be mainly responsible for high intensity REM (rapid eye movement) sleep seen after consumption of aged or fermented foods like cheese. Tyramine affects the locus ceruleus in the brain stem that is responsible for triggering dream cycles and its neurotransmitter is the stress monoamine norepinephrine which happens to be the principal transmitter potentiated by tyramine. At the same time casein in the cheese is converted to opiate-like caseino-morphine which presumably also has oneirophrenic or 'dream creating' effects.

This could be why ravers who are stoned on ecstasy, (another amine, methylene-dioxy-methamphetamine) have a craving for pizzas as they are coming down from their drug-induced high. Pizza has become known as the perfect mood food for ravers, and probably explains its popularity as a late night meal in most city centres. It is not unknown for someone coming down from a drug induced event to eat two medium size pizzas one after another, despite this being enough food for two to four normal people.

These brain-invading amines in cheese originate from the milk used to make the cheese, but we might ask ourselves what these drug-like substances are doing there in the first place?

Phenylethylamine is not necessary for nutrition, so why should it be in milk? Well, it is thought that phenylethylamine is a mood-changing substance in mother's milk designed to produce a calming effect on the infant and, in fact, may be a key factor responsible for development of the mother-infant bond. This link with mother's milk helps to protect the growth of the baby, so phenylethylamine would evolve as a benefit to the human race. The maternal-infant bonding is actually established through secretion of oxytocin and Trypsin hydrosylate decapeptide, the latter being a casein-like and hence caseinomorphin opiate-like peptide. Never thought of your mother as a drug dealer, did you? Mood-changing drugs in milk give the infant a stimulus to want more, which is good for their growth and well being, if not for their addictive tendencies. So babies develop a healthy addiction for mother's milk. These same chemicals in cows milk generate a desire to eat chocolate and drink cocoa in adults.

Milk chocolate is of course made from milk, and is a great source of phenylethylamine. A bar of chocolate produces the same kind of 'amine rush' (pronounced hay-mean) that occurs in the brain after sex, and so chocolate has become known as a sex substitute. In fact most amines are powerful sexual brain stimulants, not only those in food but also man-made amines such as methamphetamine (better known as Ecstasy) and amphetamines (better known as Speed). The slightly 'fishy' substances that are strong sexual signals emitted by women to attract males are also composed of amines.

Amines occur widely in other compounds as well, and are absolutely essential to our well being. The biggest group of essential amines are the vitamins. We've all heard so much about the need to have vitamins in our diet, but very few people know what vitamins actually are.

We have the Polish chemist Kazimierez Funk to thank for our knowledge of vitamins and their importance in health. In 1911 he was experimenting with chickens at the Lister Institute in London, trying to find out what caused nerve inflammation or 'neuritis'. He isolated a substance that prevented this disease, which happened to be an amine. Chemically an amine is any chemical that has a group of one nitrogen and three hydrogen atoms attached in a particular way.

The Body Language of Health

He called the substance Vit-amine, (short for the 'vital-amine') because it had an amine structure. It later became known as Vitamin B1, with the chemical name of Thiamine. Bet you thought that only appeared in a famous brand of cat food. Well, it is good for chickens too, and we can't do without it.

It was Kazimierez Funk, or Casimir to his friends, who put forward the hypothesis that many other diseases, such as rickets, pellagra, sprue and scurvy could be cured by vit-amine supplements.

Casimir later postulated the existence of many other essential nutrients, which became known as B1, B2, C and D. He was the first to isolate Niacin, or nicotinic acid, which has become known as Vitamin B3.

Vit-amine became Vitamin when it was realised that some of these essential compounds are closely related but are not actually amines.

Many scientists in similar fields have their discoveries named after themselves, so it is purely a quirk of history that these chemicals are known as vitamins and not Funk-amines. Imagine that - vitamin rich poultry might now be known as Funk-E chicken.

Vitamins are quite complicated molecules that appear in nature. They act as a catalyst for all sorts of biochemical reactions in our body, and without them our food can't be processed into energy, so when they are absent in our diet our bodies start to malfunction then die. Some vitamins are fat soluble, but most are water soluble. These water soluble ones are excreted all the time in urine and we have to be supplied with them regularly. All vitamins are essential to life. We can actually make a lot of them from basic substances in food, others we have to take in regularly to maintain good health.

The Vitamin B6 that is necessary to stimulate dreams has some other important benefits too. In combination with folic acid and vitamin B12, vitamin B6 lowers homocysteine levels—an amino acid linked to heart disease and stroke, and possibly other diseases as well, such as osteoporosis, and Alzheimer's disease.

So you need to take your dreams seriously. If you can't remember your dreams, you could be leaving yourself more susceptible to these diseases.

When vitamins are in short supply, the body begins to suffer. A rare but severe form of childhood epilepsy results from an inborn error in the metabolism of vitamin B6 in some children. Those with this form of epilepsy have an abnormal dependence on vitamin B6 and are usually mentally retarded. These children suffer from seizures which are reversible when the children are treated with intravenous injections of vitamin B6.

It may not be that important to you if you are unable to remember your dreams, but it is a simple sign of other much more serious consequences. This is typical of a Body Language sign. It's effects are not that important but the sign is an indicator of far more serious effects on the body or your health.

Learn to listen to your Body Language signs. Choose food that is rich in the missing elements. Take a supplement if you can't find a suitable source of the right food. Treat the Body Language symptom and you will probably protect yourself from more serious diseases.

Many of these Body Language signs are 'old wives tales' but there is much more than an element of truth in them. That is why they have been passed down throughout our history.

Here is a list of some of the vitamins and their commonest deficiency diseases

Vitamin name	Chemical name	Soluble in	Deficiency disease:
Vitamin A	Retinol, retinoids	Fat	Night-blindness, keratomalacia
Vitamin B1	Thiamine	Water	Beriberi
Vitamin B2	Riboflavin	Water	Ariboflavinosis
Vitamin B3	Niacin	Water	Pellagra
Vitamin B5	Pantothenic acid	Water	Paresthesia
Vitamin B6	Pyridoxine	Water	Anaemia
Vitamin B7	Biotin	Water	Hair loss
Vitamin B9	Folic acid	Water	Birth defects
Vitamin B12	Cyanocobalamin	Water	Megaloblastic anaemia
Vitamin C	Ascorbic acid	Water	Scurvy
Vitamin D2-D4	Lumisterol, Ergocalciferol,Cholecalciferol, Dihydrotachysterol, 7-Dehydrocholesterol	Fat	Rickets, in adults also called Osteomalacia
Vitamin E	Tochopherol, Tocotrienol	Fat	Mild anaemia in newborn
Vitamin K	Naphthoquinone	Fat	Bleeding diathesis

The Body Language of Health

You may have noticed that some letters are missing from this list, such as Vitamin F, Vitamin G etc. So what happened to them? The answer is that chemicals used to occupy these vitamin letters, but then it was found that either they had already appeared in another group, or else they were not vitamins after all. Here is a list of a few of the vitamins that very nearly made it.

Previous vitamin name	Chemical name	Current vitamin name	Reason for change
Vitamin B4	Adenine	-	Not a vitamin
Vitamin B8	Adenylic acid	-	Not a vitamin
Vitamin F	Essential fatty acids	-	Not a vitamin
Vitamin G	Riboflavin	Vitamin B2	Reclassified
Vitamins H & I	Biotin	Vitamin B7	Reclassified
Vitamin J	Catechol, Flavin	-	Not a vitamin
Vitamin L1	Orthoaminobenzoic acid	-	Not a vitamin
Vitamin L2	Adenylthiomethylpentose	-	Not a vitamin
Vitamin M	Folic acid	Vitamin B9	Reclassified
Vitamin P	Flavonoids	-	Not a vitamin
Vitamin PP	Niacin	Vitamin B3	Reclassified
Vitamin R, B10	Pteroylmonoglutamic acid	-	Not a vitamin
Vitamin S, B11	Pteroylheptaglutamic acid	-	Not a vitamin
Vitamin U	Allantoine	-	Not a vitamin

Many of these changes came about when Vitamins in the B group were reclassified as a 'complex' of vitamins. The study and naming of vitamins is fascinating in its own right but is outside the scope of this book. For example, Vitamin K came about when the German-speaking scientists who discovered it realised it was responsible for blood 'Koagulation'. The letters from F to I were more or less used up at the time so it seemed reasonable to call it Vitamin K.

The story doesn't end there for Vitamin B6 but we'll have to leave it for another chapter. Later we will talk about B6 and its role in niacin biosynthesis, which is a genetic trait that man is actually losing before our very eyes. Niacin is destined for the same genetic dustbin that claimed our ability to biosynthesise Vitamin C.

Do you have Insomnia?

You may have a Vitamin B or a Mineral Deficiency.

I suppose that one way to prevent you from remembering your dreams is to stay awake, but insomnia is a different category. Insomnia is a disruptive, debilitating problem that leaves you tired out and unable to face the next day. With insomnia, your daydreams involve imagining going to sleep.

Deficiencies of certain vitamins, minerals, amino acids and enzymes are well known to disrupt sleep, so if you have insomnia you may well be deficient, especially in calcium, magnesium, B vitamins, folic acid and melatonin.

Actually, a lot of people find that sometime in their life they have difficulty sleeping. Anyone can suffer from insomnia, although sleeping problems are more common among women (especially menopausal), the ill, the elderly, smokers, and alcoholics. Sleep problems are, however, surprisingly quite common among young people. While it is not an illness and is in no way life-threatening, insomnia can be very frustrating, exhausting, and depressing.

Insomnia is either transitory (short term) or chronic (longer lasting). Problems sleeping take different forms:

- Difficulty falling asleep – this is more common among young people with active minds.
- Sleeping lightly and restlessly, waking often, lying awake in the middle of the night - more common in people over 40. In younger people this pattern may be associated with depression.
- Waking early and being unable to get back to sleep - this is more common in older people and anyone worrying about something.
- Periodic waking and sleeping, giving the impression that you have been lying awake all night, which is rarely true, but sometimes it just seems like it.

To develop a stable sleep pattern it's important that the brain is provided with everything it needs to function correctly, and this includes not only minerals and vitamins but also amino acids and hormones for mental calm. Sometimes your brain just seems like mental anguish instead.

The Body Language of Health

Here are some nutrients you could try. I have included a fairly comprehensive list so that you can make an educated choice, and because some work better in some people than others.

Calcium, especially when contained in food such as milk, has a sedative effect on the body. A calcium deficiency in the body is known to cause restlessness and wakefulness. For adults, try a milky drink, or one of the calcium superfoods described elsewhere.

Magnesium can help induce sleep. Magnesium deficiency is responsible for nervousness that prevents sleep. Magnesium-rich foods include kelp, wheat bran, almonds, cashews, and brewer's yeast.

A lack of calcium and magnesium together can cause leg cramps during the night. This is a Body Language symptom for these deficiencies, along with a salt deficiency. Calcium and magnesium produce calming effects on the brain. They are essential for normal sleep.

B vitamins are known to have a sedative effect on the nerves.

Vitamin B6 supplements can help to prevent insomnia. And give you brilliant dreams.

Vitamin B12 is another important supplement for treating insomnia. Supplements of B12 with pantothenic acid (Vitamin B5) can serve as an effective anti-insomnia vitamin treatment. The vitamin B5 is good for relieving stress. The best food sources of the B vitamins are liver, whole grains, wheat germ, tuna, walnuts, peanuts, bananas, and sunflower seeds.

Inositol enhances rapid eye movement (REM) sleep which, while perhaps a workout for your eyeballs, is nevertheless essential for a restful night. Take this as a supplement at bedtime.

Chromium is often effective for someone with a blood sugar problem that may be keeping them awake at night. Brewer's yeast is a good source of Chromium. If you prefer supplements, take 250 to 500 micrograms twice a day with food.

Tryptophan (L-tryptophan), is an amino acid that plays a key role in the repair of protein tissues and in creating new protein. In the brain, tryptophan is converted into serotonin, a natural sleep-inducing chemical. It also enhances the brain's ability to produce melatonin, the hormone that regulates your body's natural inner clock. Tryptophan is found in foods such as milk, chocolate and turkey.

You might have heard that tryptophan supplements are risky, but this story came from America. The internet widely reports that in 1989, the then-largest manufacturer of L-tryptophan changed their manufacturing process and introduced two large batches of tryptophan contaminated with bacteria into the world marketplace. Within months, an epidemic of a bacterial disease called eosinophilia myalgia syndrome (EMS) began to develop. That's bad news, because usually, the more unpronounceable the disease is, the more serious its symptoms. Eventually, thousands of people were ill and more than a hundred died.

In the early stages of the investigation, tryptophan consumption was implicated in EMS. This prompted the American Food and Drug Administration (FDA) to temporarily block sales of tryptophan while the investigation proceeded. Eventually, researchers traced the problem to two batches of tryptophan manufactured by one company and contaminated with bacteria. The FDA, however, argued against that finding and used the EMS epidemic as a reason to ban all tryptophan from the American over-the-counter market.

Just days after the FDA banned tryptophan, the cover of *Newsweek* announced the arrival of *Prozac*, a "selective serotonin reuptake inhibitor" which became the blockbuster drug of the 90s. Unlike tryptophan, which raised serotonin levels by making more serotonin, Prozac raised serotonin levels by inhibiting the recycling of serotonin in the brain. Fortunately for Eli Lilly & Co, tryptophan's unavailability had created a serotonin vacuum that Prozac could fill. And Prozac's popularity and profitability were spectacular.

I am assured there is absolutely no risk from tryptophan, or from eating tryptophan-rich foods, or in taking supplements, and some sources still infer that two batches of faulty product were more than coincidence with Prozac waiting to find a market.

So does tryptophan work? Well, various clinical studies showed that L-tryptophan produces only modest effects in the treatment of insomnia, and not everyone who takes it for this purpose experiences the results they seek. People have to take relatively high doses of the substance, but small doses are generally not effective. More importantly, research showed that L-tryptophan can reduce REM sleep while increasing the time spent in non-REM sleep. This means you sleep well but don't feel rested. So it is not suitable for everyone. Personally I prefer to concentrate on food-derived minerals and elements than rely on supplements, though I accept that many elements are now depleted in the food we are seeking.

The Body Language of Health

Phosphatidylserine is an amino acid that helps the brain regulate the amount of cortisone produced by the adrenal glands. It is helpful for those who cannot sleep because of high cortisone levels, usually induced by stress. Cortisone is usually present in high levels in the body in the morning, where it promotes wakefulness. It is also found to be high in those who are highly stressed, and this can prevent them from getting to sleep at night. Personally, I would probably lie awake worrying about the pronunciation of phosphatidylserine.

Serotonin is an important initiator of sleep. Our body makes serotonin from the amino acid tryptophan. Taking tryptophan will raise serotonin levels and promote sleep. Tryptophan is more effective for cases of sleep-onset insomnia, since its greatest ability is to reduce the time taken to get to sleep. There is plenty of tryptophan in milk, which is why a hot milky drink last thing at night is a great nightcap. See, Granny's advice was right all along.

More effective than tryptophan is 5-hydroxytryptophan (5-HTP), a form of tryptophan that is one step closer to serotonin administration. You can buy 5-HTP supplements.

Several double-blind clinical studies have also shown that 5-HTP will also decrease the time required to get to sleep, and it reduces the number of times you wake up in the night. To increase the sedative effects of 5-HTP, take it with fruit or fruit juice near bedtime.

5-HTP increases the REM sleep by about twenty-five percent while simultaneously increasing deep-sleep Stages 3 and 4, without increasing total sleep time.

It is important to maintain adequate levels of vitamin B., niacin, and magnesium when using 5-HTP, as these nutrients serve as essential cofactors in the conversion of 5-HTP to serotonin.

Melatonin is a sleep hormone secreted naturally by the pineal gland especially at night. Being a natural hormone, it is said to induce sleep without any negative side effects. Melatonin is also found naturally in plants and in algae. Recently, it has been marketed for sufferers of jet lag or those unfortunate businessmen who get roped into long business drinking sessions with the boys that often go on most of the night. I doubt I would need anything to make me sleep under such circumstances.

In several studies, supplementation with melatonin has been found helpful in inducing and maintaining sleep in both children and adults, for both people with normal sleep patterns and those suffering from insomnia.

However, it appears that the sleep- promoting effects of melatonin are most apparent only if a person's melatonin levels are low. In other words, taking melatonin is not like taking a sleeping pill or a supplement of 5-HTP. It will only produce a sedative effect when your melatonin levels are low. So that seems to be why melatonin appears to be most effective in treating insomnia in the elderly, because low melatonin levels are common in this age group.

So, it appears that there is no 'sleep cocktail'; you just have to experiment and see what suits you best. Actually in my experience the most suitable solution is to identify the root cause and do something physical to combat the problem. As you will see below, the more physical this is the better it works.

What physical actions help combat insomnia?

It is all very well suggesting various supplements, but it seems the greatest benefits usually come from natural, wholesome foods, and natural changes to your lifestyle.

Change Your Environment

Improve your bed - put a board under the mattress if it sags, or try putting your bed in a different position. Make sure your bedding is fresh and clean, and make sure that you are warm enough, and your bed is cosy.

If light troubles you use thicker curtains or put a scarf or an eye shield over your eyes. If you feel more comfortable with some light in the room, experiment with the curtains or a lamp, or leave the light on in an adjacent room and leave the door open.

A relative of mine asked the other day why they often had headaches and woke unrested when the bedroom window was closed? When they left it open they were fine. I think it comes down to what you are comfortable with. Leaving the window open gives you fresh air and a faint background of natural sounds from the surroundings, and the satisfying knowledge you will probably hear prowlers outside. With the window closed some people have a greater feeling of internal security. Either way, it seems to affect how deeply you sleep. Headaches usually occur from poor air quality, and sleeping too soundly so that you move around less in bed and stiffen your neck muscles, which can cause headaches. The answer is to do whatever you are comfortable with.

Noise is a common cause of sleeplessness, not because the noise is too loud for you to sleep, but because noise can be intrusive so you start to listen to it and this activates your brain. When you are able to ignore it, then the noise is actually not a problem. Use earplugs if it's noise you can't do anything about - or change your attitude towards it. People can sleep through high levels of noise - it's not so much the level of noise but how you feel about it that keeps you awake. Use relaxation exercises to calm yourself and take your mind off it. Take some 'diplomatic action' - e.g. talking to noisy neighbours. Keep a radio/tape player by your bed and use it to mask other noise. I can fall asleep straight away on a plane, even when I am at the back with all the other passengers herded in like cattle. In fact I have been known to doze off while the plane is waiting to take off, despite all the mooing from those around me.

Change Your Lifestyle

Talking of physical steps you can take, here's a good one. Take some regular exercise. It is well known that exercise produces endorphins in the brain that make you feel good, relaxed and ready for sleep. These chemicals suppress the appetite too, that is mainly why athletic types are slim. In fact exercising is a poor way to burn off calories, though that's no excuse for you fatties to continue your career as a couch potato. Exercise is still the key. I heard of one overweight individual who got up out of his chair, packed a few belongings and a small tent into his rucksack, and walked the South Downs Way. That's not a style of walking, incidentally, it's a long footpath round the whole of the south coast of England. It took him a month and he lost 56 pounds in weight. And I bet he slept well at night too. Intently no doubt.

If you can't sleep, just imagine that feat of trekkery. If that doesn't work, try getting up and watching some relaxing television or read a boring book, and only go back to bed when you feel ready to sleep. But don't watch Nightmare on Elm Street or read The Shining, both of which are guaranteed to charge your body with adrenaline. Your copy of Body Language would be a safer choice.

Get into a routine that gives you a regular bedtime and 7-8 hours sleep (though individual needs do vary) If you're a late sleeper, try getting up earlier so you will be tired when it is bedtime.

Have a warm bath, do some reading or take a gentle walk before going to bed.

And, yes, it would be unfair on the general public for me to omit the fact that sex before retiring is a great way to relax and prepare for a serious night of deep relaxing sleep. Just ask any woman if sex sends her man off to sleep.

I am told it is my duty to tell men they should realise that after sex they experience an entirely different surge of hormones to women. In men the arousal level drops rapidly after sex, heart rate falls and sleep hormones flood the system. For women, hormones responsible for feelings of creativity are released in their bodies instead, making them feel the need to talk. This is a perfect way to relax together for five or ten minutes provided the man can stay awake that long. If you find that difficult, lads, just think of something exciting – you know, football, fishing; a story on 'Top Gear'; a round of golf.

Some things to avoid:

Don't take stimulants (including coffee, tea, cola, nicotine) that keep you awake, or sedatives (including alcohol) to help you get to sleep.

If you have insomnia, try not to sleep during the day no matter how tired you become.

Don't use your bed for working, watching TV, eating, telephoning or any other activity that is associated with the things you do during the day.

Don't be tempted to eat, drink or smoke when you get up during the night. Try not to drink too much towards the end of the evening. Try boosting your Vitamin B levels and take a mineral supplement. Still not sure if this category applies to you? Well, after all that advice, if you're not feeling sleepy now, you're an insomniac.

One final thing to help you to sleep, how about copying wee Willie Winkie? It is a fact that wearing socks and a nightcap in bed and sleeping in a cold room wrapped up snug in bed produces a powerful vasodilation in the extremities, and this is guaranteed to produce sleep induction. When I was a lad there was no central heating and the coal fire in the bedroom was only lit if you were ill. Winters in the Peak District of Derbyshire were harsh and we wrapped up well to go to bed. But I remember feeling snug and comfortable in bed once I had stopped shivering, and always had a brilliant night's sleep, so there must be some truth in this. Perhaps wee Willie's author William Miller suffered the same fate from the cold Scottish nights as those English swimmers, hence his choice of name for his hero.

HANDS

Do you have whorls on your fingerprints?

You might be at risk of High Blood Pressure

Fingerprints fit into four categories, arches, loops, whorls and incidentals, and each of us has a set of fingerprints that are totally unique.

The first person to solve a crime with fingerprints was a Scottish doctor called Henry Faulds. While he was working in Japan, he matched the fingerprints found on a cup at a robbery in Tokyo with those of a servant, and he described this feat in a letter to the prestigious science journal, Nature, in 1880.

Criminologists have been using the unique patterns on fingerprints to catch villains ever since. Now, scientists have started using fingerprints to solve medical mysteries too. One study in India concerned some 150 adult males, 90 of whom had duodenal ulcers. Perhaps its all that curry. The study found that there was a slight tendency for people with whorls to have more duodenal ulcers.

Another study looking at American Japanese in Hawaii showed that if men had more whorls on their fingers, they were more likely to suffer from a heart attack.

But it was Professor David Barker, head of the Medical Research Council's Environmental Epidemiology Unit at Southampton General Hospital, who found that whorled fingerprints were associated with high blood pressure in adults.

He was checking up long-term records from various maternity units in his hospital. He noticed that if babies had been born very thin, they were more likely to have whorls on their fingertips and to have high blood pressure when they became adults.

Now he and his team couldn't exactly put their finger on the reason, but it is well known that fingerprints are already laid down by the 19th week the baby is in the womb. And it is also known that if the foetus has flattened finger pads, it is more likely to have the simpler arch pattern or maybe the slightly more complicated loop pattern, but not whorls or composites/incidentals.

But on the other hand, so to speak, if the foetus had swollen finger pads, it is more likely to have a complex whorl pattern. But why would a baby who was going to be born thin, have fat finger pads?

One possible theory to explain this is that a woman who has high blood pressure produces a foetus which is in distress, and so this higher blood pressure could show itself as increased swelling in the baby's fingertips, resulting in the formation of more whorls.

Women who have higher blood pressure are probably more likely to produce offspring with higher blood pressure. So if you have a predominance of whorls, you are more likely to have high blood pressure yourself. And we already know that blood pressure is stress-related, so it seems sensible that those patients who develop duodenal ulcers and heart attacks would also be susceptible to high blood pressure, and they will also have a greater tendency to develop whorls on their fingers, explaining the Indian and Japanese studies.

Only recently, it has also been realised that our genes can be altered during gestation to prepare us for the life ahead. This process, called genetic imprinting, (not genetic fingerprinting) can switch on particular groups of genes that will be useful in later life. For example if the mother has a diet poor in nutritional value, the offspring can be genetically imprinted to have a greater appetite and store more fats, essentially to prepare it for famines ahead. Except the system goes wrong if the mother's nutritionally poor diet is simply a supply of fast food, and the offspring is born into a world of plenty.

A recent study at Edinburgh University has revealed that women who followed a low carbohydrate diet such as the Atkins plan when they were pregnant were more likely to have children that suffer from stress. The study of 86 children born in the late 1960s to mothers on a meat-rich, low carbohydrate diet found that when placed in stressful situations, the children, now in their 30s, had higher levels of the stress hormone cortisol in their systems. Lead researcher Rebecca Reynolds said: 'it may be (that) such an unbalanced diet puts stress on the foetus and that sets up the way they respond to stress in later life'.

Genetic imprinting is nature's way of preparing us for natural disasters or difficult times ahead. It is a method of speeding up natural selection when times are hard. For some reason, high blood pressure in the mother can genetically imprint the offspring to develop high blood pressure too, a process which previously we have taken to be simply hereditary.

Either way, if you have lots of whorls on the fingers of your hands, it is a Body Language indicator of high blood pressure in later life.

This could be important if you are one of those with plenty of whorls, and, incidentally, that group includes me; my I have seven whorls out of ten. Using your fingerprints to reveal your blood pressure problems will help you to control your lifestyle accordingly. Much can be done to improve your blood pressure simply by adopting a suitable diet. More of this later.

In the meantime, if detectives found a predominance of whorl fingerprints at a burglary, they could just pick out the suspects at the blood pressure clinic.

So how do you prevent your blood pressure from going through the roof? There is a special section on this later in the book. I suggest you look at 'blood pressure' in the index and review each entry, especially 292-4.

Do you have shaking hands?

You could be deficient in MAGNESIUM and VITAMIN B1

Early symptoms of magnesium deficiency can include fatigue, anorexia, irritability, insomnia, and muscle tremors or twitching. There is plenty of evidence that tremor is associated with magnesium deficiency so magnesium rich foods or even a supplement are worth trying to see if there is any improvement.

People only slightly deficient in magnesium often also become irritable, high-strung, sensitive to noise, hyper-excitable, apprehensive, or belligerent. If the deficiency is more severe, or prolonged, they may develop twitching, tremors, irregular pulse, insomnia, muscle weakness, jerkiness, and leg and foot cramps. It has even been reported that a magnesium deficient patient's hands may shake so badly that their writing becomes illegible.

Also, electro-encephalograms, electro-cardiograms, and electro-myograms, or the records of electrical waves in the brain, heart, and muscles, all become abnormal when magnesium levels are depleted.

If magnesium is severely deficient, the brain is particularly affected. Clouded thinking, confusion, disorientation, marked depression, and even terrifying hallucinations of delirium tremens are largely brought on by a lack of this nutrient and these are remedied as soon as magnesium is given as a supplement. Improvement is usually dramatic within hours after magnesium is taken.

If shaking or trembling has been present for less than 2 years, it could also be influenced by temporary conditions such as increased anxiety or stress, and excess caffeine, nicotine, alcohol or other drug excess or withdrawal. Such shaking or trembling could also be caused by endocrine, electrolyte or hormonal imbalances.

Actually, I would have thought problems with alcohol abuse were self-controlling. As the doctor said to the patient, 'Do you drink much?'

Patient 'No Doctor, I spill most of it'

There is a special section on your alcohol biotype elsewhere in the book.

As many as 1 in 20 people older than age 40 and 1 in 5 people over 65 may have essential tremor (ET). There may be as many as 10 million people with ET in the United States, and many more worldwide. Essential tremor is much more common than most neurological disease, with the exception of stroke, and is more common than Parkinson's disease – a disorder characterized by resting tremor, stiffness and slowness of movement.

Essential tremor is a very common but complex neurological movement disorder. It is called "essential" because in the past, it had no known cause. It is not caused by another neurological condition or the side effect of a medication. ET usually affects the hands, but it may also affect the head and neck (causing shaking), face, jaw, tongue, voice (causing a shaking or quivering sound), the trunk and, rarely, the legs and feet. The tremor may be a rhythmic "back-and-forth" or "to-and-fro" movement produced by involuntary (unintentional) contractions of the muscle. Severity of the tremors can vary greatly from hour to hour and day to day.

Some people experience tremor only in certain positions – this is called postural tremor. Tremor that worsens while writing or eating is called kinetic or action-specific tremor. Most people with ET have both postural and kinetic tremor.

Magnesium deficiency is the most probable cause of ET, but it can also manifest itself because of deficiency in Vitamin B1. This is a water-soluble vitamin needed to process carbohydrates, fat, and protein. Every cell of the body requires vitamin B1 to form the fuel the body runs on— a chemical called adenosine triphosphate (ATP). Nerve cells require vitamin B1 in order to function normally. Deficiency of ATP can cause tremors. Magnesium is required for the conversion of vitamin B1 to the active coenzyme thiamine pyrophosphate; hence a tremor being a feature of B1 deficiency because of hypomagnesia.

A natural decline in vitamin B1 levels occurs with age, irrespective of medical condition. But serious deficiency is most commonly found in alcoholics, people with poor absorption conditions, and those eating a very poor diet. It is also common in children with congenital heart disease. People with chronic fatigue syndrome may also be deficient in vitamin B1. Individuals undergoing regular kidney dialysis may develop severe vitamin B1 deficiency, which can result in serious complications.

When Casimir discovered the substance Vit-amine, which later became known as Vitamin B1 with the chemical name of Thiamine, he knew it was vital. Vitamin B1 deficiency causes a nasty ailment called beri-beri, which sounds, well, veriveri bad for you.

Vitamin B1 is found in very many foods, so you simply need to have a varied diet, but it is important that the food is fresh. It is surprising how much of each of the vitamins are lost in storage. Seeds and nuts are particularly good for B1 but the vitamin can be lost if the nuts are not fresh. Unfortunately nuts can be stored for a long time without deteriorating visually, so you need to make sure the source is fresh and reliable, and you should always throw away any stale seeds and nuts.

Do you have white spots on your nails?

You may have a deficiency of ZINC

Having white spots on your nails is quite a common problem, and I am sure you are aware of this Body Language sign already, but most people think that white spots on your nails are a symptom of insufficient calcium in the diet. No, it is zinc deficiency, not calcium.

Earlier I explained that Body Language signs are often trivial but can signal far more serious problems on the horizon. The signs and symptoms of zinc deficiency in nails might just be cosmetic but the effects of zinc deficiency are far more serious and very wide-ranging. The list of side effects is a long one. It includes anorexia, growth retardation, delayed sexual maturation, hypogonadism and hypospermia, alopecia, immune disorders, dermatitis, night blindness, poor sexual performance and impotence, impaired taste (hypogeusia), and impaired wound healing. The first signs of zinc deficiency in marginally nourished children and teenagers are poor growth, anorexia, and impaired taste. And white spots on nails.

The most serious manifestations of zinc deficiency were reported in Iranian dwarfs. These adolescent boys were retarded in growth and sexual development and had anaemia, underdeveloped sexual organs, hepatosplenomegaly, rough skin, and mental lethargy. After treatment with a well-balanced diet containing adequate amounts of zinc for a year, pubic hair appeared, sexual organs increased to normal size, linear growth was resumed, and the skin became normal. And their previously untreatable anaemia suddenly responded to iron supplements.

Zinc deficiency develops in some patients with liver cirrhosis because their ability to retain zinc is lost. These people need to have a zinc supplement otherwise their healing will be impaired.

There are many other biochemical signs associated with zinc deficiency and they include production of alcohol dehydrogenase in the retina (which accounts for night blindness), and decreased collagen synthesis (resulting in poor wound healing).

Clinical assessment of mild zinc deficiency is difficult because many of the signs and symptoms are non-specific. Nonetheless, if a malnourished person has a borderline-low plasma zinc level, is living on a high fibre diet containing whole-grain bread (which reduces zinc absorption), and has reduced sense of taste, then zinc deficiency should certainly be suspected, and treatment with zinc supplements should be tried.

Zinc supplementing needs care, however., because zinc and copper are interrelated in the body. Beginning in the 1940s, evidence developed to show that high amounts of zinc supplements can interfere with the uptake and metabolism of copper. The signs of copper deprivation supposedly induced by high intakes of zinc included reduction of 'good' cholesterol (HDL) in the body. However, these signs have not been consistently found with moderate zinc consumption, in fact total and low-density lipoprotein cholesterol concentrations both decreased with zinc supplementation, presumably because zinc heals so well, therefore cholesterol is not in such demand.

At least 20 percent of the population suffers from a deficiency of copper. Yet few people are aware of the health disorders that are associated with copper deficiency.

The Body Language of Health

They include osteoporosis, slipped discs, osteoarthritis and rheumatoid arthritis, cardiovascular disease, and chronic conditions involving bone, connective tissue, heart and blood vessels, and even colon cancer.

In infants and children, copper deficiency may result in anaemia, bone abnormalities, impaired growth, weight gain, frequent infections (colds, flu, pneumonia), poor motor coordination and low energy.

Even a mild copper deficiency, which affects a much larger percentage of the population, can impair health in subtle ways. Symptoms of mild copper deficiency include: lowered resistance to infections, reproductive problems, general fatigue, and impaired brain function.

You may get a copper deficiency if you eat a poor diet, suffer digestive disorders, have prolonged bouts of diarrhoea or liver problems, or take poorly balanced supplements, especially iron and zinc, because copper, iron and zinc work in harmony in the body. All you need to do to keep copper levels balanced is to eat a balanced diet, with a range of food from different food groups, which is what we are saying throughout this book. The best dietary sources of copper are seafood, (especially shellfish); meat, whole grains, nuts, raisins, legumes, chocolate (yes, chocolate); cereals, and dark green leafy vegetables and apples.

If an expectant mother has zinc deficiency it may cause anencephaly in the foetus. Secondary deficiency occurs in liver disease, in malabsorption states, and during prolonged breast feeding. Night blindness and mental lethargy may be associated symptoms.

And all these side-effects, diagnosed just from white spots on the nails due to deficiency of zinc, not calcium. But why do we get white spots?

It appears that zinc is so essential for healing our body that sticking plasters are coated with zinc oxide. Many wound dressings are also impregnated with zinc. So a deficiency of zinc will affect healing performance. In everyday life our fingernails take the brunt of knocks and bangs on our fingers, after all that is why they are there. Fingernails have evolved to protect our sensitive fingertips, not to pick our noses. These knocks and bangs damage the nail bed and when you are zinc deficient, healing is delayed, so the transparent keratin at the nail bed becomes opaque. And that is why while spots are indicative of zinc deficiency.

Good sources of zinc are lean meat, seafood (especially oysters), eggs, soya, peanuts, wheat germ, and cheese. Especially oysters, you will note, which gives us a clue to the next category which involves aphrodisiacs.

There are plenty of other Body Language signs of zinc deficiency, as well. First signs of zinc deficiency are usually one or more of the following; impairment of taste, a poor immune response and skin problems. Other symptoms of zinc deficiency can include hair loss, diarrhoea, fatigue, delayed wound healing, and decreased growth rate and mental development in infants. It is thought that zinc supplementation can help skin conditions such as acne and eczema, prostate problems, anorexia nervosa, alcoholics and those suffering from trauma or post-surgery.

Do you masturbate or have sex a lot?

You could be deficient in Zinc

Ok, I know this Body Language sign is in the section called 'hands' which I might have manipulated into the wrong category but it follows on so well from the previous topic, that I just had to make an insertion here.

There is an old wives tale that men who masturbate a lot will go blind. There is also good evidence that masturbation is a common and perfectly normal pastime of males, (and women too but this category doesn't apply to you) therefore if you happen to fit into this category, you're probably reading the Braille edition of 'Body Language'.

Actually as a religious "aside" it is understood by Christian denominations that human nature is fallen from a state of pure intellectual domination of the passions into a state where its natural instincts tend towards excess gratification.

As such, masturbation or "having sex with oneself" represents a disordered appetite in itself because it frustrates the naturally appointed function of the reproductive organs which is to procreate. This is even outlined in the Old Testament where Onan was the second son of Judah. After his older brother Er died, Onan was required by the tradition of levirate marriage to marry Er's widow Tamar. According to Genesis 38:7-10, when he had sexual intercourse with Tamar he "spilt his seed upon the ground" frustrating conception. In response to the transgression of disobedience, God killed Onan. Pretty serious stuff I'd say.

The Body Language of Health

Of course this old wives tale about going blind cannot actually be true, can it?

Well, like a lot of folk lore, there is more than an element of truth in the saying.

Semen is very rich in zinc, with each ejaculate containing around 5mg of zinc, or one third of the recommended daily nutrient intake for the average male. This is a lot of zinc for the body to lose all in one spurt. Zinc is needed to keep sperm healthy, and the body injects the zinc into the semen at the last minute, so you could say it galvanises the little tadpoles into action. Later on, I will explain in more detail why a zinc supplement could cure your infertility.

This concentration of zinc in semen indicates that three ejaculations a day could end up depleting the average male totally of his zinc requirement.

Deficiency of zinc has a number of symptoms, including poor eyesight. So if you should masturbate too much, maybe you'll go blind.

It so happens that Vitamin A is also good for eyesight, and there is a lot of vitamin A in carrots. So maybe one of the most promiscuous animals on Earth, the rabbit, is synonymous with carrots for a good reason. Maybe the rabbit is complementing its zinc loss in semen with a healthy dose of Vitamin A. I suspect, however, that a rabbit's diet must be far from healthy, otherwise why would the rabbit be saddled with the stereotype of always saying 'What's up, doc?'

There is another interesting point about zinc and sexual activity. Oysters are particularly rich in zinc, so they will help semen production and boost libido. This is probably why oysters have become known for their aphrodisiac properties. The same could be said of all seafood but I have never heard of the aphrodisiac properties of those other zinc rich foods, eggs, soya, peanuts, wheat germ, and cheese. Maybe these haven't employed such good marketing agents. But these should all be thought of as super foods if you want to be a super stud. So take this dietary advice and the world's your oyster.

Hang on, Luv, I'm just making me'self a cheese, peanut and oyster omelette. That must be the ultimate superfood for a superstud.

Do you suffer from soft or brittle nails?

You may be deficient in MAGNESIUM

Magnesium functions in more than 300 enzymatic reactions. Magnesium is also essential for the conversion of vitamin D to its biologically active form that then helps the body absorb and utilize of calcium. So a deficiency in magnesium will cause brittle nails, even if your diet is calcium rich.

The typical Western diet is frequently very low in magnesium. Many surveys have indicated that over 80 percent of Americans get less than the Recommended Dietary Intake (RDI) of this important mineral. The highest magnesium concentration is found in the tissues that are most metabolically active including the brain, heart, liver, and kidney. But these offal meats are rarely eaten nowadays as a main meat source.

Magnesium also plays a vital role in making sure your most essential muscle performs to the best of its ability. No we're not talking about sexual organs again, this is the most essential muscle of all, your heart. Magnesium can improve energy production within the heart, improve delivery of oxygen to the heart, reduce demand on the heart, inhibit the formation of blood clots, and improve heart rate. Magnesium supplementation has been used by nutritionists in many of these applications for over 50 years. But they apparently haven't told the doctors yet.

Magnesium is also effective with Chronic Fatigue Syndrome sufferers. People with CFS tend to have low red blood cell magnesium levels. A recent study in the United Kingdom conducted a double-blind experiment with CFS patients and magnesium supplements. The researchers concluded that 80% of the patients receiving magnesium reported "significantly improved energy levels, better emotional state, and less pain." If you are a CFS sufferer a supplement of magnesium is well worth trying.

Actually, we ought to shout more about Magnesium because it also plays an essential role in muscle membrane tone, even on one of our smallest membranes too. The eardrum.

On a daily average, more than 9 million Westerners are exposed to noise levels above 85 decibels, the level where the risk for permanent hearing loss increases exponentially. Since magnesium is essential in regulating cellular membrane permeability and neuromuscular excitability, researchers decided to test the hypothesis that noise-induced hearing loss and magnesium are related. The researchers were right! They discovered that magnesium supplementation is highly effective in preventing noise-induced hearing loss. Now that's something to shout about!

General Brittle Nails Information

Brittle nails are characterized by splitting or breaking at the nail tip. The nail can also appear as thin, shiny, dry or translucent. The nails can reveal much about a person's general internal health, so nail abnormalities in either the fingers or toes can indicate an underlying disorder.

Lifestyle Changes can improve brittle nails. Eat a diet high in protein, whole grains, fresh fruits and vegetables, legumes, oatmeal, nuts and seeds. And oysters, of course. Drink plenty of water and fresh fruit juices. Take two tablespoons of brewer's yeast or wheat germ oil daily. Avoid refined sugars and simple carbohydrates. Apply a mixture of equal parts honey, avocado oil, egg yolk and a pinch of salt to your nails to restore colour and texture. Treat nails gently and protect them from hot water and harmful chemicals by wearing gloves. Do not pick or pull on any flaky areas. Wear a protective base coat to help strengthen nails.

Magnesium plays important roles in the structure and the function of all parts of the human body. The adult human body contains about 25 grams of magnesium. Over 60% of all the magnesium in the body is found in the skeleton, about 27% is found in muscle, while the rest is present in other cells.

Magnesium is involved in more than 300 essential metabolic reactions. The metabolism of carbohydrates and fats to produce energy requires numerous magnesium-dependent chemical reactions. Magnesium is required by the adenosine triphosphate synthesizing protein in mitochondria. ATP, the molecule that provides energy for almost all metabolic processes, exists primarily as a complex with magnesium (MgATP). Magnesium is required at a number of steps during the synthesis of nucleic acids (DNA and RNA) and proteins. A number of enzymes participating in the synthesis of carbohydrates and lipids require magnesium for their activity. Glutathione, an important antioxidant, requires magnesium for its synthesis. Magnesium also plays a structural role in bone, cell membranes, and maintaining chromosome integrity.

In general it seems that the early signs of magnesium deficiency are mainly loss of appetite, nausea, vomiting, fatigue, and weakness. As magnesium deficiency worsens, numbness, tingling, muscle contractions and cramps, seizures, personality changes, abnormal heart rhythms, and coronary spasms can occur. Severe magnesium deficiency can result in low levels of calcium in the blood (hypocalcaemia). Magnesium deficiency is also associated with low levels of potassium in the blood (hypokalemia).

Actually, I could write a book about magnesium, it is so vital in your body. Chronically low magnesium, or hypomagnesia is associated with alcoholism, use of diuretics, antibiotic, diabetes, chronic diarrhoea, heart attacks, and chronic fatigue syndrome. More of these later.

Do you have a long index finger?

Then you probably have a large penis.

Work published in the Journal of Urology has shown that the length of a man's index finger is proportional to the length of his penis.

Dr. Evangelos Spyropoulos and his team from the Naval and Veterans Hospital of Athens conducted their investigation to gather information on how male genitalia size is related to body measurements.

Dr Spyropoulos and team measured the length of the penis as well as testicular volume in 52 healthy young males between the ages of 19 and 38 years. These measurements were then compared with other measurements of the body including body mass index, weight, height, waist/hip ratio and index finger. Disappointingly, the report didn't say why they were motivated to investigate this particular feature, or how they came up with 'testicular volume' as a measurement for this seminal report.

They found that there was no correlation with the age and body measurements of these men, nor presumably with the size of their bank balance or ego. Only index finger length showed significant correlation with the dimensions of the flaccid, maximally stretched penis according to the report.

A study group as 'small' as only 52 young men is hardly statistically meaningful, but this work indicates that there does appear to be a trend of penile length and that of the index finger.

So if women are in the least bit interested in whether a man has a long penis or not, they just have to look at a man's index finger. The longer it is, the longer he'll be. And

The Body Language of Health

any relationship with this attribute and his bank balance remains pure male exaggeration. (though there have been many occasions when my bank balance has been 'maximally stretched' I can tell you).

So there it is, the long and short of it. What else can I say? Well, any woman reading this article may find it puzzling that so many men seem to be concerned about the length of their penis, but to the average man, he sees his penis as a measure of his sexuality.

Women should bear in mind that he will take jokes or complaints about penis size very seriously, and there have been reported occasions when men have suffered from impotence (erectile dysfunction) after adverse comments about penis dimensions.

The trouble is that every man sees his own penis in a foreshortened view - the angle at which he looks down on it inevitably makes it seem shorter than it is. Of course, when he glances at another man's organ in a changing room, there's no such foreshortening effect, so very often it'll look as though the other man is better endowed than he is. A lifetime of comparison of this sort (and virtually every male does a quick mental check on each naked man he comes across) can very easily make a man feel a bit inadequate. Rather unfortunate for Dr Spyropoulos, then.

Middle age also plays its part. Every man should make a rule that he should go on a diet as soon as his penis vanishes from view below his expanding gut, and the nation's males would be a lot healthier and more satisfied with their penis size as a result.

Of course, it's true that some men have big penises and some have smaller ones, just as some men have small feet and some have big feet, but the measurement is most definitely not an index of virility.

Most women imagine that a tall, husky man will usually have a large penis, but this is not so at all. The American researchers Masters and Johnson measured the penile lengths of over 300 men. The largest organ (measuring 14 cm, or 5 ½" in the flaccid state) belonged to a slim man who was only 5' 7" tall; the smallest (measuring 6cm, or 2 ¼") belonged to a fairly heavily built man of 5' 11". Sadly, these researchers omitted to measure their subjects' index fingers or else they could now be basking in notoriety.

It's also worth pointing out that there is no correlation between penile size and race, and penis length does not seem to be a characteristic that is automatically hereditary.

But it's important for a man to realise the true facts about the length of the penis. When it is in a non-erect condition, the male organ usually measures between 8.5cm (just over 3") and 10.5cm (just over 4") from tip to base. The average figure is about 9.5cm (or 3 $\frac{3}{4}$"), but this kind of precise measurement is really rather valueless because so many factors (for instance, cold weather or going swimming) can temporarily cause a shrinkage of two inches or more. So you needn't be worried if you happen to fall short of the average figure.

The erect penis

Those measurements are for the length of the male organ in its ordinary non-erect state. But how long should it be when it's erect? Well, the interesting thing here is that most penises are very much the same size when erect. The man whose non-erect organ is smallish will usually achieve about 100 per cent increase in length during sexual excitement, while the man whose limp penis is on the largish size will probably only manage about a 50 to 75 per cent increase. In round figures, this means that the great majority of men measure between 15cm (6") and 18cm (7") in the erect position, with the average figure being about 16.5cm (6 $\frac{1}{2}$"). And if you are tempted to get the ruler out, it is difficult to measure a penis yourself because the base where you measure from is all important.

These figures show that even if a man has a small organ in the non-erect state, he's also got a built in compensating factor that will probably bring him up to average when erect.

And there's one final point that's of great importance which virtually every man forgets: it doesn't matter how long or how short your penis is, because the vagina is cunningly designed that it will accommodate itself to any length of penis.

You see, the vagina of a woman who hasn't had a child is only a mere 7.5cm (3") long when she's not sexually excited. The figures for women who have had babies are only slightly different. And even when she has been aroused, her vagina usually extends only to a length of about 10cm (4"). So it's obvious that most designs of penis will pretty much fill her vagina completely.

So, how on earth does a man with an average length penis of 6 $\frac{1}{2}$" manage to insert his penis into a normal woman's vagina at all? Well, the answer is quite simple - the vagina has great capacity for lengthening if something is introduced into it gradually. So the exceptional man whose penis is, say, 20.5cm (8") long can still make love to literally any woman, providing he excites her properly and introduces his organ slowly. If he does this, her vagina will quite happily lengthen by 150 per cent or even 200 per cent to accommodate him. After all, it is designed to accommodate a baby's head and body.

So far we haven't explained why a man's penis is related to finger length, but it is likely to be associated with the amount of testosterone available while the foetus is growing. This testosterone affects not only the penis size but the length of the fingers as well. But I am not currently aware of any pregnant woman taking testosterone supplements to try and breed a male porn star, or a concert pianist. Such actions could be dangerous to the foetus, and I suspect all she would get is a beard.

Amusingly, it seems likely that piano players and musicians who need to do a lot of fingering are likely to be well endowed. On the basis that if they are gifted at playing musical instruments they probably have long fingers, of course. So if you always wondered at the fascination women have over men like Richard Klayderman and Eric Clapton, well now you know.

When Napoleon died in 1821 doctors conducted a post-mortem that was witnessed by many people. I suppose you could say they took each bone aparte. A priest who was present, Ange Vignale claimed to have taken home a souvenir of the occasion; Napoleon's penis. His family sold what they claimed to be the penis in 1916, and in 1987 it was sold to an American for $3000. Despite such inflationary sums, the penis was described as 'looking like a shrivelled seahorse one inch long'. Perhaps it had Spirilledupoulos.

Unfortunately, we cannot verify the size of Napoleon's willy by comparing it to the length of his fingers because of his habit of putting his left hand in his pocket and his right hand inside his coat. Maybe he was conscious of his short fingers and knew the tale about finger length related to penis length.

Do you have ridges on your nails?

You may be deficient in ZINC

Zinc again; that's because zinc and nails go together like galvanising and, well, nails. The signs and symptoms of zinc deficiency make a long list, because zinc is so important to the body. If you didn't catch the list last time, here it is again. It includes anorexia, growth retardation, delayed sexual maturation, hypogonadism (small sexual organs) and hypospermia, alopecia, immune disorders, dermatitis, night blindness, impaired taste (hypogeusia), and impaired wound healing.

Nails are a substructure of the outer layer of the skin, or epidermis. They are composed mainly of keratin, a type of protein. Healthy nail beds should be pink, which indicates a rich, well oxygenated blood supply. Change or abnormalities in the nails are important indicators of poor health, which is often due to nutritional deficiencies or other underlying medical conditions. Nails can be affected by a variety of conditions. Here are the more common ones:

'Hangnails': A hangnail is a tiny sliver of skin that splits off from down the edge of your fingernail. This loose piece can catch on clothing and can become tender and inflamed. A lack of protein, folic acid and vitamin C can be responsible for hangnails.

White bands across the nails are usually an indication of protein deficiency or a previous injury to the nail bed. Often associated with deficiency of zinc.

Fragility: A deficiency of the B vitamins causes fragile nails with horizontal and vertical ridges. Often due to insufficient intake of vitamin B12 leading to excessive dryness.

'Spoon nails': nails that develop in a concave shape or have vertical ridges: Often indicative of iron deficiency. Spoon nails can also very often indicate bronchial problems such as emphysema and bronchitis. Maybe there is a link with iron deficiency and lung disease there somewhere worth investigating. Body Language suggests this link is perfectly valid and worth trying an iron supplement for a few weeks if you happen to have bronchial problems.

White spots: Zinc deficiency. See elsewhere in the Body Language signs for a full review on white spots.

Splitting nails: Often due to lack of sufficient stomach acidity, or gastric problems.

Coloured nails: Usually caused by a bacterial infection under the nail, often from pseudomonas bacteria, making the nail blue, green or grey. Keep your hands dry and it will usually recover naturally with time. Try some honey under the nail end, honey has excellent antibacterial properties, and was the wound dressing of choice in ancient times before antibiotics. Manuka honey, from the blossom of the Tea Tree is particularly good at healing or killing bacteria. Tea Tree oil is a great antifungal.

Is your index finger shorter than your ring finger?

If it is you may have an aggressive trait

For years, scientists have known that there is a correlation between finger lengths and the amount of testosterone baby boys are exposed to in the womb.

The shorter a man's index finger is, when compared to his ring finger, the more aggressive and boisterous he is likely to be, according to a study by some Canadian researchers. They say the strange connection may have something to do with the testosterone level during foetal development and early childhood. The index finger is the finger next to the thumb, and the ring finger is the finger next to the little finger.

A reader of our website tells us that this Body Language symptom is true of women too - well testosterone is not exclusive to males so it should be true for everybody. In fact recent research has shown that women who have a longer ring finger than their index finger are very good at sports. One research programme took hand x-rays and compared them to sports injuries, revealing that a high proportion of top women athletes have a long ring finger. In fact several sports coaches already secretly use this trait to spot budding athletes in college.

You could use this feature too, when interviewing for jobs that need to be filled by people who tend to be particularly aggressive at work.

You know, traffic wardens, counter staff at council offices, and car park attendants. In fact anyone eager to take a job that requires them to wear a uniform, actually. Consider looking at their index finger the next time these officious types wag it at you while telling you off.

Do you bite your nails?

You may be deficient in MINERALS

It is perhaps surprising that we bite our nails at all, considering that there are more bacteria lurking under our nails than there are down a kitchen drain. We'd never think of putting a drain cover in our mouths, would we?

The mineral content of hair or nails is similar to the mineral content of bone. Very often, because food is now depleted of certain minerals, your body is desperate to get hold of a supply of the minerals in the nail material, so the body is very grateful for the minerals you are providing when you bite your nails. Hence the reward-cycle begins and continues, and nail biting becomes a habit.

The general consensus is that people who bite their nails are nervous creatures, but mineral deficiency causes these nervous symptoms, so it is equally likely that the deficiency is causing the symptoms, which nail biting can relieve.

The human body, like everything else in nature, is made up of elements. These elements are made into complicated molecules, but elements are essential, nevertheless. The greatest volume in the body is taken up by the common elements, carbon, oxygen, hydrogen, nitrogen, calcium and so on.

These elements are the building blocks. They are the concrete, the bricks, the main structure. Together they are capable of constructing a body infinitely more complicated than the highest skyscraper.

The next group of elements in the body are present in lesser proportions. These include chlorine, sodium, magnesium, and so on. These elements are equivalent to the mortar, the plaster, the woodwork, the decorations, and the utility services such as the plumbing in the body's building.

But the body contains about another 50 or so elements. These are the trace minerals and scientists have further subdivided this group into three categories. The first of these is the essential trace minerals. These are minerals that are required in the diet for full health, and when the intake is insufficient, symptoms of deficiency will arise. These include zinc, copper, selenium, chromium, manganese, molybdenum, iodine, fluoride, and cobalt.

The Body Language of Health

The second group of elements are the essential trace elements; those required in very small amounts, and these include arsenic, boron, bromine, cadmium, lead, lithium, nickel, silicon, tin, and vanadium. In fact there is evidence that every element that exists in the periodic table below and including lead is essential to life in some form or other.

You will note in this list several minerals (arsenic, cadmium, lead) that are normally thought to be toxic. Actually, all nutrients are toxic if too much is ingested; how much is too much depends entirely on the nutrient. But we do know that if none is consumed, we develop problems, so these elements are still essential to our well being.

For some essential minerals, like copper, there is a definite gradation for health; if the intake is below the requirement, illness due to deficiency will develop; as the intake goes up, health will improve until a plateau is reached, where small increases in intake will not make any difference to health; above the top safe level (the end of the plateau), increases in intake can cause toxic illness.

In extreme cases, both deficiency at one end and toxicity at the other end of the spectrum may become so severe as to cause death. This pattern is seen for most nutrients, including, for example, vitamins, minerals, and protein. Man cannot live on bread alone.

And a few, although essential, can cause debilitating disease when present in excess. A classic example is vanadium which is essential for the metabolism of glucose, but can cause manic depression when consumed to excess.

The third category of elements and trace minerals is everything else - all the other minerals that are present in the body that do not cause any concern over toxicity or deficiency. In practice, virtually every element in the Periodic Table is essential. Elements like boron rarely feature in multivitamins and minerals formulae but boron is essential, and deficiency has been strongly linked to arthritis. Deficiency of boron also causes cloudy thinking or 'brain fog'.

These elements are the essential ingredients that make the 'building' come alive. They are the central heating, the air conditioning and temperature control, the wiring, the lighting, the lifts, the kitchens. Without these elements the building would be sterile.

Biting your nails becomes addictive because of the reward process. You're probably deficient in minerals. And what better way to replenish the body than by recycling nail material. Maybe we should encourage nail-biting.

The Body Language of Health

My geologist colleague David Thomas has studied the mineral deficiencies of plants and has come to the conclusion that we need a natural balance of all the minerals in proportion to the content of salts in the oceans. And that brings us back to our origins, as discussed earlier. We have developed a similar balance of minerals to those in the ocean because we spent a time as aquatic creatures, probably during an ice age. When our mineral balance falls below that of the oceans, we become ill. When the mineral content significantly exceeds that of the oceans, we become ill.

Some people will find the idea of an aquatic existence far-fetched, and when I have given talks, I have touched on our evolutionary past, even when addressing church meetings. To devoutly religious people, this is a particularly sensitive subject. But I believe creation and evolution can sit side by side.

At such times I have posed the question 'Why do you think that humans are split into different races – the Caucasians, the Asians, the Inuit, the Africans, the American Indians, the Aborigines, and others?

I have never really found a satisfactory explanation for this – we are all humans, but have different genetic traits and many detail differences. Like evolutionary variations on the same theme.

My own interpretation, for what it is worth, is this. It is widely acknowledged that the human race developed into the form we recognise today in the middle eastern area, the original 'garden of Eden'. [Strictly speaking from the Christian point of view we are all descendents of Noah and his family who repopulated the earth after the flood according to biblical revelation]

The human race developed and expanded, but then pockets of humans became isolated in different parts of the world, and barely managed to eke out an existence during the great ice ages. This period would be difficult to imagine, when for example much of Europe was under a blanket of ice five miles thick. Britain is still reeling from this period, the sinking of the east coast and the rising of the west coast is due to Britain and its continental plate righting itself after all that weight of ice. That is why the sea at Morecambe is miles away, and why the cliffs of Norfolk are eroding away.

Remember, for at least 120,000 years mankind endured these periodic extremes, which must have seriously limited the development of modern man as a culture, while at the same time reinforcing the survival of the fittest which endowed us with the qualities we have today. Remember also that these people were indistinguishable from modern man today, at least physiologically.

The Body Language of Health

These natural developments that happened in the past put current minor blips in climate into perspective. I imagine during the great ice ages the isolated groups of humans would develop individual features driven by the severe environmental conditions that prevailed. Any advantage would be reinforced by survival rates, leading to each isolated group quickly developing benefits. By quickly, I am suggesting thousands of years.

At this time I imagine the best source of food would be aquatic which may explain our dietary dependence on fatty acids that are most readily found in fish. In fact we could survive quite happily on marine life, rich in fish, shellfish and seaweed. Recent findings from tribes that lived in Mexico suggest they routinely swallowed clay in times of famine so that the body could go on extracting the minerals it needed even when food was scarce. No doubt these people also used to bite their nails.

Our bodies have a natural ability to store nutrients to get us over a period of famine, or a period when that particular food was not available. Many of these nutrients can be stored and used up for months. To you and me, that becomes a problem now, because our Body Language symptoms do not suddenly appear, they creep up on us as our body slowly runs out of some nutrient or other. That is all the more reason to look for the early signs that Body Language can teach us.

Civilisation as we know it is very recent, at only 10,000 years old. But we still carry these traits that were inbred into us from these isolated groups of people. Just as our digestive system and biological control mechanisms are still operating as though these times are still upon us.

I don't see these views as conflicting with religion, provided we can accept that the various religious texts and beliefs are symbolic as well as literal. And my views which combine the two are no more radical that an absolute belief in Adam and Eve which does not adequately explain how these different races came about. We are all survivors, all common men and women, in God's image. To me, the differences in evolution and creationism are simply about timing and timescales.

Recently, it has even been suggested that many of the mythological figures from antiquity originated because, very occasionally, a baby had been born with these characteristics. The mythological idea of a mermaid apparently came about because occasionally a baby would be born with both legs fused together and feet like flippers. Pixies, with pointed faces and long ears, goblins with distorted features, and numerous similar examples, have cropped up now and again throughout history. Most have died soon after birth, but the myth persists. Of course, these days, ante-natal care and medical screening of the mother largely prevents these foetuses developing into babies, and so they are never considered as anything but genetic curiosities from the past.

In the ancient past, though, genetic diversity would have been important in taking the future of the human race down a different path, via whatever form it took.

Many geneticists now believe we have reached the point of maximum evolution and are now going backwards. Evolution has given way to devolution. They argue that medicine is allowing survival of weakness that is being bred back into the human race. Survival instinct is no longer there. Our knowledge of healing plants is waning through repressive patent laws. Our instinctive knowledge of food and what is good for us has disappeared. Specialisation has removed the need for us to learn about the world around us. And of course, we no longer know what we are eating, which is a main theme of this book. Only time will tell. But fortunately our ancestors have left us with an important legacy. A superbly engineered body that just needs the right nutrients to function properly. And that bit is down to you, and you alone.

Does that thought make you nervous? Just don't use it as an excuse to bite your nails.

Do you have yellow palms?

You may have excessive BETA CAROTENE INTAKE

Beta carotene is a natural antioxidant which helps to protect the body from disease. Beta carotene is part of a larger family of nutrients called carotenoids, which are plant pigments with vitamin-like properties. Your liver can make Vitamin A from it.

Beta carotene is associated with orange fruits and vegetables and is found in carrots, broccoli, and many orange or red coloured fruits and vegetables.

What are the benefits of beta carotene?

Like other antioxidants, beta carotene, protects the body against free radicals. Beta carotene can also help to strengthen the immune system, increase lung capacity, reduce the skin's risk to sun and DNA damage as well as reduce cholesterol levels. Adequate amounts of beta carotene are essential for a healthy body and its benefits can increase when taken with other Funky antioxidants like vitamins C and E.

Reports about carotenoids, the group of compounds akin to carotene, are in the nutritional medicine journals all the time. The latest one, as this book went to press, is that mandarin oranges were found to significantly prevent liver cancer. Two studies in Japan showed that the protective effect was due to carotenoids which are akin to Vitamin A. That is what gives mandarin oranges their orange colour. The study found that patients with viral hepatitis, a liver disease, had a better success rate when drinking mandarin orange juice daily.

Am I getting enough beta carotene?

Getting enough beta carotene means eating a well-rounded diet with lots of fruits and vegetables. The American National Institute of Health recommends 9 milligrams of beta carotene daily for adult men and 7 milligrams for adult women. Foods with high levels of beta carotene include: pumpkin, sweet potato, carrots, cooked greens, apricots, sweet peppers, kale, turnip greens, broccoli, mango and squash varieties.

If you don't get enough beta carotene it can also lead to an increased risk of joint problems.

Can I consume too much beta carotene?

Only rarely. Although beta carotene is not toxic, an excess can cause some slightly unpleasant side effects like nausea, loose stools, and a yellow/ orange colouring on hands and feet. Technically, it is toxic in excess, but then so are most things.

With regards to carrots, yes you can eat so many of them that your skin will turn yellow. One large carrot contains twice your recommended daily minimum. If you eat more than 3 carrots every day you've probably saturated your body's ability to store vitamin A over a short time and so the excess shows up as an orange tint on your skin.

Broccoli and other foods high in vitamin A or carotene will do the same, but you would have to eat almost 9 broccoli spears to equal the vitamin A in one carrot. It is a very healthy habit to eat any raw vegetable that you like, especially if you try a wide variety. Writing this section on a US Airways flight from San Diego to Manchester I was impressed to find that the meal included a pack of washed, raw baby carrots, and very refreshing they were too.

But beware of carotene added to foods and drinks as a colouring. It is almost always synthetic and made from chemical precursors so it has never been near a carrot. The

The Body Language of Health

problem with synthetic products is that there can be nasty rogue chemicals in the mix where the chemical reaction has not quite progressed to completion. And there are not the complex mixtures of analogues, isomers and homologous series of chemicals that are present in natural products. It is not just carotene we need, it is the carotenoids, the whole group, and we have evolved to have this mixture in our food. That's why nature's products are best. And they are best because we have evolved with them as our food.

Good sources of beta carotene

- Carrots
- pumpkin,
- sweet potato,
- cooked greens,
- apricots,
- sweet peppers,
- kale,
- turnip greens,
- broccoli,
- mango
- vegetable squashes
- Oh yes, mandarins (in fact all oranges).

Do you have a Broccoli gene?

Experts now consider that we have evolved a 'receptor gene' that programmes our taste according to what our body needs. By testing the bitterness perceived by someone eating various foods, researchers have found we are genetically programmed to love or hate certain foods. In particular, evolution of the receptor gene dictates our avoidance of certain vegetables that can inhibit thyroid function, claim Mari Hakala and Paul Breslin of Monell Chemical Sciences Center in Philadelphia, Pennsylvania.

Compounds known as glucosinolates are present in a variety of vegetables, especially Cruciferous vegetables like broccoli. These compounds can block the formation of organic iodine and the transport of iodine into the thyroid. Iodine is necessary for proper thyroid function, and in geographic regions where inorganic iodine levels are low, people develop an enlarged thyroid, called a Goitre Neck. This is so prevalent in Derbyshire, in the middle of England that the problem is even known as 'Derbyshire Neck'. It's not surprising, because areas of low iodine, like Derbyshire, are typically those areas of land that are most remote from the sea, because iodine gets washed

The Body Language of Health

out of the soil and that is why the oceans are quite rich in iodine. The Pennines running through Derbyshire are called the backbone of England, and this ridge of hills is the 'watershed' of England from which all rainfall flows to the sea on the east and west of England, taking all the iodine with it. If you are responsible for buying food produce from a foreign country, you should consider this nutritional point when making your buying decisions.

Mari Hakala and Paul Breslin were able to show that different genetic versions of this same receptor, known as hTAS2R38, specifically determine people's perception of plants that synthesize glucosinolates.

In their experiments, the researchers found that individuals possessing two copies of a "sensitive" version of the hTAS2R38 gene rated the glucosinolate-containing vegetables as 60% more bitter than did subjects possessing two copies of an "insensitive" version of the receptor gene.

Even more interesting is that we seem to also have a 'toothpaste gene' and goodness knows what else. So we can expect food technologists to get really clever in future, with targeted products to match our genetic proclivities.

SKIN

Do you have rashes and spots on your eyelids?

You probably have an ALLERGY TO DUST MITES

Like an increasing number of people these days in the Western society, my son, James has asthma and eczema, and I will go into that in more detail later, but we had the good fortune to make the acquaintance of a local eminent expert on allergies, Dr Morrow Brown.

Dr Morrow-Brown is an amazing character now in his nineties, and as one of Britain's most eminent experts in allergies it is a great privilege to know him. These days, the Health Service has discontinued many of the earlier practices of finding the cause of the allergy, or treating the patient with desensitising injections, much to his annoyance, but he still offers his services privately. His website, www.allergiesexplained.com has some fascinating insights, some parts of which I have summarised here.

If you have a rash on your eyebrows, Dr Morrow-Brown tells us this is characteristic of allergies from dust mites. The faeces of dust mites often cause the most problems wherever they are coming into contact with the skin. So eczema of the eyebrows and round the eyes is seen quite often in children when dust mites irritate the eyes. They rub them because they itch, and this spreads the allergen.

A rash round the mouth usually suggests that that person is allergic to one food or other.

If you have a child whose mouth is often open, this is usually because the nose becomes blocked by allergic rhinitis.

Eczema on the legs or body often points to a dust-mite infested bed, and sneezing and runny nose at night often suggests a new pillow would be a good idea.

It is frequently very difficult to help eczema sufferers because there are often several reasons for the condition. This means that unless these causes are all eliminated simultaneously the eczema will not improve. Avoiding single foods such as milk will only help if milk is the only cause, and to exclude one major food in turn risks missing the other foods, because several foods together may have additive effects.

To cure these ailments you have to turn into a detective, because it is our experience that some doctors will only treat the condition, not look for the cause. We had to seek the help of an expert allergy consultant, but there are precious few of these in Britain any more.

Inhalants such as dust mite faeces and particulates from pets are often involved in allergies, as well as foods, but without skin tests, which many dermatologists will not do any more, the importance of the environment is seldom recognised.

If the eczema is allowed to persist for years, repeated infections of eczema skin sites may result in the formation of specific IgE antibodies to bacteria, thus making recovery even more difficult because bacteria are normally all around us.

Many of the side effects of eczema are debilitating. Scratching causes loss of sleep, infection is common even when the nails are kept short, cracks on the hands are very painful and limit exertion and games, victims can be teased and bullied at school and regarded as outcasts by some because they look infectious. Eczematous children put up with a great deal, and sometimes suffer all their lives. Thus there are many good reasons to investigate eczematous children for avoidable causes in the food and in the environment at as early an age as possible, rather than just put up with it somehow and wait for it to get better. Experience shows that it is unlikely to get better in fact it is more likely to change to asthma and rhinitis, unless you can do something positive about it yourself.

Dr Morrow-Brown's involvement with eczema began many years ago when he observed that the quality of life of many asthmatics was destroyed more by their eczema than their asthma. He found that when he put the patient on a restricted diet which improved the asthma, the eczema sometimes got better as well. These were patients who had also been attending the local skin clinic for years, so when there had been a remarkable improvement in the eczema he enquired if their improvement had been commented on by the Dermatologist .

To his surprise their improvement had never been commented on, or even excited any curiosity, so he became deeply interested in eczema himself as another aspect of allergy. A study of old allergy journals and textbooks, mostly American, revealed much research into finding causes for eczema at a time when there was no effective medication. These efforts had declined considerably after effective steroid creams were introduced about fifty years ago. These creams were sufficiently convenient for the doctor to prescribe, that any consideration of the cause of the eczema was conveniently forgotten. But it is just another example of the modern trend in healthcare of treating the symptoms not the cause.

Any interest in the causes of eczema by doctors has largely been restricted to 'patch testing'. Ideally, skin prick tests are the most revealing, but this practice has been discontinued in Britain. It is difficult to understand why British skin specialists often refuse to carry out skin prick tests when requested, yet routinely carry out many 'patch tests' to identify contact allergens.

Localised allergy in skin cells is a characteristic of allergy to substances like nickel and many other chemicals, where prolonged exposure is necessary to produce a reaction, therefore patch tests stay in place for two days to produce slow reactions. Positive reactions indicate what to avoid, and in recent years inhalant allergens such as dust mites and food extracts have also been found useful as patch tests in Europe, but not in Britain as far as I am aware.

But even patch testing is not always effective at identifying the cause. My mother has an allergic reaction to nickel, and tries to avoid it wherever possible. But nickel does not seem to be the real problem, it is touching nickel when she has eaten a lot of sugar. If she avoids sugar, she seems to lose her sensitivity to nickel. Really, she has a food intolerance to sugar.

It seems that many dermatologists still do not believe that allergy causes eczema, particularly food allergy. This is a very controversial subject, and it is only in recent years that even the British Eczema Society has acknowledged that foods can cause eczema, although even now they state it in a very reserved manner, with practically no reference to other allergic causes of eczema. Unfortunately GPs are programmed to refer all eczema cases to the skin department, just as they were taught in Medical School, so it is only a very persistent patient or parent who will get the allergic possibilities of eczema investigated.

Yet recent studies from USA, Australia, and New Zealand have confirmed that foods play a very dominant role in the causation of infantile eczema.

Eczema is now very common in infancy, as at least one in five infants are affected. Doctors generally give positive reassurance to the parents that their child's condition will clear spontaneously by age five or seven, or that they will 'grow out of it' in adolescence. In the meantime, steroid creams are the main method of treatment. Foods are seldom considered seriously as a cause, yet infancy is the time of life when the diet is at its most simple and easily altered. This is the easiest time to eliminate food allergy as a cause of the problem. Unfortunately when the eczema eventually subsides, as it does in most cases when left untreated, it is often replaced by asthma, rhinitis and hay fever. This progress from one sort of allergy to another is known as the 'Allergic March'. It has been suggested that if the cause is identified and avoided there is some prospect of preventing this response to allergens from becoming a persistent pattern. There is also evidence from recent surveys that if children are desensitised to grass pollen when they develop hay fever they are not so likely to develop other allergies later.

When it is foods that cause eczema the reaction is usually slow. This is because traces of the food are absorbed into the blood without causing a local reaction in the gut, and pass into the blood and then the tissue fluids to produce eczema in the sensitised skin. The same mechanism operates when the joints, brain, kidney, or any other organ system has become sensitised. Allergens such as dust mite or animal danders (flakes of skin and saliva that become airborne, particularly from cats because they lick themselves clean) may access the skin through the invisible cracks and defects which are always present in the skin, or the visible cracks from scratching, thus causing eczema to be a sort of constant ongoing skin reaction. Some allergens may also reach the skin by absorption from the respiratory system where an allergic reaction causing asthma may or may not be happening.

The itch is always worse when warm in bed, and Dr Morrow-Brown believes it is probable that traces of sweat dissolve the allergen from the tiny particles of mite faeces present in all beds. This will produce a very strong extract, much stronger than the usual skin testing solutions, which causes the continuous skin reactions.

The Allergic March

Many allergies progress from one thing to another, driving the sufferer or their parents to despair as they try one drug or over-the-counter product after another. But the answer lies in prevention, not the medication. Most treatments can only mask the problem. This progression is known as the Allergic March. I know of this from my family's experiences. Let me review our experiences in the hope that others will learn from it and make a quicker diagnosis for themselves and their children.

James, our oldest son was 9lb 2oz when he was born, and the midwife told my wife that he was so big that she clearly would not be able to satisfy his hunger if she breast fed him, although she realised too late that this is a myth. So, like most babies born it the early 1980's he was breast fed initially but as a result of little support from the nursing staff he ended up being fed with standard formula baby milk within a day or so of being born. Elsie did also continue to breast feed him, but this was not

The Body Language of Health

very successful because once baby milk has been introduced, it is all too easy for the baby to suck on a bottle teat so they tend to make a half-hearted attempt at the breast and wait until the bottle makes an appearance.

James developed eczema when he was only a few days old, and in hospital the nurses said perhaps he had a reaction to the starch in the bedsheets. He continued to have rashes on his arms, legs, face and in creases such as the backs of his knees. This is typical of Dr Morrow-Brown's theory of perspiration allowing allergens to penetrate the skin easier in creases, but we didn't know it then. James continued like this throughout childhood, and doctors prescribed E45 cream, and steroid creams to be used sparingly.

When James started taking solid food he then developed a rash round the corners of his mouth. This is a typical Body language sign of a food allergy. We didn't know that either.

The rash got worse and spread to other parts of James's body. Most people still have no idea today that foods, most particularly cow's milk in the formula baby milk can cause such an awful skin condition. And whenever we allowed him to get hot in the car his eczema could flare up and be painful and would sometimes bleed.

Traditionally the best advice for parents comes from self help groups like the Eczema Society, because general practitioners no longer specialise in these allergic conditions. The Eczema Society advise that cotton clothes should be worn as they keep you cooler, and there is more advice from the few experts like Dr Morrow-Brown, particularly from his website www.allergiesexplained.co.uk which has some fascinating pictures. Books such as 'E for Additives' contain a list of foods and additives that aggravate allergies, so that parents can control the diet. And the LaLeche League give advice on breast feeding and the hazards of cows milk in 'formula' products that bear no relation to mother's breast milk and are notorious for causing infant allergies.

GP's receive very little training in allergies so their main response is to prescribe hormones or creams, but most of these products are of little help in curing the condition, and some contain perfumes and alcohols that make the condition worse.

When James was three years old he got whooping cough and overnight it quickly developed into asthma and we rushed him to hospital where he ended up on a steroid-filled drip.

The Body Language of Health

During hospital visits the consultants continued to say that allergy tests were a waste of time because James's allergies would undoubtedly be dust mites, pets and pollen. They fobbed off any suggestions we made from our support with focus groups as not mainstream. Meanwhile James's allergies got worse. We attacked the house for any signs of dust, and took measures to prevent dust mites but it seemed to make little difference to his allergies although by this time he was on a cocktail of steroids, inhalers and ointments.

Then. when he was about four years old one night we saw a mouse run across the floor in the house, something which sounds awful but is not that unusual because we lived in the country surrounded by parkland and woods. This was a wily mouse and resisted any attempt to catch it with a trap, and when we resorted to poison bait, it refused to eat it. After a couple of weeks of futile mouse hunting we decided a cat might be a good idea. We introduced the cat to the household and monitored James's condition. We were determined to take particular note to see if it affected James's allergies, intending to get rid of the cat if there was any difference in his condition. The mouse vanished, but the allergies continued, though apparently no worse, so the cat stayed.

Many people fall into the same trap (the allergy trap, that is, not the mouse trap). They will have allergic children on so much medication that introducing a pet to the household will not really seem to have much effect to the sufferer, but this is because the allergic condition is artificially stabilised by the steroids. However the presence of an animal can elevate the base condition of the allergy so that the sufferer is now rarely well.

In later years we met Dr Morrow Brown and James became his private patient and underwent some allergy tests. These showed him to be highly allergic to moulds, certain pollens AND very allergic to CAT. But not dust mite, despite our mammoth efforts over the years to rid the house of dust. If only these tests had been available earlier they would have been such a help.

The problem with cats is that they wash their fur, and particles of saliva flake off the skin and attach themselves to everything in the vicinity. So when you have had a cat in the house, the carpets, the wallpaper, the soft furnishings, in fact everything, will have a coating of cat dander. This can only be removed by totally stripping the house, though this must be done while the asthma sufferer is living somewhere else. We threw out all the carpets, put down laminate flooring, stripped off all the wallpaper and redecorated throughout the house.

Even with all the allergens removed, an allergy sufferer will be so destabilised that it can take many weeks or even years for the allergy to subside. When you are an allergy sufferer you have to become a detective. You have to ask yourself some fundamental questions.

Are you better at the west coast, where the prevailing westerly wind has cleansed itself over three thousand miles of open Atlantic Ocean? (no pollen).

Are you better when it is frosty? (dry, clean air), are you worse in Spring? (flower and tree pollen), or Autumn? (moulds); are you worse after it has been windy? (stirs up pollen in spring/summer or moulds (autumn)).

Does cigarette smoke affect you? (particulates), does a friend's house make you wheezy? (cats, cage birds etc.), does your mouth tingle with some foods? (food allergy), do you notice any other features listed in this book? Check on other sections for 'allergy'.

There is also every possibility that some mineral imbalance is upsetting your immune system so it is worth experimenting with the Body Language book and its symptoms. I still suspect that there is a basic, underlying issue that triggers allergies, but as yet I don't know what it might be. If I was a sufferer myself I would experiment, because I am the sort of person that will persevere with everything until I find the answer. But of course it takes a book like this one to stimulate the idea that you actually can do something for yourself. I would not be surprised to find that zinc, sulphur, magnesium and some trace element deficiencies are partly responsible because not only have allergies blossomed with our sterile existence, but our food has become chronically deficient in these and so many other nutrients recently too within the same timescale that allergies have proliferated.

However I have found that others, especially parents seem oblivious to the problems of their children and the possibilities of resolving the problem themselves. No wonder so many people are walking around with sub-optimal health these days.

Maybe allergies all start because the baby is prevented from getting those essential antibodies in breast milk right from the outset. Our other children were breast fed because by then Elsie had found out about breast milk and the problems of cows milk, and they are fine. So it cannot be exclusively environmental in our case.

And I have noticed that those few allergic people I know (including James) seem to have an underlying athletes foot infection so it is worth investigating a systemic yeast infection that could be causing your allergy. A yeast infection could easily be triggering and over-stimulating your immune system.

And zinc is very important to combat allergies too. You could try a zinc supplement. Allergies don't produce stretch marks, but the next section could be relevant, because here comes zinc again.

Do you have stretch marks?

You may be deficient in ZINC

Many of the features of common chronic disorders, especially connective tissue disorders, are identical to the symptoms of zinc deficiencies. Is this a coincidence, or could zinc deficiencies be an often-overlooked factor in many disorders currently attributed to genes or other causes?

Zinc is essential to maintain the elasticity of skin so deficiency can lead to stretch marks. Zinc is essential for the replacement of skin cells and zinc is necessary in all healing processes. I would like to bet that it is probably the 'magic ingredient' in many expensive cosmetics that claim to prevent wrinkles, though zinc oxide to smear on your skin is one of the cheapest ointments and it is readily available.

When pregnant mice were fed a diet moderately deficient in zinc, their offspring exhibited a malfunctioning immune system for the first six months of life. More alarming, the second and third generations also showed signs of poor immunity - even though they were fed a zinc-plentiful diet. This is because of genetic imprinting again. What happens to the mother is instilled in the unborn young.

If zinc deficiencies can carry over from generations in mice, as noted above, could the same be true for humans? Perhaps some of the conditions in humans we currently attribute to genetic defects were actually caused by deficiencies of zinc or other nutrients occurring in past generations. And what about our children?

We already know that genetic conditioning played an important part in human adaptation to their changing environment. We explored this in the section on whorls on your fingertips.

How can genetic imprinting work? If the mother has a deficient diet that harms her immune system, how can that affect her children, and more incredibly, her grandchildren?

The Body Language of Health

I think that the answer is probably to do with the fact that a female of any species is born with a lifetime's supply of eggs in her ovaries. So this means that your Grandmother produced the eggs in your mother's womb, and you produced the eggs in your daughter's womb. When your daughter releases an egg every month, waiting to be fertilised, in effect it is your egg – your body put them there when your daughter was developing in your womb. So you in effect produce your grandchildren. Men don't have this system, as they just produce sperm daily, even though it is by the million.

So any stress, any nutritional problems you experience – including your life sustained on rubbish fast food, not only carries forward into your daughter, but into your granddaughter too. In theory this accelerates the opportunities for humans to adapt to changing environments, even when that environmental change is our responsibility. This feature has been observed many times as a consequence of war and strife which affects health and stress related illnesses. It is not just the population living through the war that is affected, it is several future generations as well, even though they never experienced the conflict.

When Darwin explained his 'Origin of the Species' he was only able to explain the slow adaptation of each offspring to their new environment. The phrase that others coined to explain his theory was 'survival of the fittest' to show that the most adapted offspring would be more likely to breed and carry that trait on to the next generation. But he was unable to explain the frequent acceleration of physical and mental attributes that enable a species to fill a void in nature. Genetic imprinting was Darwin's real 'missing link'.

If humans were to die out, another species would become top dog relatively quickly. That animal would have to be intelligent, strong for its weight, adaptable, with manipulative hands and a vocabulary of sorts. I am no biologist but I don't believe that 'top dog' would be a dog at all. I think it would be a squirrel. To my mind they have all the attributes necessary for that position. I have waged a battle of wits for years with local squirrels who delight in eating food I put out for the birds, then they invade our attic and damage roof joists and electrical wiring. Squirrels have almost the same body weight / brain size ratio to humans, incidentally, all because their metabolism produces a similar ration of fatty acids necessary for essential brain function. It would be interesting to see where they get their fatty acids from, but as far as I could tell no-one has studied the nutritional requirements of squirrels. Maybe acorns could be the next super-food.

How would it evolve into the top dog role? Genetic imprinting, probably. The life of the mother would be influential in switching on those gene patterns that benefit the offspring, while suppressing the old genetic patterns that are no longer beneficial.

The Body Language of Health

This accelerates the development of the creature when it is needed. I am surprised that genetic imprinting, which is a relatively new discovery, has not been added to Darwin's 'survival of the fittest' and heralded as the answer to the 'origin of the species'.

I happen to be a fan of old motor cars. I enjoy the engineering quality, the style, the smells and the sounds. And I like tinkering, which I cannot do on modern cars because of their computer wizardry. And old cars provide us with a fascinating example of evolution.

I used to have three Triumph Spitfires. The Mark 1 had a hard chassis, metal dashboard and solid steering column. The Mark 2 had better lights and a few safety features. The Mark 3 had a collapsible steering column, and better performance and top speed because motorways had recently been introduced when it was made. Slowly, as drivers demanded them, in came windscreen washers, disc brakes, electronic ignition, sealed-for-life bearings, air conditioning as standard, self-cancelling indicators, and a multitude of safety features. That's motoring evolution.

My little Honda Beat was designed to conform to Japanese laws that limited the size of car for those who did not have off-road parking, so it is an exercise in miniaturisation with a 660cc engine but with everything else you would expect in a modern car, including air conditioning. And it is quite fast too. It is perfectly packaged, as long as you have one for each foot. But it is a quirk of automotive engineering, with a market limited only to Japan. It was never sold in Britain and mine is an import. According to the club, there are only 49 in the country.

Now that environmental issues are becoming more topical, this is an evolutionary misfit just waiting to emerge as the dominant species. And big gas guzzling American cars and their designers are going to be the dinosaurs of the modern age. No wonder Japanese models already dominate the American market. Will we all be driving Honda Beat size cars some day? Probably. That's evolution at work again.

But this evolution requires a trigger, whether it is the overcrowding in Japan, or environmental panic in the West. In evolutionary terms, the Honda Beat is a genetic deviation, waiting for climate change to allow it to benefit and proliferate at the expense of the big gas guzzlers. And human evolution has been no different in the past, and will be no different in the future.

Back to stretch marks and zinc deficiency with all its Body Language symptoms. When we cook food, much of the zinc will go into the water, along with most of the other minerals and vitamins. So it makes sense that the cooking liquids, especially from vegetables, should be consumed as well, as a soup or in making gravy. More importantly, when foods are processed, as in the refining of grains, much of the zinc is lost, along with manganese, chromium, molybdenum, and B vitamins. Usually, only iron and sometimes vitamins B1 and B2 are added back in "enriched" foods (and this iron isn't even in the easily bioavailable form). But adding zinc, manganese, chromium, and more B vitamins such as B6, would be much better and help us avoid common deficiencies.

But a particular problem with zinc supplements is that zinc absorption may vary from about 20-40 percent of ingested zinc, depending mainly on body needs and stomach acid concentrations. Like iron, zinc from meat has been shown to be better absorbed because it is bound with proteins. When bound with the phytates or oxalates found in grains and vegetables, less zinc is absorbed. Calcium, phosphorus, copper, iron, lead, and cadmium all compete with zinc for absorption. Milk and eggs reduce zinc absorption. Fibre foods, bran, and phytates, found mainly in the outer covering of grains, may also inhibit zinc absorption. Phytic acid may combine with the zinc in the upper intestine before this mineral can be absorbed. In nutrition, nothing is simple.

The zinc-cadmium relationship is interesting too, because cadmium is considered a potentially toxic heavy metal. But when it is taken together with zinc it ceases to be a toxicity problem. When cadmium contaminates grains such as wheat, it is found in the centre of grain; zinc is found mainly in the grain covering. So eating whole grains, which have a higher amount of zinc than of cadmium, will reduce any possible absorption of cadmium. But refining of grains into flour removes the zinc rich outer layer, so the zinc-cadmium ratio is decreased, and cadmium is more likely to be absorbed and cause problems. This is just one of the reasons why whole grains are much better for you than refined grains.

In the human body, the zinc is stored in a variety of tissues. It is most concentrated in the prostate and semen, which suggests zinc's tie to male sexual function (impotence can be related to low zinc). The next most concentrated tissues are the retina of the eye, heart, spleen, lungs, brain, and adrenal glands. The skin contains a high amount of zinc, but it is less concentrated than in the organ tissues. Nails, hair, and teeth also have some zinc, and this mineral is important to these as well.

Zinc is eliminated through the gastrointestinal tract in the faeces and some is also eliminated in the urine. When you consume alcohol this stimulates the urinary system and so alcohol increases urinary losses of zinc. This means that alcoholics are often severely zinc deficient. Zinc is also lost in the sweat, possibly as much as 2-3 mg. in a day. Stress, burns, surgery, and weight loss all seem to increase body losses of zinc.

Do you have chicken skin on your upper arms?

You may be deficient in ESSENTIAL FATTY ACIDS

Keratosis pilaris (KP) is a very common genetic follicular disease that produces rough bumps on the skin that look like a turkey's backside and hence the disease is known as "chicken skin". Primarily, it appears on the back and outer sides of the upper arms, but can also occur on thighs and buttocks or any part of the body except palms or soles.

Chicken skin is affected by the level of fatty acids in your diet. Fatty acids are essential in the diet, but the recent trend of cutting down on fatty food and replacing it with junk food has reduced the amount of fatty acids we consume.

Essential fatty acids (EFA's) are needed for many physiologic processes, including maintaining the integrity of the skin and the structure of cell membranes and synthesizing hormones such as prostaglandins and leukotrienes. Considering the wealth of information about EFA's these days it is surprising that we have not encountered them before in this book. But they are not what they seem, and in 'Do you have high Cholesterol?' we are into controversy again.

EFA's are either omega-6 fatty acids or omega-3 fatty acids. These two types of fatty acids must be obtained from the foods we eat because the body cannot synthesize them. The EFA's have some complicated names; eicosapentaenoic acid and docosahexaenoic acid are two EFA's that are important components of the brain and retina.

Many studies have shown that the symptoms which are associated with a deficiency in fatty acids are precisely those that are exhibited by children with ADHD. These symptoms include thirst, frequent urination and dry skin and hair. Researchers found that children with ADHD are deficient in omega-3 fatty acids.

Attention deficit hyperactivity disorder (ADHD) is the most common behavioural disorder in children, affecting between 3 percent and 5 percent of school-age youngsters. It is diagnosed more often in boys than girls. Symptoms include an inability to concentrate for long on anything, and unruly, irresponsible behaviour.

Stimulant drugs such as Ritalin are generally used to calm children with ADHD and are effective about 75 percent of the time. But Ritalin is a derivative of Amphetamine, or Speed, and is usually prescribed long term or for life. Nutritional treatment seems to offer much better rates of success, particularly since ADHD appears to feature in those countries like America and Canada with the worst diets. And there has been great success in prisons where learning ability in job training, alertness and levels of violence have all seen great improvements when supplements of fish oils rich in EFA's were administered. For some reason, however, after the study these supplements were not widely implemented.

Omega 3 fatty acids are important for other reasons. They are healing nutrients that help prevent heart disease, depression, strokes and cancers. Some research suggests that omega-3 suppresses inflammation associated with cancer, and men with the highest level of omega-3 had the lowest incidences of colorectal cancer. Omega-3 has also been associated with protecting the heart and improving brain function.

Our bodies actually have the ability to synthesis one type of fatty acid from the other. Two common omega-6 fatty acids are linoleic acid and arachidonic acid. The body can turn the former into the latter. Common omega-3 fatty acids are linolenic acid, eicosapentaenoic acid, and docosahexaenoic acid. In the body, the last two compounds can be made from the former. So, linoleic and linolenic acids are particularly essential.

Babies fed a traditional cows milk formula can have growth failure, thrombocytopenia, alopecia, and a generalized scaly dermatitis, which resembles congenital ichthyosis, because cows milk only has about 25% of the amount of linoleic acid that is present in mothers milk. This syndrome is reversed by linoleic acid supplementation. So breast is best every time.

Although total fat intake in many developing countries is very low, most of the fat that is consumed is of vegetable origin, and this is rich in linoleic acid with some linolenic acid. For this reason the diet of the third world is often healthier than that in Western society.

Good sources of essential fatty acids are fish and fish oils, olive oil, eggs, flax-seed oil, and hemp seed oil.

OMEGA-3 FATTY ACIDS

Omega-3 fatty acids such as Eicosapentaenoic acid (EPA) are found in cold water fish. Mackerel, herring, halibut and salmon contain the most, with lesser amounts in tuna and shrimp. These are the 'good' essential fatty acids.

Flax seed oil is good source of essential fatty acids and is particularly high in omega-3 oils. It is difficult for the digestive system to break down raw flax seeds sufficiently to obtain enough essential fatty acids, so you need to buy the oil instead.

Algae can also be used, in fact EFA from algae is bound to be big in the future because of the world's reducing fish stocks and man's great appetite for essential fatty acids. Algae is more sustainable, and some manufacturers use it already for blending in with fish oils because of their fear of recriminations over fishing. Current use of fishing for omega oils is at a level where only around 10% of fish stock is used for essential fatty acid production, with the rest of the fish being used for fishmeal. Gross misuse of this valuable food resource is one of the scandals of the 21st century.

There is also an issue of lead, mercury and polychlorinated biphenols (pcbs) in marine fish, although disasters like the Japanese Minamata disaster are hopefully a thing of the past.

The essential fatty acids market has blossomed into a $3 billion industry which is expected to be worth $7 billion by 2011, and many producers feel it will be as big as the vitamin c and calcium markets are today.

OMEGA-6 FATTY ACIDS

These are the 'not so good' fatty acids. Linoleic acid, the shortest chain omega-6 fatty acid is an essential fatty acid too. Arachidonic acid is another physiologically significant omega-6 fatty acid and it is much more important because it is the building block for prostaglandins and other highly active molecules in the body. Linoleic acid is found in safflower, sunflower and corn oils.

Some research has indicated that a high level of omega-6 acids relative to Omega-3 fatty acids may increase the probability of a number of diseases and also depression. The optimum ratio is thought to be 4 to 1 or less. Modern Western diets typically have ratios of omega-6 to omega-3 in excess of 10 to 1, some as high as 30 to 1. And this causes heart disease.

Over the last century most western countries have undergone a dramatic shift in the composition of their diets in which the omega-3 fatty acids that are essential to the brain have been flooded out by competing omega-6 fatty acids, mainly from industrial oils such as soya, corn, and sunflower. In USA, for example, soya oil accounted for only 0.02% of all calories available in 1909, but by 2000 it accounted for 20%. Americans have gone from eating a fraction of an ounce of soya oil a year to slurping

The Body Language of Health

25lbs per person per year in that period. In the UK, omega-6 fats from oils such as soya, corn, and sunflower accounted for 1% of energy supply in the early 1960s, but by 2000 they were nearly 5%. These omega-6 fatty acids come mainly from industrial frying for takeaways, ready meals and snack foods such as crisps, chips, biscuits, ice-creams and from margarine. And at the same time, alcohol depletes omega-3s from the brain making the ratio of Omega 3 to Omega 6 even worse.

To test the hypothesis, researchers have mapped the growth in consumption of omega-6 fatty acids from seed oils in 38 countries since the 1960s against the rise in murder rates over the same period. In all cases there is an unnerving match. As omega-6 goes up, so do homicides in a linear progression. Industrial societies where omega-3 consumption has remained high and omega-6 low because people eat fish, such as Japan, have low rates of murder and depression.

Of course, all these graphs show is that there is a striking correlation between violence and omega 6-fatty acids in the diet. They don't prove that high omega-6 and low omega-3 fat consumption actually causes violence. Moreover, many other things have changed in the last century and have been blamed for rising violence - exposure to violence in the media, the breakdown of the family unit and increased consumption of sugar, to take a few examples. But some of the trends you might expect to be linked to increased violence - such as availability of firearms and alcohol, or urbanisation - do not in fact correlate to a rise in murder across countries.

There has been a backlash recently against the hype surrounding omega-3 in the UK from scientists arguing that the evidence remains sketchy. Part of the backlash stems from the eagerness of some supplement companies to suggest that fish oils might work wonders even on children who have no behavioural problems.

Professor John Stein, of the department of physiology at Oxford University and Joseph Hibbeln of America's National Institute of Health, with others, have been investigating what the mechanisms of a causal relationship between diet and aggression might be.

Essential fatty acids are called essential because humans cannot make them but must obtain them from the diet. The brain is a fatty organ - it's 60% fat by dry weight, and the essential fatty acids are what make part of its structure, making up 20% of the nerve cells' membranes. The synapses, or junctions where nerve cells connect with other nerve cells, contain even higher concentrations of essential fatty acids - being made of about 60% of the omega-3 fatty acid DHA.

The Body Language of Health

Communication between the nerve cells depends on neurotransmitters, such as serotonin and dopamine, docking with receptors in the nerve cell membrane.

Omega-3 DHA is very long and highly flexible. When it is incorporated into the nerve cell membrane it helps make the membrane itself elastic and fluid so that signals pass through it efficiently. But if the wrong fatty acids are incorporated into the membrane, the neurotransmitters can't dock properly. We know from many other studies what happens when the neurotransmitter systems don't work efficiently. Low serotonin levels are known to predict an increased risk of suicide, depression and violent and impulsive behaviour. And dopamine is what controls the reward processes in the brain.

Laboratory tests at NIH have shown that the composition of tissue and in particular of the nerve cell membrane of people in the US is different from that of the Japanese, who eat a diet rich in omega-3 fatty acids from fish. Americans have cell membranes higher in the less flexible omega-6 fatty acids, which appear to have displaced the elastic omega-3 fatty acids found in Japanese nerve cells.

Hibbeln's theory is that because the omega-6 fatty acids compete with the omega-3 fatty acids for the same metabolic pathways, when omega-6 dominates in the diet, we can't convert the omega-3s to DHA and EPA, the longer chain versions we need for the brain. What seems to happen then is that the brain picks up a more rigid omega-6 fatty acid DPA instead of DHA to build the cell membranes - and they don't function so well. You get Homer Simpson, not Homer the classical author of the Iliad.

Other experts blame the trans fats produced by partial hydrogenation of industrial oils for processed foods. Trans fats have been shown to interfere with the synthesis of essentials fats in foetus and infants. Minerals such as zinc and the B vitamins are needed to metabolise essential fats, so deficiencies in these may be playing an important part too.

There is also evidence that deficiencies in DHA/EPA at times when the brain is developing rapidly - in the womb, in the first 5 years of life and at puberty - can affect its architecture permanently. Animal studies have shown that those deprived of omega-3 fatty acids over two generations have offspring who cannot release dopamine and serotonin so effectively and become unruly delinquents.

"The extension of all this is that if children are left with low dopamine as a result of early deficits in their own or their mother's diets, they cannot experience reward in the same way and they cannot learn from reward and punishment. If their serotonin levels are low, they cannot inhibit their impulses or regulate their emotional responses," Hibbeln points out.

Mental health

Here too you have one possible factor in cycles of deprivation (again, no one is suggesting diet is the only factor) and why criminal behaviour is apparently higher among lower socio-economic groups where nutrition is likely to be poorer.

These effects of the industrialisation of the diet on the brain were also predicted in the 1970s by Professor Michael Crawford, currently at London's Metropolitan University. He established that DHA was structural to the brain and foresaw that deficiencies would lead to a surge in mental health and behavioural problems - a prediction borne out by the UK's mental health figures.

Two decades later, the world's first study of the effect of diet on behaviour took place in a UK prison. Bernard Gesch, now a senior researcher at Stein's Oxford laboratory, first became involved with nutrition and its relationship to crime as a director of the charity Natural Justice in northwest England. He was supervising persistent offenders in the community and was struck by their diets. He later set out to test the idea that poor diet might cause antisocial behaviour and crime in the maximum security Aylesbury prison.

His study, a placebo-controlled double blind randomised trial, took 231 volunteer prisoners and assigned half to a regime of multivitamin, mineral and essential fatty acid supplements and half to placebos. The supplement aimed to bring the prisoners' intakes of nutrients up to the level recommended by government.

Aylesbury was at the time a prison for young male offenders, aged 17 to 21, convicted of the most serious crimes. Trevor Hussey was then deputy governor and remembers it being a tough environment. "It was a turbulent young population. They had problems with their anger. They were all crammed into a small place and even though it was well run you got a higher than normal number of assaults on staff and other prisoners."

Although the governor was keen on looking at the relationship between diet and crime, Hussey remembers being sceptical himself at the beginning of the study. The catering manager was supportive, and even though prisoners on the whole preferred white bread, meat and confectionery to their fruit and veg, the staff tried to encourage prisoners to eat healthily, so he didn't expect to see much of a result.

The Body Language of Health

But quite quickly staff noticed a significant drop in the number of reported incidents of bad behaviour once their diet changed. "We'd just introduced a policy of 'earned privileges' so we thought it must be that rather than a few vitamins, but we used to joke 'maybe it's Bernard's pills'."

But when the trial finished it became clear that the drop in incidences of bad behaviour applied only to those on the supplements and not to those on the placebo.

The results, published in 2002, showed that those receiving the extra nutrients committed 37% fewer serious offences involving violence, and 26% fewer offences overall. Those on the placebos showed no change in their behaviour. Once the trial had finished the number of offences went up by the same amount. The office the researchers had used to administer nutrients was restored to a restraint room after they had left.

"The supplements improved the functioning of those prisoners. It was clearly something significant that can't be explained away. I was disappointed when the results were not latched on to. We put a lot of effort into improving prisoners' chances of not coming back in, and you measure success in small doses" said Gesch.

Gesch believes we should be rethinking the whole notion of culpability. The overall rate of violent crime in the UK has risen since the 1950s, with huge rises since the 1970s. "Such large changes are hard to explain in terms of genetics or simply changes of reporting or recording crime. One plausible candidate to explain some of the rapid rise in crime could be changes in the brain's environment. What would the future have held for those 231 young men if they had grown up with better nourishment?" Gesch says.

He said he was currently unable to comment on any plans for future research in prisons. What a wasted opportunity.

As Hibbeln says, the changes in our diet in the past century are "a very large uncontrolled experiment that may have contributed to the societal burden of aggression, depression and cardiovascular death". To ask whether we have enough evidence to change diets is to put the question the wrong way round. Whoever said it was safe to change them so radically in the first place?

Instead of governments fiddling with the penal system and building more prisons, why not legislate junk food off the menu and invest in wholesome food?

The Body Language of Health

Here is a typical young offender's diet

One young offender had been sentenced by the British courts on 13 occasions for stealing trucks in the early hours of the morning. Bernard Gesch recorded the boy's daily diet as follows:

- **Breakfast:** nothing (asleep)
- **Mid morning:** nothing (asleep)
- **Lunchtime:** 4 or 5 cups of coffee with milk and $2\frac{1}{2}$ heaped teaspoons of sugar
- **Mid afternoon:** 3 or 4 cups of coffee with milk and $2\frac{1}{2}$ heaped sugars
- **Tea:** chips, egg, ketchup, 2 slices of white bread, 5 cups of tea or coffee with milk and sugar
- **Evening:** 5 cups of tea or coffee with milk and sugar, 20 cigarettes, £2 worth of sweets, cakes and if money available 3 or 4 pints of beer.

Fish oils may lower the risk of breast cancer

Eating a low fat diet and taking a supplement rich in omega-3 fatty acids may reduce the risk of breast cancer in women, according to a study published in the Journal of the National Cancer Institute. In the study, 25 women diagnosed with breast cancer ate a low fat diet and took a daily fish oil supplement for three months. Researchers analysed their breast fat at the end of the study and found an increase in the ratio of omega-3 to omega-6 fatty acids. This may help to inhibit breast cancer, both by preventing it and reducing the risk of tumour size when cancer already exists.

Pretty powerful argument for taking notice of the chicken skin on your arms, eh?

There are many expensive cosmetic preparations available to mask your chicken skin, but what you need is oily fish. Don't be fooled by the skin cream adverts, it could turn out to be a load of codswallop.

Want to know more about avoiding cancer? There's not enough room here to go into specifics but Elsie has promised to write an article about her own research about cancer on our website at www.mybodylanguage.co.uk.

Do you sweat a lot?

You may be DIABETIC or deficient in CHROMIUM

Sometimes we are part of an experiment without realising it. My mild hypoglycaemia used to trigger a bout of getting very hot and sweaty, usually just before my hearing disappeared. So when I started to get all hot and sweaty I knew instinctively it was time to sit down and eat something sweet and sugary.

Actually, I think my thermostat is usually set wrongly, because I am invariably hotter than my family and sometimes have to go and stand outside in the winter to cool down because the central heating is set too high for me, even though it appears to be perfect for everyone else. This is another hypoglycaemic indicator.

It seems that the male side of my family has tended to have a problem in later life with this. I have a tendency to get sweaty armpits, which in my case underarm antiperspirant fails to suppress. But remarkably, since I discovered the stabilising effect of chromium on glucose metabolism, I find that the underarm perspiration vanishes like magic after I have taken a chromium supplement. So my nomination for Body Language of chromium deficiency is just that – underarm perspiration. Don't chromium plate your armpits, take a chromium supplement. It works for me and probably gives me additional benefits too like controlling my blood sugar.

People with type 2 diabetes can get sugar swings from too much, or to too little, and insufficient sugar makes them tire easily. Maybe it depends on what minerals and especially chromium they can get in their diet. Taking a chromium supplement will certainly have no adverse effect, and is well worth a try.

Incidentally my wife Elsie is now on Tamoxifen, an oestrogen blocker prescribed to women who have had oestrogen-receptive cancers. One of the side effects is that it triggers the menopause. This affects her thermostat, causing the 'hot flushes' that are associated with the menopause, so she takes the medication last thing at night so that the worst of the temperature excursion occurs while she is asleep.

I now don't need a hot water bottle in bed. But if you are on Tamoxifen, take a look at 'has your voice changed?' (Page 190).

Do you suffer from spontaneous bleeding?

You may be deficient in VITAMIN C, OR VITAMIN K

If you are deficient in either of these two vitamins you may find that spontaneous bleeding can develop from gums when cleaning your teeth, from nosebleeds, and from slight skin injuries. In my youth, we used to say that you hadn't been to a good disco if you came out without your ears bleeding, which means that discos were just as loud in my clubbing days as they are today. Of course, they don't have discos any more, nowadays they are called 'clubs' - coincidentally that's just what happens when your head comes into contact one of those.

Vitamin K deficiency exists mostly in elderly people or in teenagers who are choosy about what they eat. Chronic failure to eat sufficient amounts of vitamin K results in a tendency for spontaneous bleeding or in prolonged and excessive bleeding with trauma or injury. Vitamin K deficiency also occurs in newborn infants, as well as in people treated with certain antibiotics. Bleeding occurs because the protein in the body most affected by vitamin K deficiency is a blood-clotting protein called prothrombin.

It is a fat-soluble vitamin, which means that it will hang around in your body for a while. The vitamin K present in plant foods is called phylloquinone; while the form of the vitamin present in animal foods is called menaquinone. Both of these vitamins are absorbed from the diet and converted to an active form called dihydrovitamin K.

Spinach, lettuce, broccoli, Brussels sprouts, and cabbage are all good sources of vitamin K.

A portion of the body's vitamin K is supplied by bacteria living in the intestine rather than by dietary sources. So it is important to look after your gut. That is why vitamin K deficiency can be caused by taking antibiotics, which indiscriminately kill off all the bacteria in the gut, irrespective of whether they are friend or foe.

Vitamin K plays an important role in blood clotting. Without the vitamin, even a small cut would cause continuous bleeding in the body. Even it's name, Vitamin K is a clue, and the perceptive amongst you may remember the earlier description about 'Koagulation'. Maybe you are wondering if it was Kazimierez Funk who discovered it and named it after himself. But no, he missed out again because the German speaking discoverers realised it was crucial to Koagulation of blood after wounding. At that time most of the letters F to I were used up so they thought that Vitamin K was a reasonable letter to use.

Nowadays, most bleeding problems are most likely to be due to Vitamin K deficiency. Vitamin C deficiency also results in scurvy, a disease that involves bleeding. Although this is now rare in Britain, we should cover it anyway. You don't have to go as far as developing scurvy which is the ultimate indicator of vitamin C deficiency. But minor deficiencies of Vitamin C are more common than you would think.

Why do we need vitamin C?

Vitamin C is a water-soluble, antioxidant vitamin. It is important in forming collagen, a protein that gives structure to bones, cartilage, muscle, and blood vessels. Vitamin C also aids in the absorption of iron, and helps maintain capillaries, bones, and teeth. We cannot make vitamin C ourselves so we rely on fresh fruit and vegetables for our supply.

Smoking increases oxidative stress—and causes loss of vitamin C in the body. As a result, it is recommended that smokers consume 35 more milligrams of vitamin C per day than usual. But smoking charges up the body with nicotine, a nerve poison that can be fatal in very small doses. In our laboratory we use nicotine to make standards for tests which detect smoking levels. Nicotine is a nasty chemical to have around. It is easily absorbed through the skin, that is why nicotine patches work well. In the lab we all have to be aware that if we dropped a spot of concentrated nicotine solution on the bench and then accidentally put our hand on it, we would have only 20 minutes to live. Nicotine poisoning is a nasty way to go, it paralyses your nerves and stops your heart. In clinical laboratories, cleanliness is next to godliness in more senses than one.

Nicotine in the small quantities supplied by smoking suppresses the appetite, so most smokers have a terrible diet as well as being exposed to carcinogens. This combination makes smokers even more susceptible to cancer than smoking alone.

Benefits of stopping smoking

Stopping smoking is the best thing you can do for your health. Within five years of giving up you will have reduced the risk of a heart attack to about half that of a smoker. Within 10 years of giving up, the risk of a heart attack falls to the same as someone who has never smoked, and the risk of lung cancer falls to about half that of a smoker. The most important part in giving up smoking is your desire to stop. It is never too late in life to stop smoking.

The Body Language of Health

A new reason not to start smoking.

Recently it has been revealed that about one in 25 of the UK population carry the Alpha-1-antitrypsin (A1A) gene defect and one in 2,700 is born with the full syndrome, making A1AD the second most common genetic disorder after cystic fibrosis.

The most common effect from the A1AD gene is emphysema. Although the problem is present from birth, the effects of A1AD don't usually become apparent until someone is over 50 years old, and in many affected people there are no symptoms at all.

And the most important thing someone with the A1AD gene, or any lung disease, can do for their health is not to smoke and to avoid people who smoke around them.

Vitamin C can be lost from foods during preparation, cooking, or storage. To prevent loss of vitamin C:

- Serve fruits and vegetables raw whenever possible.
- Steam or simmer foods in a very small amount of water for the shortest time possible.
- Cook potatoes in their skins. Just wash the dirt off the outside of the potato.
- Refrigerate prepared juices and store them for no more than two to three days.
- Store cut, raw fruits and vegetables in an airtight container and refrigerate—do not soak or store in water. Vitamin C will be dissolved in the water.

Good sources of Vitamin C

- fruit – especially citrus, berries and Kiwi fruit
- vegetables (keep vegetables raw to maximise the vitamin C content)
- berries

Good sources of Vitamin K

- Green leafy vegetables

Do you get dry scaly skin with hair follicles plugged with coiled or distorted hairs and a red halo?

You may be deficient in VITAMIN C

This particular characteristic is common in people who are vitamin C deficient. Maybe it makes the hair go haywire. It is probably due to blocked pores that get infected because of low vitamin levels.

Eating a variety of foods that contain vitamin C is the best way to get an adequate amount each day. Healthy individuals who eat a balanced diet have healthy skin and rarely need supplements.

When there is a shortage of vitamin C, various health problems can arise, although scurvy is the only disease clinically treated with vitamin C. However, a shortage of vitamin C may result in "pinpoint" haemorrhages under the skin and a tendency to bruise easily, develop poor wound healing, soft and spongy bleeding gums and loose teeth.

Oedema (water retention) also happens with a shortage of vitamin C, and weakness, lack of energy, poor digestion, painful joints and bronchial infection and colds are also indicative of a vitamin C deficiency.

It is interesting to note that most animals produce their own vitamin C but only humans and guinea pigs do not have this ability. We believe this is because man evolved as a hunter gatherer and had a vegetarian diet rich in vitamin C so had no need to synthesise vitamin C in the body. This genetic trait was switched off over an extended period of evolution. Presumably guinea pigs also had a predominantly fruit diet too and their capability was also bred out.

Unfortunately this unique similarity with man has caused the guinea pig to be subjected to all kinds of experimentation over the years. Before trying it out on humans they try it out on guinea pigs. Now the very name is synonymous with experimentation.

Good sources of Vitamin C are fruit, vegetables and berries.

Vitamin C is important because it helps prevent oxidation damage to the fat-soluble vitamins A and E and also to fatty acids. Vitamin C can be beneficial in the treatment of iron deficiency anaemia and it is important to all animals, including humans, because it is vital to the production of collagen.

Why is collagen so important? Well collagen is one of the most ubiquitous (commonplace) substances in the body because it is the most abundant of the fibres contained in connective tissue. Connective tissue gives our body form and supports our organs. To give you an idea of how important collagen is, here is a list of the five types of collagen, and where they are used in the body.

- Type 1 - Connective tissue of skin, bone, teeth, tendons, ligaments etc.
- Type 2 - Cartilage
- Type 3 - Connective tissue of our organs
- Type 4, 5 - The separating layer between individual cells - for example epithelial and endothelial cells, between skeletal or smooth muscle cells, kidney glomeruli, lens capsule, and Schwann and glial cells of the nervous system. Take it from me, these are important.

As you can see, collagen is everywhere in the body, and vitamin C plays a role in the formation of collagen. So, how is vitamin C involved in collagen synthesis?

When collagen is produced, there is a complex series of events, some occurring inside the cell, and some outside the cell. Vitamin C is active inside the cell, where it hydroxylates (adds hydrogen and oxygen) two amino acids: proline and lysine. This helps form a precursor molecule called procollagen that is later packaged and modified into collagen outside the cell. Without vitamin C, collagen formation is disrupted, causing a wide variety of physical problems throughout the body.

Do you have greasy red scaly skin on your face and sides of your nose?

You may be deficient in VITAMIN B2

Vitamin B2, or 'Riboflavin' was first observed in 1879 as a green pigment found in milk. It is not stored in the human body for any period of time and it is therefore important to include a regular dietary source of this vitamin. It is pretty important for the following items too:

> It is essential for converting carbohydrate into energy
> It is essential for normal tissue respiration
> It is necessary for healthy mucous membranes

Signs of deficiency

Cracks in skin at corner of mouth, and soreness of lips, mouth and tongue
Scaling of skin around nose, mouth, scrotum, forehead, ears and scalp
Heightened sensitivity to light
Conjunctivitis and watering of eyes
Anaemia

Earlier names for this water soluble vitamin were lactoflavin, ovoflavin, hepatoflavin and verdoflavin, indicating the sources (milk, eggs, liver and plants) from which the vitamin was first isolated. Nowadays it is just plain B2.

The use of ethylene oxide in food sterilisation can destroy vitamin B2 so a lot of the 'fresh' supermarket foods will have been affected if ethylene oxide is used to prolong its life. Unfortunately there is no way of knowing whether it has been used or not.

Good sources of Vitamin B2

- Lean Meats
- Liver
- Kidneys
- Milk and Cheese
- Eggs
- Green Vegetables – especially Broccoli

Signs of deficiency also include loss of appetite, fatigue, depression, anaemia, dimness of vision, burning eyes. Some may experience decreased sensory sensitivity such as touch, temperature and vibration.

Do you have seborrhoeic dermatitis around your nose and an acne-like rash?

You may be deficient in VITAMIN B6

Vitamin B6 is not just essential for good skin condition, it is the master vitamin for processing amino acids—the building blocks of all proteins and some hormones. Vitamin B6 helps to make and modify many amino acids and is also needed to make serotonin, melatonin, and dopamine.

Vitamin B6 aids in the formation of several neurotransmitters and is therefore an essential nutrient in the regulation of mental processes and possibly mood as well.

In combination with folic acid and vitamin B12, vitamin B6 lowers homocysteine levels—an amino acid linked to heart disease and stroke, and possibly other diseases as well, such as osteoporosis, and Alzheimer's disease.

A rare, but severe, form of childhood epilepsy results from an inborn error in the metabolism of vitamin B6. Children with this form of epilepsy have an abnormal dependence on vitamin B6 and are usually mentally retarded. Seizure activity is reversible with intravenous injections of vitamin B6, which must be administered regularly by a nurse.

Vitamin B6 has a sinister side too, simply because it is the master vitamin for amino acids. This vitamin has a major role in regulating your mood disorders and is the most implicated of all the vitamins in the cause and treatment of depression. Not only that, Vitamin B6 levels are typically quite low in depressed patients and many people taking anti-depressants may well be depressed simply as a result of B6 deficiency, but end up dependent on antidepressants instead. The reason for this is that vitamin B6 is essential to the manufacture of serotonin, and low levels of serotonin are invariably linked to depression. Patients with low vitamin B6 levels usually respond well to supplements.

The Body Language of Health

Vitamin B6 deficiency also results in depressed immune function-both antibody-related and cell-mediated immunity are suppressed. This suppression is apparent as the number of white blood cells plummets, there is a tremendous reduction in quantity and quality of antibodies produced, leading to a range of ailments.

People with schizophrenia usually have peculiar nutritional profiles. Carl Pfeiffer, in the 1970's, reported B6 and zinc supplementation being 95% successful in the management of over 400 cases of pyrroluria-type schizophrenia in which kryptopyrroles have the ability to bind to vitamin B6 and then attach zinc to the complex causing an excess loss of these two vital nutrients into the urine.

Pyrroles are a worthless by-product of haemoglobin synthesis. Most people have very little if any of these pyrroles circulating in their bodies. We know this because of measured levels of pyrroles excreted via the urine. Some of us, however, are not so fortunate. Pyrroles are abnormally high in about:

- 30% of schizophrenics
- 40% of persons with psychiatric problems
- 11% of normals
- 25% of disturbed children
- 40% of alcoholics

Pyrroles do damage to us by binding to aldehydes throughout our bodies and causing their excretion along with the pyrroles. B6 (pyridoxine) is systematically removed and a severe B6 deficiency results. Equally damaging is the further scavenging done by the combination of B6 and pyrroles. Together this duo also seeks out and attaches itself to zinc and so both of these essential natural chemicals (B6 and zinc), are promptly dumped into the urine.

The loss of B6 and zinc is a psychiatric disaster. Many seemingly unrelated symptoms develop. Our interest in pyroluria is that it creates symptoms of inner tension, and bouts of nervous exhaustion and fearfulness that can be traced back to childhood or teen years. Without proper identification and treatment, pyrolurics slowly tend to become loners to avoid stressful situations. Their lives become an ongoing struggle to protect themselves from too much emotional and physical stress. It is unfortunate that these people often go undiagnosed. Pile on the zinc and B6 to effect a cure.

Zinc and vitamin B6 are critical nutrients for brain function, fertility, regulation of the menstrual cycle, maintenance of pregnancy and for the production of digestive enzymes. In addition, zinc is needed for producing stomach acid that helps to break down protein, and lots of other functions as well.

The Body Language of Health

Later on while tidying up the loose ends of this book, I found a fascinating questionnaire on the internet about diagnosing pyrroluria. Well, fascinating to me, because it mirrored much of what I have been saying in this book. Here it is in abbreviated form:

- When you were young did you sunburn easily? Do you have the lightest skin and hair in your family?
- Do you have poor dream recall or nightmares?
- Are you becoming more of a loner as you age? Do you avoid outside stress because it upsets your emotional balance?
- Have you been anxious, fearful, or felt a lot of inner tension since childhood but mostly hide these inner feelings from others?
- Do you get frequent colds or infections or unexplained chills or fevers?
- Are there white spots / flecks on your fingernails or do you have opaquely white or paper thin nails.
- Are you a nail biter?
- Do you have, or did you have before braces, crowded upper front teeth?
- Do you prefer not to eat breakfast, or even experience light nausea in the morning?
- Do you have a poor appetite, or poor sense of smell or taste?
- Do you feel uncomfortable with strangers?
- Do your knees crack or ache? (poor formation of knee cartilage)
- Does it bother you to be seated in a restaurant in the middle of the room?
- Do you have cold hands and / or feet?
- Do you tend to become dependent on one person whom you build your life around?

Now, you will probably recognise some of these questions!! I certainly do. A high positive score identifies the likelihood of pyrroluria. Perhaps you can see how valuable such questions become when interspersed with the thousand plus questions that make up Body Language. This book just covers a few of the myriad of the Body language signs I have accumulated from my research. There are a staggering one thousand four hundred signs and symptoms forming the Body Language. My next task is to compile a self-diagnostic website that everyone can use to identify their nutritional problems, and make it available on www.mybodylanguage.co.uk

So a rash round your nose could be important. You should learn to follow your nose.

Good sources of Vitamin B6 are animal products including offal , fish, eggs, vegetables especially cabbage, and fruit - especially melon, bananas and avocados.

Do you have Eczema?

You probably have an ALLERGY

An allergy is everything from a persistent runny nose, itchy eyes and palate, to severe skin rash. It aggravates the sense of smell, sight, tastes and touch causing irritation, extreme disability and occasionally fatality. It occurs when the body's immune system overreacts to normally harmless substances.

Allergy is widespread and affects approximately one in four of the population in the UK at some time in their lives. Each year the numbers are increasing by 5% with as many as half of all those affected being children. It is the modern epidemic of the West.

What causes Eczema? Substances in the environment known as allergens cause allergic reactions. Almost anything can be an allergen for someone. The most common allergens are:

- Pollen from trees and grasses,
- House dust mite faeces
- moulds,
- pets such as cats and dogs, or their dander (dust)
- insect stings such as wasps and bees,
- industrial and household chemicals,
- medicines,
- Foods such as milk, eggs, lupin flour, potatoes, peanuts.
- less common allergens include nuts, fruit and latex.

Virtually all irritants causing allergies happen to be proteins. There are a few non-protein allergens which include drugs such as penicillin, but for these to cause an allergic response it is thought that they need to be bound to a protein once they are in the body.

Eczema is often worse at night, because the skin gets moist in bed, and the surface allergens turn into a concentrated liquid that aggravates even more. The skin is literally bathed in concentrated allergen.

An allergic person's immune system has been foiled into believing that allergens are damaging and so it produces a special type of antibody, Immunoglobulin E (IgE) to attack the invading material. This causes other blood cells to release further chemicals (including histamine) which together cause the symptoms of an allergic reaction.

The most common symptoms are:

- sneezing
- runny nose
- itchy eyes and ears
- severe wheezing
- coughing shortness of breath
- sinus problems
- headaches (migraine)
- sore palate
- eczema
- nettle-like rash

It should be understood that all the symptoms mentioned can be caused by factors other than allergy. Indeed some of the conditions are diseases in their own right. Asthma, eczema, headaches, lethargy, loss of concentration and sensitivity to everyday foods represent a huge problem in society today

Where do you start - especially with Asthma and Eczema?

- Remove pets - cats are particularly troublesome because they wash their fur and emit 'dander' that even sticks to the wallpaper, and comes off as an invisible cloud as you walk past.
- Remove carpets because they are dust contaminated
- Try exclusion diets to determine the problem food and keep a diet diary.

Try an exclusion diet

An exclusion diet doesn't mean that you give up food. Just most of it! This may sound drastic but it is much better to identify the allergen than put up with it for life or mask the condition with creams and steroids.

To start an exclusion diet, first of all cut out all foods/drinks except rice, fruit, (but cut out citrus and apples), vegetables (cut out potato) and water. It's not that hard, just remind yourself you are doing an experiment that will give you better health than you can possibly imagine, but for the rest of your life.

Take this bland diet for two weeks and be sure to stick to it. No snacks, no chocolate, no fizzy drinks – nothing except the simple diet. You won't starve and two weeks will soon pass. Remind yourself that half of the world's population survives on only one plate of rice or sorghum a day (if they're lucky!).

After two weeks start to introduce one thing at a time. Try a small dose, wait two hours and then if there is no reaction, complete the portion. Wait at least a couple of days between each new food before you introduce another. That way, if you get a reaction, you know which food caused the reaction. Keep a diary so you can work back over those foods that are OK and those which spark off problems. If you want to be thorough, you could classify foods as causing mild, average or severe reactions.

NO dairy, grains or flour, nuts or potato. Leave those until the very last because they are the most likely culprits of all.

Make sure you stick to single foods, because mass-produced food often contains dozens of strange substances.

Obviously if you get a reaction, you're allergic to that food.

If you're reading this and think that's a lot of trouble, or are in the middle of an exclusion diet and are thinking of giving up, just look at the pictures on Dr Morrow-Brown's website at www.allergiesexplained.com to remind you of the problems that allergies give. Persevere and you may be able to look forward to the rest of your life free from the debilitating troubles of allergies. And remember, most health care experts treat skin disorders in a different category altogether, so don't be put off by negative opinions from the experts. It's just that their training dealt with allergies from a different angle altogether – they are trained to treat the condition, not to look to prevention.

Disease prevention will be something that will revolutionise health in the future, but we are not in that position yet. Perhaps in future we will look back at healthcare in the twentieth century with the same disdain we apply today to the strange blood-letting and weird antics of the nineteenth century.

The Body Language of Health

Strange but true - Dogs may prefer fleas

It is said that there are many perfectly happy and healthy dogs with fleas galore, but many other dogs that are religiously kept flea-free suffer from massive itchy skin problems.

Recent research supports this observation. Studies have shown that the presence of a small number of fleas may, in the long run, actually help a dog. Apparently, a dog with fleas develops an immune response that a dog kept flea-free never has a chance to muster.

Allergies are a disease of the latter part of the twentieth century. Perhaps our ancestors evolved in harmony with the human flea, (we know humans were troubled by fleas because that is how epidemics such as the bubonic plague were carried!!) and developed an immune system to match, which is now out of step with the modern, sterile world. No-one has yet been so bold as to suggest hospitals should issue a flea prescription. Would anyone suffering from eczema possibly jump at the chance?

People with peanut allergy may risk severe allergy to lupin flour

Researchers have found that people with peanut allergy - about 1% of the UK population - should avoid any products containing lupin flour because it can trigger serious allergy effects.

Lupin flour is used in some European countries as a replacement for soya in speciality breads and catering foods, some of which are now reaching the UK. One in 50 children in the UK is allergic to nuts, so they could have allergic reactions to lupin flour used in their baby food manufacture.

The following study by the Royal Free Hospital, London, has been published in The Lancet. The study highlighted the case of a 25-year-old woman who, in August 2004, had an allergic reaction after eating a restaurant meal of chicken, French-fried potato, and onion rings. During the meal, her mouth itched and her lips and tongue started to swell. Fifteen minutes later she was having difficulty breathing, her throat had narrowed, and she felt very weak.

An ambulance was called, anaphylaxis - a life-threatening allergic reaction - was diagnosed, and she required emergency hospital treatment. Once the effect wore off she made a full recovery.

The woman knew she had a severe allergy to peanuts after a reaction to a peanut sweet when she was 15. However, peanut contamination of her food was considered unlikely. Lupin flour, an ingredient of the onion ring batter, was eventually identified as the cause of her attack.

The prevalence of lupin allergy has increased markedly in some countries, especially France, which permitted the addition of lupin flour to wheat flour in 1997. Although the food use of lupin has been permitted in the UK since 1996, few lupin-containing foods are so far on sale.

A new directive on food labelling came into force in Europe in November 2004, requiring food manufacturers to specifically list 12 potential allergic ingredients. However, lupin flour was not included on this list, despite recommendation from the UK-based Institute of Food Science and Technology.

David Reading, of the Anaphylaxis Campaign, told the BBC News website it was important the potential problem was flagged up now, before lupin flour-based products became more widespread in the UK.

"We are aware of a handful of cases where people have almost certainly reacted to lupin flour, but thankfully it is small problem at the moment because only a small number of products contain the flour," he said.

This story puts added meaning to the Monty Python sketch which featured a parody on Dick Turpin who announced 'Your Lupins or Your Life!!'

Do you have dark rings under your eyes?

You may have an ALLERGY

Most people who have dark rings round their eyes will tell you that they haven't felt 'really fit and bursting with vitality for as long as they can remember'

Are you one of them? Why is that, you may ask? Well, Assuming you haven't been given two black eyes through fighting or walking into a lamp post, dark rings round the eyes are usually associated with allergies.

Of course, some people with olive skin often have a tendency to darker pigmentation round the eyes, but that's not what we are talking about in this topic. You will only get these if the rest of your family have them. But rings round eyes that should be bright and sparkling are different.

The previous Body Language symptom describes allergies, but it is not often realised that dark rings under the eyes can be the first indicator of allergies, even before you start to sneeze or develop a rash.

Dark rings are usually caused by vascular dilation, a fancy name for enlargement of blood vessels under the loose skin that is round your eyes. Allergies produce IgE that causes inflammation and the area round the eyes is usually where you will see the effect first. And environmental pollutants have the same effect to a lesser extent. That's why dark rings often identify a smoker – actually not quite true – they identify a smoker whose body is saying 'enough is enough – please oh please change your habits for my sake!!"

In fact, for a smoker, it doesn't even need to be dark rings, either. The same problem can cause puffiness round the eyes with or without the dark rings.

Many allergies are debilitating because your immune system is working on double-time, just as it does when you have a bad cold. These allergies make you tired, so dark rings are also associated with tiredness, not necessarily because lack of sleep causes them, but because they are symptomatic of poor quality sleep!

There are many cosmetics claiming to treat dark rings but they will only mask the problem. If you really want to do something about it, sort out your allergy. There is advice on how to achieve this elsewhere in the book.

Does sex with a Milkman cause painful joints?

You may have a semen allergy.

Dr Morrow-Brown's website on allergies contains some fascinating stories, and I have extracted the cream off the site to bring you this bizarre–but-true story about milk that I suspect may be more common than you would think.

The Body Language of Health

Yes, you can have an allergy to just about everything, and you could certainly be allergic to semen. But the title is misleading, we don't mean sex with a milkman, although that is supposedly more common than you would think if you've watched many Ealing comedies. No, what I mean is that if you have a milkman, then you almost certainly have milk deliveries, your husband will drink milk, and your husband's semen will therefore contain milk-derived proteins. And as you now know, most allergens are proteins. So if you are allergic to milk, sex in a household visited by a milkman could have painful consequences.

The story behind this Body Language sign goes as follows.

Dr Morrow brown had a patient who had worsening arthritis in many of her joints. He realised through an exclusion diet that she had a milk allergy, so she adjusted her diet to exclude milk. Her arthritis subsided, as it so often does when milk is excluded totally from a sufferer's diet.

She was delighted, and felt a new woman. Except that she noticed her previously arthritic joints ached the morning after intercourse the previous night. She was advised to use a condom and this effect ceased. So was she allergic to semen?

Dr Morrow Brown has a special skin prick needle he has developed. It pierces the outer layers of skin, without drawing blood, and he pricks the skin through a droplet of the allergen. When he suspects dust or a particular irritant is the problem he makes up a solution and pricks through that. If the substance is an allergen the skin forms an allergic 'hive' which looks like a little beehive on your skin. He can even do a control 'prick' using histamine, that I can assure you itches like hell.

A skin test on this woman's arm performed by pricking the skin through a droplet of her husband's semen caused a delayed action itching of the skin, and so Dr Morrow Brown concluded that her husband's semen probably contained milk-derived proteins, that produced an adverse arthritic reaction in the woman after intercourse.

The husband was advised to give up milk too, and he discovered to his astonishment that his chronic eczema in his ears that had been a nuisance for thirty years cleared up completely!!

The couple then discovered that intercourse without a condom no longer caused any aches and pains in the woman's joints. It was also apparent that whenever the husband had food with even a trace of milk in it, the woman developed her painful joints after intercourse. It was a clear case of allergy to semen because of milk proteins.

Now an interesting point of this story is that for this evidence to be acceptable to the medical profession it would have been necessary to carry out a double-blind trial.

A blind trial is where someone is given either a drug or a placebo (dummy) and they don't know which one they have been given. A double-blind trial is where not only does the patient not know which he has been given, but the doctor also does not know which he has prescribed either. So with a double-blind trial there is no risk of suspicions as to what they were given interfering with the result.

For the medical profession to accept that semen allergy exists, this woman would have to undergo sexual intercourse a statistically meaningful number of times (probably at least fifty occasions) with random males some of whom would be taking milk, and some of whom would not. So that there could be no risk of bias, all participants would have to be unknown to the woman to avoid any possibility of her inadvertently reacting to someone she knew. In this case it would mean that not only the woman but all her sexual partners would have to be blindfolded. That is a new definition of a 'double blind trial' though it does not usually mean that literally, it simply means the participants have no knowledge of what product they are given. I think she would be in no doubt what she had been given after that lot.

Not surprisingly, the couple did not feel they could participate in such an experiment, and instead they sacked the milkman and lived happily ever after. But clinical trials or not, I think you will agree the facts speak for themselves. Where common sense and reasoning comes in, who needs double blind trials?

This must be one of the most unusual allergy stories ever put into print.

Sexually Transmitted Coca Cola

Not quite. Here is one that is certainly as bizarre, and shows just how much of a Private Dick you have to be to work out just what is driving your allergy. Of course the only real solution is to find the cause and prevent the problem. It pays to persevere with your detective work, and it is very satisfying when you get to the bottom of the problem.

This particular patient of Dr Morrow-Brown's was keen on horse riding. She began to experience extreme pain in the genital area after riding, especially when wearing thin riding pants in the summer. This directed Dr Morrow-Brown to inspect the saddle, which had been treated with a special polish containing 'Balsam of Peru' which happens to be a well known skin sensitiser. Sure enough, when he did skin prick tests with

The Body Language of Health

Balsam of Peru the woman had a very intense skin reaction. The problem was apparently solved by avoiding this particular type of saddle polish.

Some months later she returned with a different, but related problem. This time, more serious reactions were occurring with her genitalia after intercourse. This clearly indicated she was reacting to seminal fluid, though in this story her partner was not a milkman. It seemed curious that she did not react in this way every time, and her prick tests using semen from her partner were sometimes positive, sometimes negative.

Now Dr Morrow-Brown is also a detective to equal Sherlock Holmes, and after carefully recording her history he found her partner had an intense love of Coca-Cola. He also found that her allergic reaction occurred whenever he had drunk more than usual before intercourse. Elementary, my dear Dr MB.

Enquiry revealed that Balsam of Peru is a very complex product, and that it is sometimes present in chocolates, chewing gum, various toilet articles and – yes, you've guessed it – Coca Cola. Tiny traces of Balsam of Peru in his semen from drinking a lot of Coca-Cola was giving her a reaction.

Dr Morrow-Brown does not tell us if this inflamed partnership resolved itself, but it does show you what a complicated subject allergies are and how you have to be a true detective to sort it out. But you really have to persevere because to produce a cure you have to find the cause. To treat the area with steroid is really not the answer, and it is a treatment for life that does not treat all of the allergy that is affecting your basic health. Remember, most people who have dark rings round their eyes (i.e. an allergy) will tell you that they haven't felt 'really fit and bursting with vitality for as long as they can remember'. Masking the itch with a medical product won't take that away, you need to find the problem and remove it from your life.

Hopefully with these two sexual tales I have aroused your desire to investigate and tackle your allergy once and for all. And hopefully I haven't inadvertently alerted the whole world to that 'vital ingredient' in coca cola which has been held a secret at all costs on pain of death for over a century.

Bear in mind also that it must even be possible to develop an allergy to coca cola, or at least one of its (now not so) secret ingredients.

Do you have Pale Skin?

If you do, you may be deficient in IRON, FOLIC ACID, OR VITAMIN B12

Pale skin is a common symptom of anaemia. Even blondes who have pale skin should still have a reddish glow, due to a plentiful supply of oxygenated blood (see 'Do blonde's have more fun?' Page 323).

Anaemia is a condition in which the blood cannot carry enough oxygen, either because there is a low number of red blood cells or because each red blood cell is less able to carry oxygen than normal. Symptoms of anaemia include feeling tired or faint and getting breathless easily. And pale skin, of course.

Everyone automatically thinks of iron and anaemia, but iron deficiency is not always the only problem. There are many different types of anaemia with different causes. Vitamin B12 deficiency is just one of the common ones. This is because Vitamin B12 is needed to make red blood cells, and it is also essential for the nerves and brain. Other nutrients that are needed to make red blood cells include folic acid (Vitamin B9).

Common causes of iron-deficiency anaemia

- A common cause of iron-deficiency anaemia in women is heavy periods (menorrhagia). About 1 in 10 women become anaemic at some time in their life due to heavy periods.
- Stomach ulcers, piles, ulcerative colitis (inflammation of the colon) and bowel cancer may cause bleeding in the gut and result in anaemia. Often the bleeding is not obvious because the blood is passed unnoticed in the stools. (see Do you crunch ice cubes?).
- Kidney or bladder disease can cause bleeding that can result in anaemia. The blood may be passed unnoticed in the urine.
- Some bowel conditions, such as coeliac disease (gluten sensitivity) or chronic diarrhoea, cause poor absorption of foods containing iron.
- Low dietary iron can lead to anaemia. There are many sources of iron, including meat, green vegetables, milk, wholemeal flour and eggs, but anaemia can occur in the UK due to a poor diet, especially in children and 'faddy eaters'.
- Pregnancy can lead to iron-deficiency anaemia, because the growing baby needs iron and takes its supply from the mother. Naturally, iron deficiency

is more likely to develop during pregnancy in women whose diet does not contain plenty of iron.

- Certain medical conditions, such as rheumatoid arthritis or even cancer, can lead to iron-deficiency anaemia. In this case adequate iron is present in the diet, but the developing red blood cells in the bone marrow cannot use the iron properly.
- Long-term aspirin-taking is associated with iron-deficiency anaemia because it can cause bleeding in the stomach.
- Hookworm infection can cause iron-deficiency anaemia, and this is one of the most common causes of anaemia worldwide. People who live in or travel to tropical countries are at risk of hookworm infection. Hookworms feed off blood inside the intestines, leaving the host (i.e. you) short of iron.

Causes of vitamin B12 deficiency leading to pernicious anaemia

In most cases, vitamin B12 deficiency happens because the stomach cannot produce enough of a substance called intrinsic factor (IF), which is needed for vitamin B12 to be absorbed. This is called pernicious anaemia.

Pernicious anaemia is an autoimmune condition. Normally cells called antibodies, produced by the body's immune system, attack foreign substances such as viruses and bacteria. With autoimmune conditions, the immune system mistakes the person's own tissue as foreign and attacks it. Mostly, this is due to smoking.

With pernicious anaemia, antibodies damage the cells in the stomach that produce intrinsic factor. Pernicious anaemia usually develops in people over the age of 50, and tends to run in families. If left untreated, pernicious anaemia can become life-threatening.

Other causes of B12 deficiency

- Poor absorption of vitamin B12 can be caused by parasites or certain bacteria that interfere with absorption in the small intestine. Crohn's disease (a condition of the small bowel caused by TNF alpha usually started by smoking) can also interfere with vitamin B12 absorption.
- Vitamin B12 deficiency can be associated with a poorly functioning pancreas; liver damage, caused by excess alcohol intake; gastrectomy (surgical removal of part or all of the stomach); and taking some medications for stomach ulcers on a long-term basis.

- Dietary-related vitamin B12 deficiency is rare, but strict vegans may be at risk because their diet excludes the foods that provide this vitamin. Vitamin B12 is the only vitamin that is not found in vegetables.

Symptoms

People with vitamin B12-deficiency anaemia have symptoms caused by a low level of oxygen in the body. These include:

- Breathlessness
- Tiredness
- Dizziness
- Rapid, weak pulse rate
- Palpitations – irregular or strong heartbeats
- Headaches
- Pale skin and numbness in certain parts of the body

As well as the symptoms of anaemia, vitamin B12 deficiency may cause neurological symptoms such as inflammation of the nerves (neuritis) which can affect movement and sensation, tinnitus (ringing in the ears), colour blindness, light-headedness, confusion, depression, poor concentration and forgetfulness. There may also be loss of appetite, diarrhoea and weight loss, or numbness in parts of the body. Sometimes B12 deficiency can cause numbness right down one side of the body.

Diagnosis

Anyone with symptoms that suggest anaemia, such as pale skin, weakness and fatigue, should visit their GP. They will ask about your symptoms, medical history and current eating habits, and perform a physical examination.

A simple blood test can count the number of red blood cells and measure the amount of haemoglobin. The level of vitamin B12 can be measured with a blood test, if necessary. The antibodies which cause pernicious anaemia can also be tested for and a blood test can also identify coeliac disease or rare blood conditions such as thalassaemia.

The size of the red blood cells will also be examined. Enlarged red cells, called megaloblasts, are caused by vitamin B12 deficiency and folate deficiency. If they are present the condition is called megaloblastic anaemia. Finding megaloblasts in the blood can help to diagnose anaemia but does not determine the cause.

Your doctor may recommend further tests to identify the cause of B12 deficiency. One test looks at how well vitamin B12 is absorbed by the body. This involves fasting overnight and then having a vitamin B12 injection and taking radioactive-labelled vitamin B12 tablets. The amount of vitamin B12 that comes out in the urine is measured. This is called the Schilling test but it costs rather more than that to conduct.

Treating vitamin B12 deficiency

Treatment for vitamin B12 deficiency anaemia, especially in the case of vegetarians usually involves injections of vitamin B12. The frequency of injection depends on the exact type and severity of the anaemia, but is usually every one to three months, after an initial two weeks of more frequent injections.

In severe cases of B12-deficiency anaemia, a blood transfusion may be required. If the deficiency is caused by low dietary intake, vitamin B12 tablets may solve the problem.

Prevention

The best way to prevent B12-deficiency anaemia is to eat a diet containing plenty of vitamin B12. It is found in meat and animal products, particularly liver, salmon, cod, cheese and eggs, yeast extract, seaweed and spirulina algae.

Strict vegetarians should consider taking a regular vitamin B12 supplement to prevent this type of anaemia. Anyone who is worried about vitamin B12 intake should speak to their doctor or a dietician.

Good sources of iron include meat, liver, wholegrain cereals, raw green vegetables, and fortified foods such as some breakfast cereals.

Despite iron from plant foods being less readily absorbed research has shown that vegetarians are no more likely to suffer from iron deficiency than non-vegetarians. It's a good idea to eat foods containing vitamin C at the same time as eating non-meat sources of iron because this helps with iron absorption.

Good sources of vitamin C include peppers, Brussels sprouts, Sweet potatoes, oranges, and kiwi fruit.

Do you suffer from scaly red skin round the eyes, nose, mouth and genitals?

If you do, you may be deficient in BIOTIN (Vitamin B7)

Biotin is a water-soluble vitamin, generally classified as a B-complex vitamin, B7. After the initial discovery of biotin, nearly forty years of research were required to establish it as a true vitamin. Biotin is required by all organisms but can only be synthesized by bacteria, yeasts, moulds, algae, and some plant species.

Although serious biotin deficiency is very rare, the human requirement for dietary biotin has been demonstrated in two different situations: prolonged intravenous feeding without biotin supplementation, and consumption of raw egg white for a prolonged period (many weeks to years).

This is because Avidin, a protein found in egg white, binds to biotin and prevents us from absorbing it in our digestive system. Cooking egg white denatures avidin, so we are safe with cooked egg but not raw egg. Curiously, egg yolk contains biotin but egg white destroys biotin.

Symptoms of biotin deficiency include hair loss and a scaly red rash around the eyes, nose, mouth, and genital area. Neurological symptoms in adults have included depression, lethargy, hallucination, and numbness and tingling of the extremities. The characteristic facial rash, together with an unusual facial fat distribution, have been termed the "biotin deficient face" by some experts. Individuals with hereditary disorders of biotin metabolism resulting in functional biotin deficiency have evidence of impaired immune system function, including increased susceptibility to bacterial and fungal infections.

Function of Biotin

In its physiologically active form biotin is attached at the active site of four important enzymes, known as carboxylases. Each carboxylase is a catalyst for an essential metabolic reaction.

Acetyl-CoA carboxylase catalyses the binding of bicarbonate to acetyl-CoA to form malonyl-CoA. That is required for the synthesis of fatty acids.

Pyruvate carboxylase is a critical enzyme in gluconeogenesis, the formation of glucose from sources other than carbohydrates, for example, amino acids and fats.

Methylcrotonyl-CoA carboxylase catalyses an essential step in the metabolism of leucine, an indispensable (essential) amino acid.

Propionyl-CoA carboxylase catalyses essential steps in the metabolism of amino acids, cholesterol, and odd chain fatty acids (that is, fatty acids with an odd number of carbon molecules).

Good sources of biotin are egg yolk, yeast and liver.

We normally also have our own 'manufacturing plant'. The bacteria that normally colonize the colon (large intestine) are capable of making their own biotin. In order to obtain these bacteria it seems we need to eat a healthy dose of soil now and again. This trait will have been inherited from our recent ancestors who were around before the invention of the kitchen sink.

Diabetes mellitus

It has been known for many years that biotin deficiency results in impaired utilization of sugar. In a trial, blood biotin levels were significantly lower in 43 patients with type 2 diabetes than in non-diabetic control subjects, and lower fasting blood glucose levels were associated with higher blood biotin levels. After one month of biotin supplementation of 9 mg/day fasting blood glucose levels decreased by an average of 45%. Reductions in blood glucose levels were also found in 7 insulin-dependent diabetics after 1 week of supplementation with 16 mg of biotin daily.

Several mechanisms could explain the glucose-lowering effect of biotin. As a cofactor of enzymes required for fatty acid synthesis, biotin may increase the utilization of glucose to synthesize fats. Biotin has been found to stimulate glucokinase, an enzyme in the liver, resulting in increased synthesis of glycogen, the stored form of glucose. Biotin has also been found to stimulate the secretion of insulin in the pancreas, which also has the effect of lowering blood glucose. An effect on cellular glucose transporters is also currently under investigation.

Biotin and brittle fingernails

The finding that biotin supplements were effective in treating hoof abnormalities in horses and pigs led to speculation that biotin supplements might also be helpful in strengthening brittle fingernails in humans. Three uncontrolled trials examining the effects of biotin supplementation (2.5 mg/day for up to six months) in women with brittle fingernails have been published. In two of the trials, subjective evidence of clinical improvement was reported in 67-91% of the participants available for follow-up at the end of the treatment period. As trial results go, this is pretty impressive. It would have been nice to have seen a correlation between biotin levels and gut bacteria, but this was not studied.

Biotin and hair loss

Although hair loss is a symptom of severe biotin deficiency, there are no published scientific studies that support the claim that high-dose biotin supplements are effective in *preventing or treating* hair loss in men or women.

Does your skin have a yellow tone to it?

You could have an underactive thyroid.

A slightly yellow tone to the skin all over your body will often point to an underlying problem. This is different to yellow palms, a topic that we have already covered, which relates to too much carotene in the diet. With yellow skin we often assume that there is a problem with jaundice, that can indicate liver disease, but there is another more common and less threatening condition that produces a yellow tinge to the skin, and that is an underactive thyroid.

The Body Language of Health

Hypothyroidism is not diagnosed by the usual suite of blood tests so you will have to discuss the matter with your doctor if you suspect this is the problem. Other symptoms of an underactive thyroid include feeling cold, (especially cold hands and feet) tiredness, dry skin, poor hair quality and brittle nails.

Iodine deficiency has lots of other Body language symptoms too. The three that immediately spring to mind are memory loss ......er

Oh, and cold hands and feet. And weight gain. And a sluggish mental capacity that makes you unable to add up correctly.

Seriously, the number of symptoms of hypothyroidism are huge, not to mention the Spanish Inquisition. It is an extremely common condition and is responsible for an enormous amount of morbidity. Apart from causing obvious symptoms like fatigue, overweight (though 40% of hypothyroid subjects are underweight), and sensitivity to the cold, it ensures that almost every system in the body is at a low ebb. The list of possible symptoms include (but are not limited to):-

- Weight gain
- Heat and / or cold intolerance
- Headaches and migraines
- Low motivation and ambition
- Irritability, anxiety and panic attacks
- Depression
- Fluid retention
- Decreased memory and concentration
- Unhealthy nails, brittle nails,
- Low sex drive
- Insomnia
- Hives
- Asthma and allergies
- Slow wound healing and acne
- Carpal tunnel syndrome
- Low blood sugar
- Attention deficit disorder (ADD)
- Pancreatitis (from hypothermia)
- Adrenal exhaustion from excess secretion of adrenaline
- Gallbladder disease (six times higher in women with excess estrogen or on birth control pills or ERT)

- Female problems (fibroids, ovarian cysts, endometriosis, PMS, cramps, dysmenorrhea, amenorrhea, spontaneous abortion, cyclic seizures, dry vagina and infertility)
- Osteoporosis (from excess eostrogen leading to excess adrenaline and then to excess cortisol).
- Poor appetite
- Intestinal symptoms which can include irritable bowel syndrome, dysphagia (swallowing problems); poor digestion (low acid and pancreatic enzymes, decreased gall bladder motility); nutrient malabsorption; gas and wind; colic; decreased peristalsis; and especially chronic constipation.

There is a very good test for iodine deficiency and you will be amazed at how well it works. The skin is actually rather porous, as I have recently found out while doing transdermal patch development. And here is a graphical experiment to prove the point.

The 'iodine tincture 2.4% test' involves painting a patch of standard iodine solution on the soft tissue of your belly and observing any colour change over 24 hours. If the yellow patch fades you need more iodine and you have a sluggish thyroid. If the patch stays the same your iodine level is OK. It is that simple, this is that old diffusion/osmosis thing working again to balance out the levels in your body and the surrounding environment. Be careful not to get the iodine on your clothes, it stains and they don't work the same as your body does in balancing out the iodine and putting it where it is needed.

Dr Broda Barnes demonstrated in the early 70's that supporting the thyroid improved diabetes symptoms (but not the blood sugar imbalance), namely improved wound healing, weight loss, energy levels improve, and most importantly of all reduced atherosclerosis. To you and I that is called 'hardening of the arteries' but its medical name is much more graphic; it comes from *atheroma* which is Greek for "lump of porridge"

You can also try the **Barnes Temperature Test** to make a provisional home diagnoses of hypothyroidism. According to one source, this test will sometimes pick up a sluggish thyroid that was not even spotted by a blood test.

Underarm temperature should be recorded for ten minutes *before arising in the morning*. This means as soon as you wake up. Not after making a cup of tea, or having a shower! This procedure should be followed for at least three mornings in a row (seven would be better) and the average temperature calculated. The correct temperature should be within the range 97.8 - 98.2 degrees Fahrenheit (36.6 - 36.8 degrees

Celsius). An average temperature of below 97.8 degrees Fahrenheit (36.6 degrees Celsius) is suggestive of hypothyroidism. A mean temperature of below 96.4F (35.8C) usually indicates severe hypothyroidism.

Note for women: Premenopausal women should not perform this test during their periods when their temperature is higher than normal.

Although it is not absolutely foolproof, failing the temperature test and having about 5 or more of the typical low thyroid symptoms listed above may indicate hypothyroidism.

The underarm temperature test can be used to monitor progress in treatment, too, and the goal of treatment is to normalize this temperature. Bear in mind that this condition does not come on overnight and is not resolved overnight. Be willing to increase your iodine level over 12 weeks or more. Please note if you are taking conventional low thyroid medication (thyroxine) you definitely should not stop your medication, (at least not without thorough discussion and the agreement of your doctor).

Do you have coloured sweat?

You may have a bacterial infection of the skin.

Remember how chromium was associated with lots of coloured things except technicolour pee? Well, here's that 'chromo' name again.

Chromohidrosis is a condition characterized by pigment on the skin that appears to be coloured but is actually local sites of active pigment-forming bacteria. *Chromohidrosis* or *Pseudochromhidrosis* may manifest itself as different coloured patches around the areas of sweat glands.

The average person has a staggering 2.6 million sweat glands in their skin. Assuming you are average that means you. No wonder we are obsessed with personal odours. Sweat glands are distributed over the entire body -- except for the lips, nipples and external surfaces of genital organs.

The Body Language of Health

The sweat gland is in the layer of skin called the dermis along with other pong equipment, such as nerve endings, hair follicles and so on. Basically, the sweat gland is a long, coiled, hollow tube of cells. The coiled part in the dermis is where sweat is produced, and the long portion is a duct that connects the gland to the opening or pore on the skin's outer surface. Nerve cells from the sympathetic nervous system connect to the sweat glands. There are two types of sweat glands:

- Eccrine - the most numerous type that are found all over the body, particularly on the palms of the hands, soles of the feet and forehead.
- Apocrine - mostly confined to the armpits (axilla) and the anal-genital area. They typically end in hair follicles rather than pores.

The two glands differ in size, the age that they become active and the composition of the sweat that they make. Compared to apocrine glands, eccrine glands are smaller, are active from birth (Apocrine glands become active only at puberty), and produce a sweat that is free of proteins and fatty acids.

The apocrine glands are at locations where we have hair growth - particularly the genitals and armpits. Why is the hair there? Why to spread the sweaty, musky odours to attract a mate of the opposite sex. This odour is vitally important, because our noses unknowingly are programmed to prefer the odour of a partner who has a different immune system to ours. Pairing with someone who has a different immune system helps to maximise the immunity of our children. If we pair with someone who has the same immune system, there is a good chance that our children will have a compromised immunity. It has even been suggested that the increase in allergic diseases in modern society has something to do with the introduction of deodorants, which prevents us from choosing a genetically suitable partner by his or her smell.

Women will tell you they dislike the smell of a male at any time, but research has shown that women dislike male odours except during the time when they are fertile, when they are attracted only to males that have the correct complimentary immune system. These odours are programmed by the particular species of bacteria that thrive on the male's body. And of course these species are allowed to culture on the body by virtue of the intricacies of the body's immune system, so it all makes sense.

Chromhidrosis is apocrine in origin. Although apocrine glands are found in the genital, axillary, areolar, and facial skin, chromhidrosis has only been reported on the face, axillae, and breast areola.

The Body Language of Health

Eccrine chromhidrosis is rare and only occurs with ingestion of certain dyes or drugs, and pseudochromhidrosis occurs when clear eccrine sweat becomes coloured on the surface of the skin as a result of extrinsic dyes, paints, or chromomeric bacteria.

Lipofuscin pigment is responsible for the coloured sweat. This pigment is produced in the apocrine gland, and its various oxidative states account for the characteristic yellow, green, blue, or black secretions observed in apocrine chromhidrosis. It is nothing to worry about and does not signify an underlying medical problem.

The ear connection

Did you know that the lining of your outer ear has modified apocrine glands called ceruminous glands? These modified sweat glands produce ear wax.

Ear wax is thought to prevent foreign material and insects from entering your ears, and a steady production of ear wax allows the ear to slowly get rid of debris from within its confines.

The canine connection

Chromohydrosis sometimes develops in dogs too, but not in sweaty places because dogs don't have sweat glands in places we do. Dogs sweat through their pads and feet, but their main cooling method is by panting.

However, some dogs tend to develop stains round their eyes, and these stains are often brown or red, so they are most often noticed on white dogs such as terriers. The minerals and proteins in the tears allow bacteria to develop, forming a chromohydrosis stain. I noticed the other day someone has even developed a product to add to the dog's food that stops this problem. My guess is that it may contain tryclosan, the antibacterial product that is in toothpaste. So maybe you should buy your dog a toothbrush instead.

LEGS AND FEET

Do you suffer from burning feet or heels?

You may have a deficiency in VITAMIN B5

Vitamin B5, or should we say Funky B5, is the chemical called Pantothenic Acid. Unlike the early vitamins that Kazimierez Funk detected, this is an acid, not an amine.

Known as "the anti-stress vitamin", pantothenic acid plays a role in the production of the adrenal hormones and the formation of antibodies, aids in vitamin utilization, and helps to convert fats, carbohydrates, and proteins into energy. It is required by all cells in the body and is concentrated in the organs. It is also involved in the production of neurotransmitters.

This vitamin is an essential element of coenzyme A, a vital body chemical involved in many necessary metabolic functions. Pantothenic acid is also a stamina enhancer and prevents certain forms of anaemia. It is needed for normal functioning of the gastrointestinal tract and may be helpful in treating depression and anxiety. A deficiency of pantothenic acid may cause fatigue, headache, nausea, and tingling in the hands. Pantothenic acid is also needed for proper functioning of the adrenal glands. Wow that is quite a multitude of important roles.

Sources of Vitamin B5

Pantothenic acid is widely distributed in plants and animal tissues and is found in the following foods: meat (for example, beef, pork, liver, kidney), yeast, eggs, fresh vegetables (for example legumes broccoli, cauliflower, sweet potatoes, tomatoes), mushrooms, nuts, royal jelly, saltwater fish, whole rye flour, and whole wheat.

Vitamin B5 Deficiency

Vitamin B5 provides adrenal support in high stress situations and deficiency causes atrophy of the adrenal glands, which leads to fatigue, headache, sleep problems, nausea, and abdominal discomfort. People suffering from chronic stress or those using corticosteroids continuously may benefit from vitamin B5 supplements of 100-500 milligrams a day. Patients who had these symptoms had to wait seven to 14 days before seeing any effect of the supplementation, so don't expect immediate results.

Neuromuscular degeneration may also occur in the absence of vitamin B5. Patients fed a diet low in pantothenic acid for just ten weeks reported tiredness, headache, sleep problems, nausea, abdominal cramps, some vomiting, and impaired coordination.

Do you often have cold hands and feet?

You may have a deficiency in MAGNESIUM and IODINE

Magnesium is the fourth most abundant mineral in the body and is absolutely essential to good health. Approximately 50% of total body magnesium is found in bone. The other half is found predominantly inside cells of body tissues and organs. Only 1% of magnesium is found in blood, but the body works very hard to keep blood levels of magnesium constant. If it is in short supply, the body will rob your bones of magnesium, because it is so important that the blood magnesium level is maintained.

Magnesium is needed for more than 300 biochemical reactions in the body. It helps maintain normal muscle and nerve function, keeps heart rhythm steady, supports a healthy immune system, and keeps bones strong. Magnesium also helps regulate blood sugar levels, promotes normal blood pressure, and is known to be involved in energy metabolism and protein synthesis. There is an increased interest in the role of magnesium in preventing and managing disorders such as hypertension, cardiovascular disease, and diabetes. Dietary magnesium is absorbed in the small intestines. Magnesium is excreted through the kidneys and must be topped up continuously in our diet.

What foods provide magnesium?

Green vegetables such as spinach are good sources of magnesium because the centre of the chlorophyll molecule (which gives green vegetables their colour) contains magnesium. Some legumes (beans and peas), nuts and seeds, and whole, unrefined grains are also good sources of magnesium. Refined grains are generally low in magnesium. When white flour is refined and processed, the magnesium-rich germ and bran are removed, so bread made from whole grain wheat flour provides more magnesium than bread made from white refined flour. Tap water can be a source of magnesium, but the amount varies according to the water supply. Water that naturally contains more minerals is described as "hard". "Hard" water contains more magnesium than "soft" water. Recent trends to filter tap water may be removing substantial amounts of the essential magnesium we get from our water source, so be sure to eat plenty of green vegetables to avoid a magnesium shortage.

Magnesium and heart disease

According to Dr. Brodsky, associate professor of medicine at the University of Medicine and the director of the Cardiac Arrhythmia Service at the University of California, mineral imbalances interfere with the heart's normal nerve function. When you sweat, a significant amount of magnesium is lost. Magnesium is said to be the most under-recognized electrolyte disorder in America. Dr. Mildred Seelig, one of the country's leading authorities on magnesium suggests that 80%-90% of the population of America is deficient is magnesium.

While most athletes have been conditioned to drink a potassium rich drink after sweating, very few have been educated on the dangers of a magnesium deficiency, even though it has been implicated as a cause of many sudden heart attacks on the sports field. Dr. Brodsky says that arrhythmia therapy should focus on replenishing two key minerals: potassium and magnesium.

Almost all physicians have known for some time just how vital potassium is for normal heartbeat. Magnesium is an entirely different story, however. According to Carla Sueta M.D., Ph.D., assistant professor of medicine and cardiology at the University of North Carolina at Chapel Hill School of Medicine "apparently, many doctors still don't realise how important a role this mineral can play in some heart patients. In fact, most never check the magnesium level. She has shown through her research that magnesium reduced the incidence of several types of ventricular arrhythmia by 53 to 76 percent.

Magnesium deficiency can even be induced by the very drugs meant to help heart problems. Most diuretics, or 'water tablets' cause the body to excrete both magnesium and potassium, as does digitalis too. And magnesium deficiency is often at the bottom of what's called refractory potassium deficiency. The amount of magnesium in the body determines the amount of a particular enzyme that determines the amount of potassium in the body. So if you are magnesium-deficient, you may in turn be potassium-deficient, and no amount of potassium is going to correct this unless you are also getting enough magnesium.

Iodine and your thyroid

Cold hands and feet are most often caused by iodine deficiency. Iodine deficiency is the leading cause of mental retardation, producing typical reductions in IQ of 10 to 15 IQ points. It has been speculated that deficiency of iodine and other micronutrients may be a possible factor in observed differences in IQ between ethnic groups. Curiously, the most obvious physical indications from birth that the mother was iodine deficient is that the baby is born without thumbs.

But the condition most often associated with iodine deficiency and goitre is cretinism. Cretins are commonly characterised by mental deficiency, deaf-mutism, squint, disorders of stance and gait, stunted growth and hypothyroidism

The word 'Chretien' is the old French for Christian, and the link probably came about because religious refugees in the Pyrenees retired into remote valleys because of religious persecution. As a result of restricted diet poor in iodine, as well as isolation, intermarriage, etc., children often had peculiar stunted bodies and retarded mental faculties, a condition we now know to be associated with thyroid deficiency. The term "chretien" for this kind of Christian seems to have developed as a term of contempt and was applied to other children of the same kind in other localities.

Certain areas of the world are still severely affected by iodine deficiency. It is particularly common in Asia, Africa and India, where 500 million suffer from iodine deficiency, with 54 million from goiter, and two million from cretinism.

Iodine is readily lost from the soil, so watershed regions in acountry often lose their iodine as it is washed out of the soil by rainwater. Even Derbyshire has its own type of iodine deficiency, where elderly inhabitants brought up on local produce have a goitre that is called 'Derbyshire Neck'.

You will find more information on Iodine elswehere in this book by referring to the index.

Do you have Tender Calf Muscles?

You may be deficient in MAGNESIUM

Calcium and magnesium are usually found together in the earth's crust, and these elements are in the same group of the Periodic Table, so these elements act like brother and sister.

The irony of the calcium-magnesium story is that without magnesium, calcium will not work properly. Our current diet tends to over-supplement with calcium, but this makes getting enough magnesium almost impossible. It is a typical brother and sister relationship actually, always fighting together. Research shows that the ratio of calcium to magnesium in the caveman diet — the ancient diet that had evolved with our bodies — was 1:1, compared with a ratio of between 5:1 and 15:1 in present-day diets. With an average of ten times more calcium than magnesium in our current diet, it is not surprising we have widespread magnesium deficiency in modern times.

This is also why osteoporosis is such a big problem of today. Until we correct our diet, no amount of expensive drugs will rectify the problem. What most of us need is magnesium, not calcium. Or, more accurately, less calcium.

Good sources of magnesium are brown rice, soya beans, nuts, wholemeal flour, fish, green vegetables, and pulses.

All the muscles, including the heart and blood vessels, contain more magnesium than calcium. If magnesium is deficient, calcium floods the smooth muscle cells of the blood vessels and causes spasms leading to constricted blood vessels and therefore higher blood pressure, arterial spasm, angina, and heart attacks. A proper balance of magnesium in relation to calcium can prevent these symptoms. A high calcium ratio, stimulating the cells in the muscular layer of the temporal arteries over the temples, can cause migraine headaches. Excess calcium ratio can constrict the smooth muscle surrounding the small airways of the lung, causing restricted breathing and asthma. Finally, too much calcium, without the protective effect of magnesium, can irritate delicate nerve cells of the brain. Cells that are irritated by calcium fire electrical impulses repeatedly, depleting their energy stores and causing cell death.

To understand how you can create a calcium/magnesium imbalance in your own body, try this experiment in your kitchen. Crush a calcium tablet and see how poorly it dissolves in a little water. Then crush a magnesium tablet and slowly stir it into the calcium water. When you introduce the magnesium, the remaining calcium dissolves very quickly; it becomes more water-soluble. The same principle occurs in your bloodstream, heart, brain, kidneys, and all the tissues in your body. If you don't have enough magnesium to help keep calcium dissolved, you may end up with calcium-excess muscle spasms, fibromyalgia, hardening of the arteries, dental cavities, and even calcification of tissue in the breast, one of the conditions that triggers breast cancer and the worry of this can occasionally convince healthy women to undergo double mastectomies. Another problem focuses on the kidneys. If there is too much calcium in the kidneys and not enough magnesium to balance it, you can get kidney stones. Magnesium supplements may even dissolve them.

So all these big problems suggest that if you have tender calf muscles you shouldn't take the condition lying down.

Do you have Brisk Knee Reflexes?

You may be deficient in MAGNESIUM

Here is another condition that indicates magnesium deficiency. Most Body Language symptoms can be dressed up in medical terms, and this Body Language sign is called 'deep tendon reflex'. This is triggered when the doctor strikes the upper or lower part of the knee with a rubber hammer or the edge of his hand. This is commonly performed to test reflex in the legs, especially where there could be nerve damage from diabetes or from an injury. Technically, the test is carried out with the lower leg hanging freely with the upper leg supported horizontally on a bench or table. Deep tendon reflex is quite difficult to trigger with your own actions, so it works best when the light impact is applied by a helping hand.

A very powerful deep tendon reflex is considered to be associated with magnesium deficiency.

Since we already covered magnesium deficiency in the preceding chapter, let's have a look at a few different characteristics of this light metallic element.

Inadequate dietary intake of magnesium is often caused by chronic alcoholism or malnutrition, or eating an inadequate diet based on junk food. Other causes include use of a diuretic. Symptoms of low magnesium levels cover a magnitude of symptoms including:

- Leg and foot cramps
- Weight loss
- Vomiting
- Muscle spasms, twitching, and tremors
- Seizures
- Muscle weakness
- Arrhythmia

Involuntary convulsions can occur when the body is low in magnesium, particularly at times of stress such as during childbirth. One major trial has shown that risk to the mother is significantly reduced when magnesium sulphate is used as anticonvulsant therapy rather than using anticonvulsive drugs.

There is no harm in trying a magnesium supplement at any time, because it is very unlikely that you will overdose, and it might give your body a kick-start. (in medical terms a brisk tendon reflex-start) as well as possibly preventing kidney stones.

Do you get muscle cramps?

If you do, you may be deficient in MAGNESIUM

If you have read the two previous chapters, you'll probably have guessed the main cause of this Body Language sign. Magnesium again. Many people experience cramps when they sleep, and this can be associated with excruciating pain. Athletes, on the other hand, tend to develop muscle cramps when they are exercising. A wide variety of factors can cause muscles to contract painfully. The following are common causes:

- A mineral deficiency involving potassium, calcium, magnesium and/or sodium.
- Dehydration, particularly in athletes who exercise hard in hot conditions and do not drink sufficient liquid.
- Excessive intake of fluid, for example drinking 2-3 litres or more of water in addition to your daily fluid intake - this can 'wash' the above-mentioned minerals out of your body and lead to cramps. Excessive sweating will also remove valuable magnesium from the body.
- Lack of fitness - well-trained muscles are less likely to cramp. Although this mainly applies to athletes, people who are not fit and get too little exercise often develop cramps because their muscles are not used to exertion.

The Body Language of Health

- Wearing tight constrictive clothing, especially in bed. Try to wear comfortable, loosely fitting clothes at all times. Aim to be comfortable, rather than stylish if you are plagued by cramps. The constriction of the blood supply to muscles from tight clothing can cause the muscles to contract painfully.

Minerals that play a role

There are four minerals that can influence how a muscle contracts, namely calcium, potassium, sodium and magnesium.

Calcium. You are probably not aware of the fact that calcium is essential for the normal contraction of muscle tissues, including those of the heart. Patients with extremely low blood calcium levels can develop a condition called tetani where the muscles fibres contract continuously. When this occurs, there could be a risk of heart failure.

Fortunately, such severe calcium deficiencies are rare, but on the other hand, sub-optimal calcium intakes are relatively common, especially in teenagers and young women who diet excessively because they are afraid of gaining weight. For this reason, people with eating disorders are particularly at risk from heart failure.

Magnesium. People eating a poor western diet that lacks fresh fruit, vegetables, legumes and unprocessed grains and cereals, may well have inadequate intake of magnesium. If you suffer from muscle cramps, you can try increasing your intakes of the foods listed above (especially green, leafy vegetables such as spinach, cabbage, lettuce, broccoli) or take a calcium and magnesium supplement (remember, taking these two minerals together improves their mutual absorption).

Potassium. This is one of the most abundant minerals available in common foods and most people should not develop a deficiency. However, eating sparsely or eating monotonous diets to lose weight, or cutting out all fruits, vegetables, grains and cereals can cause a potassium deficiency. Drinking too much water can also deplete your potassium reserves.

The easiest way of ensuring that you have abundant potassium is to eat five or more servings of fruit and/or vegetables a day. If you think you lack potassium, you could buy a variety of fresh vegetables and boil them lightly in chicken stock to make a delicious, fat-free soup that will be loaded with potassium. If you have a juicer, make an apple or grape and carrot drink to boost your potassium intake. Bear in mind that if you boil vegetables the potassium will end up in the water, so don't throw it away, use it to make the stock or soup. Great for making gravy too.

As you know, I am not generally in favour of supplements willy-nilly, because there is plenty of potassium in fresh wholesome fruit and vegetables. Potassium supplements should preferably only be taken if your potassium levels have been checked by a doctor and have been found to be low. Medical or nutritional experts will only prescribe potassium supplements under supervision, because a number of medications can influence the potassium levels in the body - for example, there is a group of so-called 'potassium-sparing diuretics' that help to prevent loss of potassium from the body. If you take a potassium supplement, you could develop hyperkalaemia (excess potassium in the blood), which is also harmful. So you are better to eat fruit and vegetables and whole grains to top up on potassium, rather than take supplements.

Sodium. Most people on a western diet, which is based on processed foods, won't develop a sodium deficiency. However, drinking too much water, sweating a lot, and certain imbalances in kidney function can lead to sodium depletion, which in turn can cause cramps. If you do a lot of exercise in hot weather or if you are an athlete training hard, you need to make sure that you are getting enough salt in your diet.

People who develop cramps and don't eat any salt or use salt substitutes (which are rich in potassium) should consider that they might have a sodium deficiency. You should refer to 'Do you crave butter?' to check up on your natural 'salt to taste' salt balance system.

Do your legs have brown or yellow skin?

You may risk diabetes

A brownish or yellowish discolouration of the skin on the front of your legs is very often an early warning sign that you could be insulin tolerant and heading for diabetes type 2. But it's not too late to act. Refer to the Body Language section under 'diabetes' in the index.

This Body Language sign probably came about because insulin tolerance and diabetes can reduce the efficiency of blood flow especially to the legs. This can result in discolouration.

When people talk about diabetes, they generally mean diabetes mellitus and some people have type 1 diabetes (in which they need insulin) but by far the biggest majority of people have type 2 diabetes, also called NIDDM (or, non-insulin dependent diabetes mellitus).

Potassium is valuable in treating hyperinsulinism, insulin resistance, and type two diabetes or NIDDM by preventing a trigger-happy pancreas from secreting insulin inappropriately.

Do you entwine your legs together or stand cross-legged?

You may have low blood pressure

Most men will read this Body Language sign displayed by a woman as a classic sign that she doesn't want her space invaded. Or it might be a sign that a woman needs the toilet. But there is a more sinister meaning to this body language sign for some people.

Experiments have shown that standing cross legged or entwining one leg round the other is very effective in limiting the fall in blood pressure at the brain that naturally occurs when people are standing up. Crossing legs prevents blood from pooling in the abdomen and the legs by reducing the amount of blood that will drain into the lower body. You don't realise it, but your brain may have decided that it is happier with its blood supply when you stand cross-legged.

Some people, especially women, can also sometimes be found sitting on their legs. This may be another body language symptom of low blood pressure. Considering the low cost of reliable personal blood pressure meters these days, it is good practice to check your blood pressure from time to time, compare your values and refer any unusual values or variations to your doctor. Entwining legs can be a sign of low blood pressure and your blood pressure meter will give you your reading; but only if you are sitting comfortably.

To take your blood pressure you should get your meter ready and then sit down for ten minutes and relax. Then put the meter on your wrist or your upper arm depending on which model you are using. Avoid any tightly fitting sleeves or other clothing. Turn on the machine, and record your blood pressure according to the machine's instructions.

MOUTH

Do you have a pale, fissured tongue?

You may be deficient in IRON

The tongue is richly supplied with blood close to the surface, so the tongue of a healthy person should always be a bright red colour and fairly free from white deposits. If your tongue is pale, that is an indication that you are anaemic.

Iron is a metal that happens to be a key element in haemoglobin, the red portion of the blood. A shortage of iron causes anaemia.

Anaemia is the most common nutritional problem in the world and mainly affects women of child-bearing age, teenagers and young children. The condition also affects one in six women over the age of 85.

While it is not usually a threat in its own right, it may be an indication of a more serious underlying problem. One in five people over 65 years of age diagnosed with iron deficient anaemia - the most common form of the condition - also have a serious problem with their gut. That is why anaemia should always be referred to your doctor.

There are several causes of anaemia. They include:

- Defective bone marrow
- A shortage of iron in the diet
- A shortage of the vitamins B12 or folic acid, both needed to produce red blood cells
- Loss of blood, through heavy menstruation, or internal bleeding.
- An infection

The problem is most commonly due to a lack of iron in the diet combined with some other factor such as menstruation in women. It may also be that the gut is unable to effectively absorb iron from the diet. This may be due to coeliac disease, a disorder that impairs digestion, which in turn could be due to a poor diet. These days we don't know what a 'good diet' is any more, because food manufacturers go to extreme lengths to increase the volume of their food or find ways to cut costs or extend its life. Good sources of iron include fruit, wholemeal bread, beans, and lean meat.

The Body Language of Health

Basically speaking, iron-deficiency anaemia is due to the loss of iron at a greater rate than it can be replaced. If your food is deficient in iron or you are losing iron, you'll end up with anaemia.

The diseases most commonly responsible for loss of iron are those associated with loss of blood through the digestive tract, such as gastritis, peptic ulcer, stomach cancer, inflammatory bowel disease, haemorrhoids, and also bowel tumours. Use of aspirin and similar nonsteroidal anti-inflammatory drugs can also cause gastrointestinal bleeding especially when taken over an extended period.

There are very simple bowel tests called faecal occult blood (or FOB) tests which can be bought from your chemist or ordered on the internet. These tests look for signs of blood in your stools. You can't see this with the naked eye, because blood that has leaked into the gut turns brown and is hidden from view by the natural colour of the faeces. If you do discover any red blood on the surface of the stool, then this is usually a clear indication that you have bleeding from haemorrhoids.

The FOB test is a very useful home screen, and is the test that would have detected the ice cube cruncher mentioned earlier. To carry out a home FOB test you simply familiarise yourself with the test instructions, then collect some faeces on a paper tissue or a disposable plastic tray when you next go to the toilet. Use the collection stick that comes with the test to collect a representative sample of the stool, collecting from several places if you can. Put the stick back in the liquid, shake, and then put a spot of this liquid on the test cassette at the position indicated. With most tests, you will have to wait for the liquid to be absorbed, then add another drop, wait again for absorption, then add a third drop.

The liquid will run along the test membrane and most tests will give you an indication of a line to say whether the test is negative or positive.

At one time these tests would detect any kind of blood, so you had to refrain from eating meat for several days before you carried out a test. But modern tests use an antibody that will only detect human haemoglobin, so it is safe to eat meat, unless you happen to be a cannibal, that is.

Faeces are brown because they include a chemical called Bilirubin, which is excreted in bile to digest food.

Bilirubin shot to notoriety with non-medical people when Hannibal Lecter used Billy Rubin as an anagram of Buffalo Bill's name to taunt Agent Starling in the novel, The Silence of the Lambs. This was presumably too subtle for cinemagoers, and its complexities never quite reached the big screen. Lecter even jumbled Bilirubin's formula of carbon, hydrogen and nitrogen to spell CHILTON, a clue to his next victim, his prison governor Dr Chilton.

The author of 'the Lambs' Jonathan Demme would know all about bilirubin because he studied to be a vet until he realised he could make more money writing. Maybe the same thing could happen to a forensic scientist someday. We all live in hope.

Are there any other symptoms?

Yes. The first symptoms of anaemia are usually tiredness and sometimes there are palpitations. Other common symptoms include shortness of breath and dizziness. If the anaemia is severe there is a risk of angina (chest pain), headache and leg pains. The body's ability to fight infection is also impaired if you are anaemic.

Long-term anaemia can also result in a further range of symptoms including:

- A burning sensation in the tongue
- Dryness in the mouth and throat
- Sores at the corners of the mouth
- An altered sense of touch
- Difficulty in swallowing
- Brittle hair

Some more useful Body Language signs there!. Anaemia is not just a problem for the elderly. Young people can also develop severe anaemia too, but because they are generally more active and alert they may not really have any classical symptoms. A pale tongue is a good Body Language for such people. Older people have less reserves in their muscles and brains and other organs, so they will feel the effects much more.

How is anaemia treated?

The most common way to treat anaemia caused by iron deficiency is to prescribe an iron supplement. Some hospital patients may even be given injections, and if iron depletion is very severe blood transfusions may be necessary.

Do you have a white coating on your tongue?

You might be dehydrated or have a yeast infection.

A 'furry tongue' is surprisingly common amongst today's modern population. Some people seem to have a slightly furry tongue for no apparent reason and they can often clear it by scrubbing their tongue in exactly the same way they clean their teeth, with toothbrush and toothpaste. But mostly a furry tongue is a symptom of dehydration or a Candida (yeast, or 'Thrush') infection.

Don't worry, it is perfectly harmless to have a white tongue as long as the overgrowth is not excessive. Virtually all of us have a yeast infection of some sort because of our diet that includes fermented dairy products like yoghurt, and bread made with yeast. It is not a problem as long as there is no risk of a yeast overgrowth.

But a furry tongue may also be the cause of bad breath, and that's not quite as nice for other people. Really pungent bad breath is usually caused by the bacteria in your mouth, throat and on your tongue. The aroma often contains sulphur compounds which are particularly distasteful, often with a 'bad eggs' smell. So dental hygiene is essential if you want to improve your breath. Toothpaste generally contains triclosan, an antiseptic that kills bacteria, though there is evidence its use leads to bacterial resistance, which could be storing up a halitosis war in future. But it is not very effective on yeasts.

Some years ago I worked on several products that contained triclosan, and helped a team at work to develop antibacterial paint that had the miraculous property of killing all the bacteria that landed on it, including those little buggers E coli, C difficile and MRSA. Unfortunately the NHS were not interested even though they could then have been confident that any nasty contaminated hand-prints would have been rendered harmless in seconds. It could also be used to paint door handles and virtually anything inanimate that doctors come into contact with. I think it would have made a big contribution to preventing MRSA. In Britain as many people are killed from MRSA infections in hospital as are killed on the roads, but there is no money to be made in saving lives in hospital, while there is a fortune to be made in penalising innocent motorists travelling at 34 miles an hour in a 30 mph zone. Maybe they could spend some of the speeding fines on buying my antibacterial paint.

Developing antibacterial coatings seemed a good idea at the time but you can lead a mule to water but you cannot make him drink. But at least we went on to develop antibacterial/antifungal grout and that has now been adopted widely by manufacturers. There is a bit more triclosan in these products so that it also prevents black mould, Aspergillus niger, from forming round the grout or silicone sealant at the edge of the bath and wash basin.

Drink more Corporation Pop

Current recommendation for water consumption in the West is said to be eight glasses per day. This amount should be sufficient for most healthy people who are not in a hot, humid environment or sweating from physical work or exercise. Those who are should drink more water more often. Be sure to drink water, not soft drinks which are loaded with sugar. Sugar and yeast go together like beer and ....yeast. Not sure about that analogy, but I am sure you know what I mean.

Unfortunately most of the hot countries in the world happen to have the worst water supplies in the world. Many women walk over 10 miles (15 kilometres) a day just to carry home some water for their family. That's why a share of profits from this book is going to charities that include Water Aid, the organisation that provides fresh water to third world countries.

How can you tell if you are dehydrated? The easiest way is to pay attention to the colour of your urine each time you urinate. Urine that has accumulated in your bladder during sleep will be more concentrated, so you have to ignore the first urine of the morning.

Afterwards, your urine should be light coloured and odourless for the remainder of the day, assuming that you have normal functioning kidneys and no bladder disease or infection. If your urine is dark, you're not drinking enough.

Some foods will affect urine smell and colour. For example Asparagus produces a strange smell to your urine, due to two chemicals in asparagus called methylthioacrylate and methylthiopropionate. And turmeric found in curries and piccalilli turns the urine bright yellow.

Thrush, or Candida

Thrush in the mouth is an infection caused by the fungus *Candida albicans*, the same little bugger responsible for vaginal yeast infections. The disease is common among babies, who may be exposed to the micro organism as they pass through the birth canal. Thrush is also common in people who take antibiotic or steroid medication, and in people with compromised immune systems. In all of these cases, the healthy balance of bacteria in the mouth can be disrupted, making it easier for *Candida albicans* to grow and spread. Smoking is a risk factor, too, since it also upsets the balance of bacteria in the mouth.

When people take antibiotics, the good bacteria are killed along with the disease-causing ones. This leaves yeasts, such as Candida which is not affected by antibiotics, to grow unrestrained, proliferating and overrunning the intestinal tract. The consequence is a yeast overgrowth or infection. Such infections can last for years causing a wide variety of symptoms ranging from headaches to digestive problems and even ME.

Visual symptoms of thrush can include:

- White patches on the tongue and insides of the cheeks
- Creamy, cottage-cheese-like sores, also on the tongue and in the mouth
- Pain or burning in the mouth and throat
- Lessened ability to taste food or an unpleasant taste in the mouth

Sometimes, thrush can be a sign of a more serious, underlying condition, especially if you're not in one of one of the higher-risk groups mentioned earlier in this topic. Diabetes and HIV are two possible candidates. If you're concerned, or if you have been in sexual situations that have placed you at risk, it might be a good idea to see a health care professional if you have developed a white tongue.

Several non-thrush conditions can also cause a white tongue, including:

- *Scarlet fever.* The tongue has a white coating for the first two days of the disease.
- *Kawasaki disease.* A white coating and prominent red bumps appear on the tongue.
- *Herpes simplex virus — type 1.* Cold sores that are caused by the herpes virus can also be responsible for a white coating on the tongue.
- *Lichen planus.* A skin disease that causes lacy white patches on the tongue and inner cheeks if the mouth is infected.

Most of these conditions, however, come with a variety of other symptoms. If you suspect something more serious than yeast or dehydration, you should see your doctor. There is a good home test for detecting a yeast infection on P265.

Do you have a sore, fissured tongue?

You may be deficient in VITAMIN B2

Vitamin B2, or Riboflavin, is necessary for healthy skin and eyes. It is vital for converting proteins, fats and carbohydrates into energy. Vitamin B2 is also necessary for red blood cell formation, antibody production, and cell growth. It is also important in the prevention and treatment of cataracts. Vitamin B2 also takes part in the utilisation of oxygen by the tissues of the skin, nails and hair.

Are there other Body Language symptoms?

Yes, lots. Symptoms of vitamin B2 deficiency include sensitivity or inflammation of the mucous membranes of the mouth; cracks or sores at the corners of the mouth (which is called cheilosis); a red, sore tongue; eye redness or sensitivity to light, burning eyes, eye fatigue, or a dry, sandy feeling of the eyes; fatigue and/or dizziness; dermatitis with a dry yet greasy or oily scaling; nervous tissue damage; and retarded growth in infants and children. But don't expect to get all these at once, like most Body Language signs, you may only get one or perhaps two together. Cataracts may occur more frequently with B2 deficiency, so a fissured tongue is not to be taken lightly. Hair loss, weight loss, general lack of vitality, and digestive problems are also possible with depletion or deficiency states of vitamin B2.

Where can I get Vitamin B2?

Deficiency of B2 is almost always due to eating diets that do not include riboflavin-rich foods. These include special diets for weight loss, ulcers, or treatment of diabetes; or the latest food fad or crash diet may be to blame. Some people who have bad eating habits and consume mostly refined foods and fast foods are living on a shockingly poor diet that is deficient in many of the essential vitamins. So expect to see many problems like these in the fast food cultural centres like American cities.

Many of these diets are so nutritionally poor that you almost might as well eat nothing – maybe that is where the title 'fast' food came from? Hence the slogan 'Nothing is as good as so-and-so's burger' (so you might as well eat nothing).

Vitamin B2 deficiency is also more commonly seen in people with alcohol problems, in the elderly and the poor, and in depressed patients who notoriously live off an unimaginative diet.

The Body Language of Health

If we eat a varied diet of fresh, natural food there is no reason why we should develop this deficiency or any other for that matter. Foods rich in Vitamin B2 include liver, yeast, meat, fish, eggs, vegetables, dairy foods and grain products. Vegetables containing particularly high vitamin B2 levels include leafy green vegetables, asparagus, artichokes, avocados, broccoli, Brussels sprouts, watercress, spinach, kelp, peas, beans, pumpkins, and sweet potatoes.

Vitamin B2 is so important because it functions as the building block for two coenzymes that are essential in energy production. Flavin mononucleotide (FMN) and flavin adenine dinucleotide (FAD) act as hydrogen carriers to help make energy as adenosine triphosphate (ATP) through the metabolism of carbohydrates and fats. Vitamin B2 is also instrumental in cell respiration, helping each cell utilize oxygen most efficiently; it is helpful in maintaining good vision and healthy hair, skin, and nails and it is necessary for normal cell growth.

B2 supplements are popular to treat and help prevent visual problems, eye fatigue, and cataracts. It seems to help with burning eyes, watery eyes, and decreased vision resulting from eye strain. Vitamin B2 is also used by nutritionists for many kinds of stress conditions, fatigue, and vitality or growth problems. For people with allergies and chemical sensitivities, riboflavin-5-phosphate may be more readily assimilated than B2.

Vitamin B2 is also given for skin difficulties such as acne, dermatitis, eczema, and skin ulcers. It is also used in the treatment of alcohol problems, ulcers, digestive difficulties, and leg cramps, and supplementing it may be advantageous for prevention or during treatment of cancer. There is, however, very little published research to support the benefits of its use in these conditions. You have to judge for yourself if you suffer from these conditions. Try it and see.

Like all the advice here, it pays to focus on the foods rich in that nutrient. If you decide on a supplement, take it for at least a few weeks because you shouldn't expect the result to be instantaneous, your body has a 'buffer' for most nutrients. After that, if you don't see an improvement, chances are that is not what you are deficient in, and you should review other sections of the book to help you.

Considering these linked ailments, deficiency of B2 in common with most of the B-vitamins, is of significant concern to us all. Some authorities claim that vitamin B2 deficiency is the most common nutrient deficiency in America. However, because some B2 is produced by intestinal bacteria, it may not cause actual symptoms as severe as those seen in other vitamin deficiencies.

Do you have peeling lips and a burning tongue?

You may be deficient in VITAMIN B2

Vitamin B2 again. I have just developed a burning desire to refer you to the previous topic. Vitamin B2, or Riboflavin, is necessary for healthy skin and eyes, and a deficiency can cause burning sensations. And a multitude of other symptoms.

Do you have a swollen tongue?

Suspect FOOD INTOLERANCE or a FOOD ALLERGY

This problem occurs when specific adverse effects occur after eating a particular food or food ingredient. A genuine food reaction is different from psychologically based food aversion, which is when a person strongly dislikes a food or believes that a food produces a particular reaction. Food intolerance usually takes a while to act, while a food allergic reaction is usually quick acting.

What foods are involved?

This book is too short to list them, but the most common foods, in order of frequency are milk, eggs, nuts, fish/shellfish, wheat, chocolate, artificial colours, pork, chicken, tomato, soft fruit, cheese and yeast. There are many other foods that we could list here.

With **food intolerance**, food chemicals such as many additives and some natural food chemicals are also often involved. For example, asthmatics are most likely to be affected by sulphite or nitrite preservatives in a wide range of foods and drugs including fruit flavoured cordials and drinks, wine, bread, sausages, bacon, dried fruit and even some medications. Many sufferers seem to have intolerance to artificial food colourants and flavourings too.

Whilst not all food intolerances are related to meat and dairy products, it can be seen from the above list that vegetarians, and particularly vegans, will suffer less from food intolerance because they already eliminate some of the most common causes of intolerance. This suggests that if you are affected by food intolerance and find it difficult to stick to an exclusion diet, you could at least go vegan for a while and see if it improves your condition.

Symptoms

The most common symptoms include asthma, gastro-intestinal symptoms (nausea, vomiting, and diarrhoea), eczema, urticaria (hives), rhinorrhea (that's heavy discharge from the nose, not heavy discharge from a Rhinoceros' bottom), wheeziness after eating, and swelling of the blood vessels and tongue. Other longer-term symptoms can include depression, anxiety, fatigue, migraine, sleeplessness and hyperactivity in children.

Food intolerance is a pharmacological reaction (like the side effects of a drug) to the chemicals in foods. **Food allergy** is usually an immunological reaction to food proteins. The two reactions are very different. Intolerance is typified by migraine, irritable bowel symptoms, and behaviour problems, while allergy is typified by hay fever, eczema or asthma

Family history may be helpful in identifying a food intolerance or allergy because there is some evidence that these conditions are hereditary.

Who is affected?

An Allergy is most likely to start while someone is a baby or a young child because of their underdeveloped immune system.

An intolerance is also likely to affect a child because dose for weight they consume a higher dose of food chemicals than adults, but intolerance does often start in later life. Women of child-bearing age are especially vulnerable because of hormonal influence. The elderly become more vulnerable because older livers and kidneys are slower to excrete chemicals from the body. Exposure to toxic chemicals, pharmaceutical drugs or illness such as gastrointestinal infection can also trigger food intolerance, and these can build up as we get older.

How common are they?

Food allergies (not airborne allergies such as pollens) are considered to be relatively uncommon - affecting up to 8% of babies under 12 months, 3% of children under five, and less than 1% of adults.

Food intolerance is much more common. Some experts suggest 10% of the population is affected by food intolerance.

Timing

Allergic reactions are quick. They usually occur within 30 minutes and are often easy to identify.

Food intolerance reactions can be delayed up to 48 hours or more. Identification of reactions can be difficult. When problem foods are consumed frequently, symptoms can appear to be a chronic condition rather than a food reaction.

Dose- relationship

Allergic reactions can develop even when there is a small amount of an allergen. Sometimes trace amounts can set off anaphylactic shock, if sensitised to the substance, for example peanut allergies can work in this way.

Intolerance reactions to food chemicals are dose-related. Some people are more sensitive than others. In theory, most people will react to food additives if they consume enough. One study involving monosodium glutamate confirmed this, although a few of the subjects only reacted to very high doses which were highly unlikely to be consumed in a normal diet.

Symptoms

Allergic reactions can be itching, swelling, rash, spreading hives, vomiting, diarrhoea, breathing difficulties and in the most severe of the allergic disorders, anaphylaxis can lead to collapse and death. By definition, anaphylaxis is an allergic reaction which involves two of the body's systems (e.g. respiratory and gastrointestinal or skin). Anaphylactic deaths as a result of insect bites or penicillin are usually very quick - within minutes - and due to cardiac arrest. Anaphylactic deaths due to food allergies are usually due to suffocation (breathing difficulties due to restrictions in the airways). These conditions are very rare.

The Body Language of Health

Food intolerance reactions can be the same as above, as well as:

- *Skin* (rashes, swelling)
- *Airways* (asthma, stuffy or runny nose, frequent colds and infections)
- *Gastrointestinal tract* (irritable bowel symptoms, colic, bloating, diarrhoea, vomiting, frequent mouth ulcers, reflux, bedwetting, poor bowel control over faeces)
- *Central nervous system* (migraines, headaches, anxiety, depression, lethargy, impairment of memory and concentration, panic attacks, irritability, restlessness, inattention, sleep disturbance, restless legs, mood swings, PMT).

Symptoms of food intolerance can come and go, and may change throughout life.

Diagnosis

Food allergies: Diagnosis involves an immunoglobulin IgE response and can be identified by skin prick tests or RAST blood tests and confirmed with avoidance and challenge tests.

Food intolerance: There are no foolproof laboratory tests, though some are helpful. Those that are available look for food-specific IgE test results, but the only way to identify provoking foods is through a comprehensive elimination diet and careful challenges, by introducing foods one at a time several days apart to give each new food time to trigger a reaction.

Treatment

Food allergies: scrupulous avoidance of the food that causes the allergy. Life-threatening peanut allergies in particular are increasing. This is thought to be due to exposure through the use of peanuts in many Western-style processed foods. In allergic families, complete avoidance of peanuts, peanut-containing products and also cows milk is recommended for pregnant women for the last six weeks of pregnancy and throughout breastfeeding. Some schools have banned peanut butter.

Food intolerances: an elimination diet with challenges to pinpoint the culprits, gradual reintroduction of certain foods and chemicals to ascertain tolerance, and subsequent avoidance to that limit. For an occasional antidote to a reaction, a pinch of sodium bicarbonate in half a glass of water is said to be helpful when drunk.

THE EXCLUSION DIET

Since many allergies, and, by definition, all food intolerances involve what we shovel into our mouths, the only way to identify what food or food additive is causing the problem is to remove it from our diet. But usually we have no idea what is causing the problem, and we have to survive on something. The answer is the exclusion diet. This is the only sure way to identify and alleviating food intolerance. I have described an exclusion diet elsewhere, please refer to P139.

Do you have a smooth, sore tongue?

You may be deficient in FOLIC ACID

It is estimated that 88 per cent of all North Americans suffer from a folic acid deficiency, and the statistic is likely to be similar elsewhere in the world.

Folic acid is vitamin B9 and is an essential nutrient for proper growth and development. Folic acid has been shown to reduce a woman's risk of having a baby with a neural tube defect when it is consumed before conception and during the early weeks of pregnancy. It is prescribed to pregnant women for this reason.

You will find many references in this book to folic acid and folates, the salts of this acid. There are important differences between these. Folic acid is the synthetic form of the vitamin that is used in supplements and fortified foods. Folate is the natural form that is found in many foods, such as beans and other legumes, leafy green vegetables and orange juice. However as far as we are concerned the two names are synonymous, so I will use the term folic acid here.

You should get enough folic acid by eating a healthy diet that includes fresh fruit and vegetables.

Who should take folic acid supplements?

Prospective mothers should be taking folic acid as soon as they decide to have children, but at least half of all pregnancies are believed to be unplanned or incorrectly timed, and neural tube defects occur before most women know they are pregnant. For this reason, you should be consuming foods that are rich in folic acid if you are:

- In your reproductive years
- Capable of becoming pregnant
- Sexually active

Good sources of folic acid

- Lentils, peas, chickpeas, asparagus, broccoli, collard greens
- Papaya, strawberries, oranges

But it's not just pregnant women who should be making sure they have enough folic acid though. Health starts with the individual cells of our body. If our cells are healthy so are we. Healthy cells, in turn, depend on the continued, faultless replication of our DNA. And DNA can be seriously damaged through attacks by free radicals. So an adequate supply of antioxidants is essential to cell health. However, it is becoming clear that antioxidants alone are not enough to protect our DNA; more and more research points to folic acid as being equally or perhaps even more important in ensuring proper DNA replication.

It is therefore not surprising that a folic acid deficiency has been implicated in a wide variety of disorders from Alzheimer's disease to atherosclerosis, heart attack, stroke, osteoporosis, cervical and colon cancer, depression, dementia, and hearing loss, as well as the more well known cleft lip and palate, and of course, other neural tube defects.

The reason for this is that folic acid has been found to be essential for the synthesis of two of the nucleic acids that make up our genes, our DNA and our chromosomes; adenine and thiamine. It is also required for the proper metabolism of the essential amino acid methionine that is found primarily in animal proteins.

A folic acid deficiency has also been clearly linked to an elevated level of homocysteine, a sulphur-containing amino acid. High homocysteine levels, in turn, have been linked to cardiovascular disease and a host of other undesirable conditions such as schizophrenia.

So don't be in two minds about it, you should be listening to what your tongue is saying, quite literally.

Do you have cracked lips?

You may be deficient in VITAMIN B2

We just can't stop talking about vitamin B2 at the moment. Vitamin B2, Riboflavin, is not stored in the human body for any period of time and it is therefore important to include a regular dietary source of this vitamin. It is essential for converting carbohydrate into energy, essential for normal tissue respiration, and necessary for healthy mucous membranes.

Some signs of deficiency

- Cracks in skin at corner of mouth
- Soreness of lips, mouth and tongue
- Scaling of skin around nose, mouth, scrotum, forehead, ears and scalp
- Heightened sensitivity to light
- Conjunctivitis and watering of eyes
- Anaemia

Good sources of Vitamin B2 are lean meats, liver, kidneys, milk, cheese and green vegetables - especially broccoli and spinach.

Vitamin B2 deficiency and Cataracts

If you want to avoid cataracts you should pretend you're Popeye. A Harvard University study found that women who ate spinach more than five times a week had a 47 percent decrease in risk of cataract surgery compared with those who ate spinach less than once a month. (Yes, eating spinach five times a week adds up to a whole lot of spinach, but some women in the study were apparently eating it that often. The study didn't say whether Olive was involved in this study.) Spinach may beat carrots when it comes to cataract protection, but more than five times a week does sound like a Popeye fixation. In fact, it's always a good idea to eat a variety of fruits and vegetables, and not an exclusive spinach diet, I suspect this was just a university study to demonstrate how powerful spinach is. Any more and they'd be pop-eyed.

Do you have bleeding gums?

You may be deficient in VITAMIN C

Gum disease is one of the first symptoms of vitamin C deficiency, which in clinically deficient cases eventually results in a disease called Scurvy.

Early symptoms of Scurvy are malaise, lethargy, myalgia and arthralgia. Other symptoms include skin changes with easy bruising, gum disease , loosening of teeth and poor wound healing.

Then the gums become swollen, purple, spongy, and friable. The skin shows papules and haemorrhages around hair follicles, petechiae and multiple bruises. Nail splinter haemorrhages may occur. In the later stages, jaundice, generalised oedema, oliguria, neuropathy, fever, and convulsions may occur. These are followed a few days later by death.

Ask someone in Britain if they have heard of a disease that is connected with a vitamin deficiency and they will probably say Scurvy. That is because Scurvy was prevalent in the British Navy and Britain has a long history as a seafaring nation. Ask someone in America the same question and they will probably say Pellagra, a debilitating disease which was the scourge of the Southern States for many years. The history of these diseases and the hunt for a cure is fascinating in its own right but is outside the scope of this book.

Vitamin C (Ascorbic acid) is essential for collagen formation and helps to maintain the integrity of connective tissue, bone and dentine. It is essential for wound healing and promotes recovery from burns. Vitamin C also promotes the absorption of iron. Severe deficiency results in Scurvy, but the adverse effects of more mild degrees of vitamin C deficiency are not so well publicised, but are equally harmful. Vitamin C is an anti-oxidant and helps to minimise cell damage in the body. Without it, your body suffers.

Vitamin C is found in a wide variety of fruit and vegetables. Good sources include:

- Fruits: especially grapefruits, lemons, blackcurrants, oranges and kiwi fruit
- Vegetables: e.g. broccoli, green peppers, tomatoes, cabbage, sprouts, and sweet potatoes
- Fresh milk

The Body Language of Health

Vitamin C deficiency is potentially worst in children aged 6-12 months who are fed a diet deficient in citrus fruits or vegetables at a time when diet is most important. Deficiency also occurs in the elderly who find it increasingly difficult to prepare a balanced diet and may have problems chewing and digesting fruit.

Other risk factors include the following:

- Alcoholics and people with food fads
- Elderly
- Low income families tend not to buy foods high in vitamin C
- Vitamin C deficiency has been noted in refugees
- Increased need for Vitamin C due to increased utilisation in pregnant and lactating women, thyrotoxicosis, surgery, and burns
- Chronic diarrhoea increases deficiency of Vitamin C.

Jacques Cartier in 1536 described the symptoms of what is now known to be scurvy. It was one of the earliest descriptions of vitamin deficiency disease. However, it was not until 1753 that James Lind, a Scottish physician, documented a way to prevent this disease by supplementing the diet with lemon or lime juice, which subsequently led to the British sailors being nicknamed 'limies'. Of course the active ingredient that had such a powerful anti-scurvy effect was vitamin C. Scurvy is fatal if it goes untreated, but patients respond quickly to oral therapy.

The clear view on cataracts

It is claimed that people with low vitamin C levels have 11 times the normal risk of developing cataracts. A recent study investigated the relationship of supplements and cataract formation. The study involved 350 men and women who were given supplements of both vitamin E and vitamin C. Results showed that the consumption of these supplementary vitamins reduced the risk of senile cataracts by about 50%. That makes supplementation of these two vitamins relevant to us all.

A clear case of suck it and see.

Do you have trouble swallowing (dysphagia)?

If you do, you could be deficient in MAGNESIUM

This body language sign originated from stories like the problems of a 41 year old woman who had a 4 month history of throat spasms set off by eating, yawning or talking. They were so severe that she worried she would choke to death and she had virtually stopped eating or talking as a result.

She complained of tingling in her mouth, and throat spasms. She'd also had severe diarrhoea over the preceding year and had lost 15 kilograms of weight. When her biochemistry was analysed the results suggested hypomagnesaemia-induced hypocalcaemia. In other words, low magnesium, causing low calcium too.

Due to her severity of symptoms she was sent to hospital. Fortunately her doctor knew about the link between magnesium and dysphagia and she was given magnesium injections to relieve her hypomagnesaemia. She improved dramatically within 24 hours. In other words she was back to the usual female trait of talking nineteen to the dozen. The doctor would have asked her to record her story for this book, but he couldn't get a word in edgeways.

Trembling and spasms (known as neuromuscular hyperexcitability) are also a feature of low magnesium. See 'essential tremor and shaking hands'

Do you have mercury fillings in your teeth?

If you do, you may be deficient in SELENIUM and GLUTATHIONE

There is a very strong interaction between some trace elements. A surplus of mercury causes a diminishing of selenium in the body. Why is that important? Here is an internet article I found written by a doctor.

"Most of our cancer patients have a lot of amalgam dental fillings. 1 remember a study we made few years ago at the University of Vienna. One group of students with amalgam fillings had to chew a chewing gum for twenty minutes, and the other group had to sip hot lemon juice for twenty minutes. We wanted to know what happens with the mercury level in their blood. By chewing the gum, with dental fillings of amalgam, or by drinking hot and acid juices, there was always a big mercury intake in the blood.

In the same way, the level of selenium was lowered, because a lot of selenium was needed to detoxify the mercury. Selenium mops up mercury by forming a new compound, mercury selenite, therefore it was not available any longer as an antioxidant in the body. What we didn't expect was that the immune status showed us a small decrease in the immune-competent cells after this test." *Transcript of a lecture delivered to the Proceedings of the First World Congress on Cancer by Professor W Kostler (President of Austrian Society of Oncology, Austria.)*

The internet has lots of information about mercury toxicity from amalgam fillings. What is less publicised is that essential selenium in the body is being used up to flush out mercury, so anyone with amalgam fillings is likely to be selenium deficient.

Why is that important? Because a deficiency of selenium is associated with cancer. For that story see 'Do you have a family history of cancer?'

Amalgam fillings also seem to be implicated in chronic fatigue syndrome, autism and foetal birth defects.

Thimerasol (Thimerosal in USA) is a mercury based preservative that was still used in Britain in child vaccines until a strategic withdrawal by U.K. Government a few years ago. Britain, I understand, was the last country to ban mercury preservative in vaccine. This has been documented on a number of websites as the possible link between child autism and vaccination, though I have seen no confirmed evidence of this in medical journals. On a recent trip to Sweden I asked if anyone had mercury fillings and everyone was surprised and shocked because they said mercury fillings were banned in Sweden a long time ago. But they are still being used in Britain.

The most clearly illustrated incidence of selenium deficiency stems from China, where selenium soil levels are extremely low in some areas. A widespread fatal heart disease in children called Keshan's Disease was shown to arise from selenium deficiency, because their foods were selenium deficient, and Keshan's has now been successfully treated with sodium selenite, a common salt of selenium.

It has also been revealed that selenium contributes as an antidote to heavy metals, by forming compounds with them, thus enabling them to be excreted from the body. Hence the link with mercury. Selenium acts as a chelating (pronounced 'key-late-ing) agent, enabling the body to get rid of toxic heavy metals like mercury. Glutathione status has also been shown to have an impact on the ability of the body to handle heavy metals such as cadmium, arsenic, lead and mercury.

Glutathione.

Glutathione is an enzyme made up of a chain of amino acids that controls the status of cell life, including detoxification of oxygen free radicals and carcinogens in cells. If glutathione is depleted, that person can be predisposed to incur stress from pollutants. Glutathione and glutathione-related enzymes are important antioxidants and these enzymes appear to play an especially important role in detoxifying carcinogens.

Selenium has been shown to be an important component of the enzyme glutathione peroxidase which is of crucial importance to the immune system and to the protection of the cell walls. This appears to be the magic link between selenium and cancer resistance – since the enzyme and selenium itself are both important antioxidants. When the body is deficient in selenium, the immune system may be affected.

So mercury fillings may cause depletion of selenium, which can cause a similar reduction in immunity.

Glutathione can be taken as a supplement, but when taking glutathione, vitamin C is also recommended because vitamin C assists glutathione in maintaining its powerful free radical-suppressing effects.

Considering the high proportion of people in Britain with mercury fillings, and the possible links with cancer, perhaps everyone should be taking selenium supplements with a daily orange.

See also 'Do you have a family history of cancer?'

Do you suffer from recurrent mouth ulcers?

If you do, you may be deficient in IRON, ZINC, FOLIC ACID AND VITAMIN B12

You may be one of the unlucky 1-2% of the population who gets recurrent, ordinary mouth ulcers. The medical term for these is 'aphthous ulcers'. Usually the problem starts in childhood or adolescence, and seems to improve in the 40s. Typically, the ulcers come in crops of one to five at a time. The mouth is remarkably good at healing, so the ulcers last for only 1-2 weeks. Then, a few weeks later, they can flare up again.

Recurrent mouth ulcers are often due to anaemia or shortage of iron, folic acid or vitamin B12. A few women find that mouth ulcers are more likely before their periods, so hormones might perhaps have an influence too.

A survey found that mouth ulcers stopped more than 50 per cent of people from kissing. Many of those stopped because it was too painful, but also many stopped because they thought they were contagious - which in fact is not true. If you want to be kissed, practice good dental hygiene taking care not to damage your teeth and gums, and visit your dentist every six months for a check up.

The same survey confirmed that mouth ulcers made it difficult to eat, drink, and even talk. Particularly difficult for women, then. Many people with mouth ulcers don't want to socialise either.

To stand the best chance of avoiding mouth ulcers, eat a healthy diet that's rich in vitamin C from fresh fruit; B vitamins from wholegrain bread and potatoes; iron from lean red meat and leafy green vegetables; and zinc from sea-foods, wholegrain bread, seeds and cereals. This enables your immune system to stay strong and resist unwanted approaches by infections. Avoiding food and drinks that are too hot is essential and of course relax and reduce your stress. Take a zinc supplement, perhaps.

And avoid garlic and strongly flavoured vegetables like cabbage immediately before a snog.

Good sources of Vitamin B12 are dairy produce, eggs, yeast extract, seaweed, spirulina algae; good sources of iron include meat, cereals, raw green vegetables, and fortified foods such as some breakfast cereals. Despite iron from plant foods being less readily absorbed research has shown that vegetarians are no more likely to suffer from iron deficiency than non-vegetarians.

It's a good idea to eat foods containing vitamin C at the same time as eating non-meat sources of iron because this helps with iron absorption. Good sources of vitamin C include peppers, Brussels sprouts, sweet potatoes, oranges, and kiwi fruit.

Good sources of folic acid are lentils, collard greens, chickpeas, papaya, peas, asparagus, broccoli, strawberries, and oranges.

Has your voice changed?

It could be hormonal or something you should check out

Anyone who regrets the fact that they have never had the chance to learn a musical instrument should rejoice in the fact that they have already mastered the most complicated musical instrument of all – the human voice. Even if they are not a singer – even if they are tone deaf, the ability to control any sort of a sound from a few bits of stretched skin is remarkable in the extreme.

The vocal chords are an amazingly complex structure.

If your voice develops a persistent hoarseness you should discuss it with your doctor. Mostly this is quite harmless but there can be some serious causes that warrant quick attention by a qualified medical expert. In extreme cases it can indicate cancer of the throat, and these days that is operable with success but must be caught early.

Mostly, the reasons for vocal changes are hormonal.

Elsie sings in a church choir and has taken part in several elaborate Roger Jones musicals. So when her voice began to get hoarse a few years ago, and she developed a feeling that she wanted to clear her throat when she was singing, she got worried, especially since when she did clear her throat it didn't make much difference to her voice. If you started at the beginning of this book, you'll appreciate the reason for her concern, though this time it didn't involve lettuce.

Her voice has also deepened a little, she can't sing soprano any more and is firmly in the alto group. She still doesn't sound like Rod Stewart, but she says that while on the telephone at work people occasionally ask her if she has a cold. Hopefully her answer to them is to discuss 'Handbags and Gladrags' rather than asking 'Do you think I'm sexy?'

She discussed her vocal changes with her doctor and he referred her to a speech therapist. But I think I already had the answer.

Since her lettuce addiction, which is where this book began, she has been on a hormonal blocker called Tamoxifen. This drug has some success in preventing breast cancer from returning, though Elsie puts her own remission down as much to good old fashioned research of the subject (aided by her good old fashioned husband) and the influences of Professor Jane Plant, who has repeatedly shown the link between breast cancer and consumption of dairy products, especially in hormone-linked cancers.

Although her medical contacts had never heard of it, just take a look on the internet at Tamoxifen + voice and you will find a number of links that demonstrate that the voice can deepen in some women who are on Tamoxifen. It is hormonal.

Nevertheless you should still discuss this with your doctor since you should not assume anything if your voice changes.

Do you suffer from skin cracks at the corners of your mouth?

If you do, you may be deficient in VITAMIN B2 and B6

Symptoms of vitamin B2 and B6 deficiencies include painful cracks in the corners of the mouth and on the lips and a sore mouth and tongue. The tongue may turn magenta, and greasy (seborrhoeal) patches may appear around the nose and in the area between the nose and the lips.

A good source of B2 is cheese, and I am always reminded of the fact when I come across cases of cracked skin by Wallace's immortal lines 'Cracking cheese, Grommit'

EYES

Have you become sensitive to bright lights?

*You may have a deficiency in **Vitamin B2***

Vitamin B2, or Riboflavin, is necessary for healthy skin and eyes. It is important in the prevention and treatment of cataracts. B2 also facilitates the use of oxygen by the tissues of the skin, nails and hair.

Symptoms of vitamin B2 deficiency include sensitivity or inflammation of the mucous membranes of the mouth; cracks or sores at the corners of the mouth, called cheilosis; a red, sore tongue; eye redness or sensitivity to light, burning eyes, eye fatigue, or a dry, sandy feeling of the eyes; fatigue and/or dizziness; dermatitis with a dry yet greasy or oily scaling; nervous tissue damage; and retarded growth in infants and children.

Cataracts may occur more frequently when you are B2 deficiency. So don't overlook these symptoms, because they could have long term consequences. Hair loss, weight loss, general lack of vitality, and digestive problems are also possible with depletion or deficiency states of vitamin B2.

Deficiency of vitamin B2 occurs with diets that are low in B2, in crash diets for weight loss, poor eating when you have ulcers, or treatment of diabetes. Nowadays we should include the diets of people who have bad eating habits and consume mostly refined foods and fast foods. B2 deficiency is also more commonly seen in persons with alcohol problems, in the elderly and the poor, and in depressed patients.

Foods rich in vitamin B2 include liver, yeast, meat, fish, eggs, vegetables, dairy foods and grain products. Types of food containing vitamin B2 include the following:

- Liver, beef kidneys, chicken, turkey, fish.
- Eggs, cheese, milk, yoghurt.
- Leafy green vegetables, asparagus, artichokes, avocados, broccoli, Brussels sprouts, dndelion greens, watercress, currants, spinach, kelp, peas, navy beans, lima beans, pumpkins, sweet potatoes, cayenne, parsley, sage, rose hips.
- Whole-grain breads, enriched breads, fortified cereals.
- Mushrooms, nuts, molasses.

The Body Language of Health

Strange but true

Pirates used to wear an eye patch not because they had eye damage, but in order to make their covered eye more sensitive for navigating at night on the high seas. At night they would remove their eye patch to expose their sensitised 'night vision' eye to hunt out wealthy merchant vessels. Modern soldiers are taught the same technique to improve their night sight, even though most sophisticated armies now have infra-red night goggles.

Pirates often seem to be associated with parrots, and I wondered whether the eye patch was to protect them from the beak of the parrot sitting on their shoulder. A reader of the Body Language website put me right on that score, apparently the parrot was worth a lot of money when the pirate king returned back to shore, that is why pirates were often associated with parrots. It was their extra perk at the end of the voyage to raise more money; useful because the sale of his parrot could pay for the cleaning bill for his jacket.

The eye's response to light is remarkable. It can now be used to diagnose many medical conditions, such as diabetes, schizophrenia etc. A new device called an Eyecheck pupillometer monitors the eye response to a flash of light, and diagnoses a number of medical conditions from the response. It is also accurately able to detect the effects of drugs, alcohol, and even fatigue. Apparently the effect of 18 hours without sleep is equivalent to the legal driving limit of alcohol. In other words if you have been up for 18 hours and are driving you have a similar speed of response to a drunken driver. Police take this so seriously that they are considering using pupillometry as a measure of fitness to drive.

I have been looking down microscopes all of my career and when I used a pupillometer I found the mechanism that dilates and contracts the pupil was faulty in my left eye. Maybe that is something to do with the fact that my earlier microscopes had a single eyepiece so I had to screw the faulty eye up and use only the other one. I assume Patrick Moore has a similar problem from looking through a telescope because he now wears a monocle and has a permanent squint.

Supplemental riboflavin is commonly used to treat and help prevent visual problems, eye fatigue, and cataracts. It seems to help with burning eyes, excess tear formation (watery eyes), and decreased vision resulting from eye strain. Riboflavin is also used for many kinds of stress conditions, fatigue, and vitality or growth problems. For people with allergies and chemical sensitivities, riboflavin-5-phosphate may be more readily assimilated than riboflavin.

Do you have cataracts?

You may be deficient in CHROMIUM or have excess FREE RADICALS

We've already talked about cataracts and how you can help to prevent them. Here, we look at your deficiencies if you have cataracts. Before we start, let's have a look at what a cataract is.

A cataract is a cloudiness in the lens of the eye caused by damage to the protein of the lens. This damage impairs vision. Cataracts are more likely to occur in those who smoke, have diabetes, or are exposed to excessive sunlight because all of these factors lead to oxidative damage. Oxidative damage to the lens of the eye appears to cause cataracts in people and also in animals, though I have never seen an animal wearing sunglasses yet.

Vitamin C is one of the strongest antioxidants, so that is probably why people with low vitamin C levels have 11 times the normal risk of cataracts. A recent study investigated the relationship of vitamin supplements and cataract formation. The study involved 350 men and women who were given supplements of both vitamin E and vitamin C. Results showed that the consumption of these supplementary vitamins reduced the risk of senile cataracts by about 50%

Although it may sound obvious, age is the biggest risk factor in age-related eye disease. As we get older the changes in our body processes also affect our eyes and this may be cumulative.

Oxygen is essential for the human body, but it can also be harmful. Just as steel gets oxidised and forms rust, so oxygen produces free-radicals in the body which damage cells or prevent them from regenerating properly. This cell regeneration process is affected progressively as we get older due to free radicals and other age-related factors.

A free radical is simply a chemical that has free bonds so it is very active, attaching itself to anything convenient, like a cell wall. Oxygen free radicals want to 'oxidise' whatever they come into contact with.

Our bodies do have natural protective systems against the effect of free radicals, but under certain conditions this protection is not good enough.

The Body Language of Health

Free radicals damage the retina, a light sensitive layer at the back of the eye. They also affect the lens, a clear tissue found behind the coloured part of the eye known as the iris. The lens helps to focus light onto the retina which then sends an image of what we are looking at to our brain. This is how we see. Mostly, these free radicals are neutralised by the body's defences. Many vitamins and minerals can help the body and our eyes to combat the effects of free radicals.

A recent study showed that substances found in leafy green vegetables helped to protect eye cells from damage by ultraviolet (UV) light. UV light is thought to be a major cause of cataracts. This study found that two antioxidants called lutein and zeaxanthin, as well as vitamin E, protected the eyes from UV light.

Lutein and zeaxanthin are found in green vegetables such as kale, spinach and collard greens. So you should include them in your diet to help protect your eyes.

Do you have dark rings under your eyes?

You may have an ALLERGY

This Body Language sign appeared under 'skin' but is worth reiterating here, not least because allergies are so common these days.

Allergies are widespread and affect approximately one in four of the population in the UK at some time in their lives. Each year the numbers are increasing by 5% with as many as half of all those affected being children. At this rate we will soon all be allergic to something.

Allergic reactions are caused by substances in the environment known as allergens. Almost anything can be an allergen for someone. Allergens nearly always contain protein; this is not surprising since antibodies are proteins too. There are some non-protein allergens which include drugs such as penicillin. For these to cause an allergic response they usually need to be bound to a protein once they are in the body.

The most common allergens are pollen from trees and grasses, house dust mite, moulds, pets such as cats and dogs or cagebirds, insects like wasps and bees, industrial and household chemicals, medicines, and foods such as milk and eggs. Less common allergens include nuts, fruit and latex.

The most common symptoms are: Sneezing, runny nose, itchy eyes and ears, severe wheezing, coughing shortness of breath, sinus problems, a sore palate and nettle-like rash.

It should be understood that all the symptoms mentioned can be caused by factors other than allergy. Indeed some of the conditions are diseases in themselves. Asthma, eczema, headaches, lethargy, loss of concentration and sensitivity to everyday foods represent a huge problem in society today. You should try an exclusion diet to identify your allergens; this is explained in the 'Do you have Eczema' section.

Do you have BLONDE HAIR AND BLUE EYES?

You may be deficient in ZINC, MAGNESIUM, Vitamin B6 and ESSENTIAL FATTY ACIDS

Genetically, blue-eyed blondes have a greater tendency towards hyperactivity and certain deficiencies unless the diet is well balanced. This lack of pigment seems to be genetically linked to particular dietary deficiencies. (Hyperactive boys are often blonde with blue eyes)

The diagnosis for hyperactivity that appears to work best is to do a Connor's score. This is a very simple check list which works well in clinical practice and has been widely used for research purposes. You can do this test at home. In fact it has been found that if the parents do the scoring, then make the diagnosis, they are more trusting of the result, whereas if the doctor does the scoring the parents are more likely to deny that a positive result relates to their offspring.

All you do to calculate your Connors score is to answer the following questions. Score 0 for not at all, score 1 for sometimes, score 2 for quite often, and score 3 for a lot.

Would you say yes or no to the following statements about your child:

- Restless or overactive
- Excitable or impulsive
- Disturbs other children
- Fails to finish things
- Short attention span

- Constantly fidgeting
- Inattentive, easily distracted
- Makes demands that must be met right away
- Easily frustrated
- Cries often and without provocation
- Mood changes quickly and dramatically
- Temper outbursts
- Explosive and unpredictable behaviour

A score of 15 or more suggests that hyperactivity is likely

Hyperactive children always appear to be zinc deficient so add plenty of zinc rich foods and get rid of the junk food. They are also often thirsty which can be a sign of deficiency of essential fatty acids. Another Body Language sign is 'chicken skin' over the elbows and back of the upper arms.

Elimination diets are essential to help you identify what is causing this effect. But if you think this is too drastic for your troublesome child, you can try a step by step progression:

- Cut out all sugar in the diet. Don't forget to cut out sweetened drinks, added sugar in cereals, cakes etc
- Cut out all artificial colourings, flavourings, additives, E numbers, preservatives etc. This was the basis of the Feingold diet which has already helped many hyperactive children.
- Cut out all stimulants particularly caffeine in tea, cola, chocolate and all 'sports drinks' such as Red Bull.
- Cut out foods which the child has a particular liking for. For some reason concentrated blackcurrant juice is a common offender.
- Do an elimination diet such as the stone age diet described elsewhere.

Expect a response within a week for any dietary change except in the case of wheat and dairy products. Often these cause delayed reactions and the diet must be enforced for one month. It will be hell, but remember your child has the rest of their life in front of them. Do a good chemical clean up as chemical sensitivity is a common cause of hyperactivity. This means avoiding any processed foods, and exposure to toxins.

Some children are sensitive to salicylates and respond to a low salicylate diet (there is a section on salicylates in this book to help you identify foods containing salicylates).

Consider an anti-fungal regime - many children seem to react in an almost allergic way to yeast in the gut. Do this by cutting out all yeast, fermented products and sugar.

After this regime for a month try the Conor's score again, being honest about any changes that you have seen. Then if you really want to you can introduce certain things one by one and see if you notice any difference, though your child will actually be much better off without the things you have persevered to remove from their diet.

Do you have dry eyes?

If you have, you may be deficient in VITAMIN A

Globally, 3 million children suffer clinical Vitamin A deficiency, exhibiting the signs and symptoms of eye damage and xerophthalmia. However, the full magnitude of Vitamin A deficiency often remains hidden: an estimated 140-250 million children under five years of age are at risk of sub-clinical Vitamin A deficiency, mainly in Asia and Africa. Though showing none of the ocular signs or symptoms at this age, these children suffer a dramatically increased risk of death and illness, particularly from measles and diarrhoea, as a consequence of Vitamin A deficiency.

Long known to be a principle cause of childhood blindness (250,000 to 500,000 children lose their sight each year), Vitamin A deficiency is now recognized as a major contributing factor in an estimated 1-3 million child deaths each year.

In the developing world, the simple provision of high-dose vitamin A supplements every 4-6 months not only protects against blindness but also has been repeatedly shown to have a dramatic and multiple impact on the health of young children in the age range 6 months to 5 years:

- Overall, all-cause mortality is reduced by 23%
- Measles mortality is reduced by 50%
- Diarrhoeal mortality is reduced by 33%
- 85% coverage can result in a 90% reduction in severe xerophthalmia

The Body Language of Health

Vitamin A and Malaria: A recent study in Papua New Guinea found that when young children were given vitamin A supplements three times a year they had 30% fewer malaria attacks and the number of malaria parasites in their blood dropped by 36%.

Vitamin A and HIV/AIDS: Trials are currently on-going to determine if vitamin A supplementation can reduce the mother-to-child transmission of HIV during lactation.

How can this be?

Most of us in the West have no idea just how poor the diet is for the majority of people in the world, who survive on one or two simple staple foods like rice, sorghum or millet and usually nothing else. I remember travelling to China for the first time. Not the tourist centres like the Great Wall, but the developing industrial areas out in the country. I travelled with a colleague from work and we were the first Europeans that most people had seen and they just stood and stared at us. At that time their meagre diet was anything that grew, moved or squeaked. And the greeting that one peasant gave to another was the Chinese equivalent of 'are you hungry?' at a time when people still starved to death. This is still the daily situation for millions of people.

Good sources of Vitamin A are eggs, milk, liver and fresh, colourful vegetables

Vitamin A is a family of fat-soluble vitamins. Retinol is one of the most active, or usable, forms of vitamin A, and is found in animal foods such as liver and eggs and in some fortified food products. Retinol is named after the vitamin that improves eyesight.

Retinol is often called 'preformed vitamin A'. It can be converted to retinal and retinoic acid, other active forms of the vitamin A family. Some plant foods contain darkly coloured pigments called provitamin-A carotenoids that can be converted to vitamin A.

Beta-carotene is a provitamin-A carotenoid that is more efficiently converted to retinol than other carotenoids.

Vitamin A plays an important role in vision, bone growth, reproduction, cell division and cell differentiation, which is the process by which a cell decides what organ or type of tissue it is going to develop into. This is clearly vital if you are pregnant, but we are all having our cells regenerated all the time throughout our lives. In fact this process ensures we get a new body every seven years or so. I'm hoping to get mine next week.

Vitamin A helps maintain the surface linings of the eyes and the respiratory, urinary, and intestinal tracts. When those linings break down, bacteria can enter the body and cause infection. Vitamin A also helps maintain the integrity of skin and mucous membranes that function as a barrier to bacteria and viruses.

Vitamin A also helps regulate the immune system. The immune system helps prevent or fight off infections by making white blood cells that destroy harmful bacteria and viruses. Vitamin A may help lymphocytes, a type of white blood cell that fights infections, function more effectively.

Some carotenoids, in addition to serving as a source of vitamin A, have been shown to function as antioxidants in laboratory tests. However, this role has not been consistently proven in humans. Antioxidants protect cells from free radicals, which are potentially damaging by-products of oxygen metabolism that may contribute to the development of some chronic diseases.

So overall, deficiency of vitamin A could be something to cry about.

Dry eyes may also be indicative of an allergy. Review further information under 'Do you rub your eyes?'

Do you have poor vision and night blindness?

You may be deficient in VITAMIN A and ZINC

It is said that just a single raw carrot a day reduces a person's risk of macular degeneration by 40 percent. Evidence suggests that more is even better.

Reading this Body Language sign now could save your eyesight later, if it convinces you to eat a raw carrot every day.

We've all known since we were toddlers that "carrots are good for our eyes." What's staggering is that nearly one in four of us in the Western world won't have eaten even a single serving of any vegetable today. That alone would rectify most of the 10 million cases of macular degeneration in America.

A lack of antioxidants in the diet puts the retina at risk, causing premature aging and deterioration. Therefore, consuming generous amounts of the body's principle protective antioxidants, namely vitamins C and E, the carotenes, and small amounts of the mineral, selenium, will help protect your sight. Start now, for macular degeneration is the number one cause of vision loss in the elderly.

Our body gets vitamin A only when we eat foods containing this vitamin. Lack of vitamin A causes eye diseases, and it has been claimed that vitamin A is the single greatest preventable cause of childhood blindness in the world. People most at risk are children between six months to six years, pregnant women, and women who are breast feeding.

Why is Vitamin A important?

Vitamin A maintains healthy cells in various structures of the eye and is required for converting light into nerve signals in the part of the eye called the retina. When vitamin A is not available to the body, gradual changes begin to affect the eye. The first sign of a problem is when a child or a pregnant or a breast feeding woman finds it difficult to adjust to seeing in the dark. This condition is called night blindness.

What are the symptoms of lack of Vitamin A?

Vitamin A deficiency progresses slowly, causing more and more damage to the eye as the days go by. This condition is called Xerophthalmia, a name which describes a range of disorders affecting your eyes.

The symptoms are as follows:

Night blindness:
>   Vision is very poor in the dim light or twilight. Night blindness is also found in pregnant women, especially during the last trimester of pregnancy when vitamin A requirements are increased.

Bitot Spots:
>   These are foamy and whitish cheese-like tissue spots that develop around the eye ball, causing severe dryness in the eyes. These spots do not affect eye sight in the day light.

Blindness:
>   In severe cases, once dry eyes set in, the eye becomes very sensitive and begins to scratch and scar. The eyelids become swollen and sticky. This eventually leads to blindness. Once blindness occurs, it cannot be reversed.

Other symptoms of deficiency:
> When the body lacks vitamin A, the systems that resist infection and disease do not work very well. That is why children with Vitamin A deficiency fall sick more often, take much longer to recover and are more likely to die. Problems with bones and teeth can also frequently occur.

How common is Vitamin A deficiency?

Vitamin A deficiency is believed to cause 350,000 children to go blind each year. About 140 million children in 118 countries are Vitamin A deficient and 1 in 4 child deaths are caused by Vitamin A deficiency. It is estimated that 30% of the world's blindness is due to vitamin A deficiency. In addition to this, 600,000 women die during child birth due to complications from vitamin A deficiency.

What are Vitamin A-rich foods?

Sources of vitamin A can be divided into two groups: one is animal source, and the other is vegetable source. Vitamin A is better absorbed from an animal source, but when it is not possible to buy meat, or for vegetarians, vitamin A derived from vegetable sources are sufficient to supply our daily needs.

Examples of animal food sources are as follows:

- Liver
- Fish liver oil
- Egg yolk
- Milk and milk products
- Breast milk
- Butter
- Small fish

Examples for vegetable sources are as follows:

- Dark green leaves
- Natural plant oils
- Yellow and orange vegetables (like carrot, sweet potatoes, yellow yam)
- Yellow and orange fruits (like papaya, mangoes)

The Body Language of Health

With so many foods available, why is it that so many people are deficient? Well, we have to appreciate that half of the world's population is starving to death while statistics show the other half throw away 40% of the food they grow or buy.

If you have already been diagnosed with the condition, your doctor has probably told you that there is no medical treatment that can help you. If so, then there is no reason not to try nutrition. If antioxidants can prevent macular degeneration, larger amounts of them may help reverse it.

The theory is easy enough to test, and safe enough to trust. There are no toxic levels whatsoever for Vitamins E and C and carotene. (Too much Vitamin C is indicated by very loose bowels, that's all). Excessive carotene, which is the orange colour in carrots, is indicated by orange coloured skin. Vitamin E is so safe that premature babies are given it to prevent oxygen damage of their retinas.

Selenium increases the effectiveness of Vitamin E in the body. Only a little selenium is needed. If you have mercury fillings your probably depleted in selenium (see 'Do you have mercury fillings?'). But like all the other trace elements, too much selenium can be toxic, so limit the amount you consume to no more than 600 micrograms daily.

Zinc is another important mineral for the retina. Up to 660 milligrams of zinc a day has been used in some retina studies, but there is an eventual risk of copper deficiency and anaemia if such a high level is maintained. Just one-fifth of that amount, about 100 mg per day, may be enough to slow or stop the process of macular degeneration. The amino acid chelate form of zinc is very well absorbed and is probably the one to go for. Or you could eat a lot of molluscs (oysters in particular) and pep up your sex life as well.

Zinc deficiency in America is the rule, not the exception, because most Americans don't even consume the recommended minimum of 15 mg per day. Zinc deficiency is especially prevalent in older people. The signs of too little zinc in the diet are, curiously enough, a weak immune system, poor wound healing, loss of taste and smell, psoriasis-like skin lesions, prostate problems, rheumatoid arthritis, and senility. Have you visited a nursing home recently? The idea of zinc supplementation certainly hasn't.

Instead of beta carotene supplements, I would recommend carrot juice. Not only does it contain a great deal of beta carotene, but it also contains numerous other carotenes, not just the common beta-carotene which is what everybody is referring to when they call it carotene. Freshly made from your own juicer, raw carrot juice tastes good and provides many other valuable nutrients and plenty of fibre. All health maniacs drink carrot juice, so you are in good company.

In addition to carrots, really intense consumption of fresh, raw foods may help much more, and there have been astonishing reports of eyesight returning to near-blind people after this treatment. The internet records the following story.

'I know of a person whose degeneration of the retina was very severe and sadly she had lost much of her sight. In desperation, she began a nearly 100% raw food diet. She ate mostly salads and a helping or two of home-grown sprouts a day. I won't say that she loved doing it, but she loved the results. Over a period of a year or so, her ophthalmologist confirmed her improvement. Not only was she no longer losing her sight, she was actually gaining it back. Her recovery was remarkable and, medically speaking, impossible.'

Incidentally, the story was put about in the last world war that the British Royal Air Force was so good at shooting down enemy aircraft at night because the Spitfire pilots ate a lot of carrots. It gave them exceptionally good eyesight. But this was a smokescreen to hide the fact that Britain had invented Radar – giving the pilots super night-vision and the ability to see planes approaching many miles away. However even though the carrots story was a smokescreen, carrots are still nevertheless jolly good for eyesight.

Do you rub your eyes?

You could have a stress or a sleep problem

When you rub your eyes it stimulates the ocularcardio reflex, applying pressure around the rectus muscles that move the eyeball. This causes a response in the vagus nerve, through their close association. This stimulation lowers heart rate.

So we rub our eyes in order to slow our heart and metabolism down to prepare our body for sleep. Producing a vagus response in this manner from pressure round the eyes is used in martial arts, massage, hypnotism, and is a method of disabling violent prisoners/patients (sometimes even to the degree of inducing a faint).

The Body Language of Health

For most people, this relaxation technique feels good, and may be why stressed people often gain benefit from rubbing their eyes and face with their hands, especially after a stressful telephone call, meeting or uncomfortable confrontation. It is a calming, relaxing action. You could try practising this technique if you are an insomniac.

Eyes and allergies

Many people with eye-rubbing problems also have dry eyes, that can be associated with an allergy. The more inflamed any tissue gets, the more it itches - this is called the itch/scratch/itch cycle that doesn't stop until damage has been done and in extreme cases the skin starts to bleed if the itch is in an exposed area.

In a recent survey 42% of eye care professionals said they have seen an increase in the number Age Related Macular Degeneration sufferers in the past five years. The survey revealed just how importantly optometrists and dispensing opticians regard the role of nutrition and a good diet in maintaining eye health.

An overwhelming 90% of respondents believe that good diet/nutrition is crucial in maintaining eye health, with 58% attributing the general deterioration in eye health to factors that could be linked to poor nutrition.

Over 50% of those opticians surveyed confirmed they do discuss the importance of nutrition and a good diet with patients who suffer from age-related eye conditions.

Despite this, no-one seems to be telling us EXACTLY what we need to eat. As we have seen, 'a healthy diet' is not good advice. So what do we need to eat to maintain good eyesight?

Primarily, we need plenty of Vitamin A, chromium, and zinc. Plenty of greens, and orange or red fruits and vegetables. Tiny amounts of selenium, and all the other trace elements. In fact, the prehistoric diet we talked about earlier.

It is worth taking a leaf out of the US Airways in-flight manual, which lists 'Superfoods' American style. The descriptions are theirs.

Salmon. This is a great source of omega 3 fatty acids which can help prevent Alzheimer's, obesity, sunburn and even depression.

The Body Language of Health

Blueberries. This fruit is rich in fibre, vitamin C, and antioxidants. Studies show consumption may improve motor skills and memory.

Cinnamon. This can help reduce blood sugar levels in diabetics. It's also an antibacterial. And smelling it is said to result in a 'brain boost'.

Kale. Loaded with beta carotene to keep eyes healthy, this leafy green also contains organosulphuric compounds that help fight off certain cancers.

Pumpkin. The potent antioxidants in this vegetable have been found to reduce the risk of several types of cancer as well as heart disease and cataracts. And it is high in vitamin A and carotenoids.

Soya. This bean's protein has been hailed for lowering cholesterol and the risk of osteoporosis, Alzheimer's, certain cancers, and kidney disease. It is also said to reduce the effects of the menopause.

Walnuts. The monosaturated (good) fats found in walnuts are believed to reverse some of the effects of eating food that is high in saturated (bad) fats. Plus, they are loaded with plant-based omega 3 fatty acids.

Avocado. The combination of fat, protein and carbohydrate is ideal in this fruit. It is also high in glutathione, which blocks up to thirty different carcinogens.

Oats. They're full of both types of fibre. Soluble fibre helps reduce cholesterol and keeps the heart healthy, and insoluble fibre supports the digestive system.

Dark chocolate. Rich in flavonols that boost the production of nitric oxide in blood vessels, this type of chocolate can lower blood pressure and improve circulation.

Good advice from an American source, for a change.

NOSE

Do you have a crease on the end of your nose?

You probably have an Allergy

In infants and young children, nose congestion may appear as mouth-breathing, sniffing, snuffling, snorting or snoring, and nose rubbing. I have noticed many young children these days habitually breathing through their mouth, most probably due to milk allergy.

The habitual nose rubbing that usually accompanies this problem is sometimes known as "the allergic salute" - pushing the nose up with the palm of the hand until a crease develops across the skin of the nose. Doing this often enough results in a turned up nose with a crease above the tip.

The nose is the most sensitive part of your body to allergens because 2,000 gallons of air pass through this tiny passageway every day.

Congestion or inflammation of the nose (rhinitis), sinuses (sinusitis), and throat (pharyngitis) may be due to airborne irritants and allergens; however, food allergy is also likely to be supplying the underlying allergen and will be the undiagnosed cause of all these common problems.

Nasal stuffiness, snoring, increased mucus flow in nose and throat and recurrent sore throats are often due to allergies. Recurrent middle ear "infections" are very common in young children and have been successfully treated by removing milk, wheat, and eggs from the diet.

More about Allergies

Many studies have reported that a majority of Chronic Fatigue Syndrome (CFS) patients have allergies to foods, pollen, metals (such as nickel or mercury), or other substances. One theory is that allergens, like viral infections, may trigger a cascade of immune abnormalities leading to CFS. (Most allergic people, though, do not appear to have CFS.)

The Body Language of Health

Some research indicates that people with both allergies and emotional disorders, such as anxiety or depression, may be more vulnerable to the effects of the inflammatory response, a harmful overreaction of the immune system that can cause fatigue, joint aches, and fever as well as hormone and brain chemical disturbances.

One theory that may help tie in some of the various factors common to CFS suggests that allergies, stress, and infections may deplete a chemical in the body called adenosine triphosphate (ATP). This chemical stores energy in cells, and studies have reported a deficiency in many CFS patients.

Supporting this theory was a study in which patients reported reduced CFS symptoms after they took a vitamin-like supplement called NADH, which increases ATP levels.

Do you have poor sense of smell and taste?

If you have, you may be deficient in ZINC

Zinc deficiency suppresses taste and smell and leads to loss of appetite. The reason is that zinc is essential for the taste perception is because taste is mediated through a salivary zinc-dependent polypeptide called gustin, therefore low salivary zinc levels invariably leads to a reduction of taste.

Zinc is known to alter taste and smell and zinc deficiency is thought to be a factor in some cases of anorexia and bulimia, because a deficiency removes the appeal of food. Fortunately zinc deficiencies are generally short-term, and symptoms can be quickly relieved by restoring adequate zinc in the diet. But of course anyone with an eating disorder won't receive this. So these people should be encouraged to try a zinc supplement.

If on a long term basis you don't smell things as well as you once did, there could be many explanations. Advancing age can be a contributing factor, possibly because infection has taken its toll or because you've sniffed too many noxious fumes (such as sewage works) over the years. Moreover, you shouldn't be surprised if you temporarily lose your sense of smell because you've had an infection such as a bad cold.

A head injury is another possible cause of loss of smell if the delicate nerves leading from your nose to your brain are damaged. Also, certain prescription drugs can rob you of some ability to enjoy subtle fragrances such as flowers, perfume, or fresh-baked food.

As smell diminishes, your sense of taste may suffer, too. The two senses are so closely related that people who complain of not being able to smell often say that they also have trouble tasting. I am sure we are all too familiar with the problems of a stuffed up nose when we have a cold, during which time everything seems to taste very bland, showing that smell and taste are closely linked.

Do you have nasal polyps?

You may be sensitive to SALICYLATE

Salicylate is the basis of aspirin, or *acetylsalicylic acid*. But salicylates occur naturally in many plants used as foods (e.g., strawberries, almonds, tomatoes) as well as the witch hazel bark from which aspirin was first isolated and used medically. Before that, witch hazel was widely known as nature's painkiller. Methyl salicylate is the main component of wintergreen, sweet birch, gaultheria, and betula oils; the compound is used in rubbing liniment to soothe muscular aches as well as being used as a flavouring in mentholated sweets.

Sodium salicylate, traditionally used in the treatment of arthritis, is also used in dyes and as a non-edible preservative. Salicylates act as preservatives to delay rotting, that's why many plants manufacture them to protect the plant against harmful bacteria and fungi. Salicylates are stored in the bark, leaves, roots, and seeds of plants.

The use of salicylate dates back 2500 years to when Hippocrates recommended the use of willow bark to relieve the pain of childbirth. Salicylic acid is the extract from willow bark that produces the analgesic effect. Today, salicylate is used in many over-the-counter and prescription medications for their analgesic, anti-inflammatory, and antipyretic properties.

Salicylate ingestion of over-the-counter medication was a common cause of poisoning and death in children in the United States prior to the 1970s, when legislation was passed requiring childproof packaging on medications. Despite the reduction of poisonings because of repackaging, salicylate toxicity remains a significant cause of death.

Some people develop a sensitivity to salicylates. This is more usually due to the body's inability to handle more than a certain amount of salicylate at any one time. A salicylate-sensitive person may have difficulty tolerating certain fruits, vegetables, or any products which contain salicylate, but they are much more likely to have intolerance to the wide range of manufactured products that currently use salicylates as preservatives.

Symptoms of Intolerance

Salicylates sensitivity can manifest itself in a huge number of ways:

- Anaphylaxis (very rare)
- Asthma
- Breathing difficulties
- Changes in skin colour
- Congestion
- Fatigue
- Headaches
- Hyperactivity
- Itchy skin, rash, or hives
- Itchy, watery, or swollen eyes
- Lack of concentration or memory
- Mouth ulcers or raw hot red rash around mouth
- Nasal polyps
- Persistent cough
- Sinusitis
- Some cognitive and perceptual disorders
- Stomach aches or upsets
- Swelling of eyelids, face, and lips
- Swelling of hands and feet
- Urgency to pass water or bedwetting
- Wheezing

Sources of Salicylates

Here is a list of the many products that may contain aspirin or salicylate compounds. Most have salicylates as preservatives in their formulation.

- Acne products
- Breath fresheners
- Bubble baths
- Cosmetics
- Fragrances and perfumes
- Chewing gums - mint flavoured
- Hair shampoos, conditioners, or sprays
- Herbal remedies
- Lipsticks
- Lotions
- Lozenges
- Medications
- Mouth washes
- Muscle pain creams
- Pain medications
- Medicated razors
- Shaving creams
- Skin cleansers or exfoliants
- Sun screens or tanning lotions
- Supplements derived from rose hips or bioflavonoids
- Topical creams
- Toothpastes
- Wart or callus removers

Quite a list, isn't it? Now some people know they are salicylate intolerant – they can't take aspirin or any pain killer product that contains aspirin (Acetyl salicylic acid). But these people are not usually aware that salicylates are in so many manufactured products that come into contact with the skin. Just goes to show it always pays to read the label.

Do you get a blocked nose after drinking red wine?

If you do, you may be deficient in MOLYBDENUM

The reason for this Body Language symptom may be sulphites. Sulphur-containing compounds called sulphites are used as a preservative in wines. Molybdenum helps convert potentially harmful sulphites into taurine, a beneficial amino acid. But if you are deficient in molybdenum, these sulphites become bronchial irritants.

Molybdenum deficiency may be implicated in asthma or other symptoms associated with sulphite sensitivity because of its involvement with sulphur. Molybdenum deficiency may also be responsible for sulphite sensitivity since it is a cofactor for sulphite oxidase. Sulphite oxidase catalyses the last step (sulphites to sulphates) in the breakdown of sulphur amino acids.

It may be wise to balance molybdenum supplementation with copper supplements, since one can cause a deficiency of the other. It should be noted that if your copper level is too high this can drive molybdenum levels down. Note also that copper can be harmful in excess.

Sulphites in the urine are claimed to be indicative of molybdenum deficiency.

VITAMIN D and ASTHMA

Researchers in this field say that Vitamin D could be used to prevent thousands life-threatening asthma attacks in the event that steroid treatments do not take effect, after research showed that vitamin D3 could substantially improve a patient's responsiveness to steroid treatments.

Conversely, if you are an asthmatic, how about taking a high dose of Vitamin D and seeing if your asthma is more manageable?

EARS

Do you have a crease on your earlobe?

You may be susceptible to cardiovascular disease

At least 30 different studies have shown that a diagonal crease across the earlobe is a highly accurate sign of increased risk for heart attack. Typically the presence of a crease across one earlobe was associated with a 33% increase in the risk of heart attack and this rose to 77% if both earlobes were creased.

It appears that chronic circulatory problems cause the blood vessels in the fleshy part of the earlobe to collapse. This then causes swelling of the tissue and creates a crease in the earlobe. In fact in most people a diagonal earlobe crease is a more accurate predictor of sudden death from heart attack than age, smoking, weight, high cholesterol, or lifestyle factors. Incidentally, be sure to read the section on cholesterol as it busts a few myths about low cholesterol being bad for you.

You should therefore definitely take notice of your own ears, and try to take steps to improve your risk factors if you do happen to have an earlobe crease or two.

This Body Language sign doesn't quite apply to everybody, however. For some reason a creased earlobe doesn't indicate an increase in the risk of heart attack in Asians and Native Americans.

There is some conflicting research that seems to suggest that earlobe creases become more common in older people, and that increasing age, not the presence of creases, accounts for this increased risk of heart disease. Other genetic factors such as race and earlobe shape may also determine the ease with which the earlobe creases and whether it appears in childhood or adulthood. Nevertheless, taking notice of your earlobe creases and doing something about it won't do any harm and could be the biggest health step you ever take in your (freshly extended) life.

Cardiovascular disease is a major killer in the West and there has been more written about it than any other disease. You would think this should make research of the subject for this book child's play. Not so, this has been one of the more difficult sections to compile. I must have researched around 200 websites and at least as many 'high quality' professional links in journals and medical and nutrition books on heart disease. The variations in advice makes it difficult to judge what is right. Low salt, high salt, low sodium, high sodium, low cholesterol, high cholesterol, homocysteine; the list is virtually endless.

In the finish, I took the middle ground to tell you the low down on heart disease, diet and cholesterol.

Confused about what food is best for health and stable weight?

I would suggest you follow this golden rule. The more natural the food, the better. Natural food is not absolutely perfect, nor is it likely to be 100 per cent natural, but it's LESS likely to be fattening and MORE likely to be healthy.

'Natural' Foods include:

- Fresh fruit
- Fresh vegetables, including potatoes
- Fresh fish
- Wholegrain muesli (no sugar)
- Nuts, seeds
- Whole meal or wholegrain bread
- Brown rice
- Bottled water
- Cheeseburgers (Whoops! Just kidding)

Diet is of primary importance to your well-being, together with regular exercise. The Western diet is often criticised as being too low in fibre, folic acid, fruit and vegetables, and too high in saturated fats and refined carbohydrates and sugar. Even adolescents are showing a worryingly high proportion of cardiovascular damage due to their inappropriate diet and lack of exercise.

A sensible diet to contribute to heart health is generally accepted as being one based on the Mediterranean model, which is also found to be ideal to avoid insulin resistance and diabetes. This diet includes plenty of leafy green vegetables, unsalted nuts, seeds, pulses, soluble fibre, antioxidants and monounsaturated fats. Traditionally prepared Asian diets are also rich in fish, vegetables and cardio-protective spices, though this may not be true of the typical Indian takeaway, nor unfortunately the pizza parlours most of which use synthetic cheese and are a thousand miles away from a traditional Italian dish.

Cholesterol - the facts

I am afraid this advice is bound to be controversial. The fact is that we all need cholesterol. It plays a vital role in cell membranes and transports nutrients round the body. High cholesterol may or may not necessarily be a problem in the body, but the medical profession appears to have been driven by the pharmaceutical companies to focus on cholesterol reduction as a treatment using a drug group called statins.

Are Statins a good idea?

People are becoming increasingly aware of their cholesterol levels because doctors have been putting a lot of effort into reducing levels with statin drugs. But high cholesterol does not seem to be the real problem, just an indicator of the problem.

The main class of drugs currently used to reduce cholesterol in the body are the statins, but they have problems which are not generally voiced by the drug companies for obvious reasons. The main problem is that in many trials, while statins reduce the cholesterol level, they do not significantly reduce overall mortality - that is to say, people do not particularly live any longer when given statins. And the internet is awash with advice that tells us statins cause other health problems.

Researchers have also found that high cholesterol is not a risk factor for older people. On the contrary, many studies have found that elderly people with high cholesterol live the longest. So what on earth is going on here?

Statins work by inhibiting the enzyme that creates cholesterol, but it also incidentally inhibits the enzyme responsible for creation of selenium proteins. Selenium proteins such as glutathione peroxidase (a major antioxidant which protects against cancer), are essential for muscle function (selenium deficiency in sheep causes white muscle disease), and for heart function (selenium deficiency in humans causes Keshan's disease - a type of cardiomyopathy).

Statin use may also lead to muscle weakening, which is not a good thing for our most essential muscle, the heart. Muscle loss occurs because statins block the production of co-enzyme Q10, which is vital for the production of cell energy. Research shows marked reduction of coQ10 in patients on statin drugs. And statins appear to be particularly bad for chronic fatigue syndrome (CFS) sufferers because of their harmful effects on muscle metabolism.

The Body Language of Health

Where does Cholesterol come from?

Cholesterol is an essential constituent of the body. Around 80% of cholesterol in the blood is manufactured in the liver, only 20% comes from diet, so it is impossible to make much difference to the cholesterol levels simply through eating food low in cholesterol. A raised cholesterol is a bio-chemical symptom. That means it is indicative of a problem elsewhere in the body.

Cholesterol is a *lipid* which is just a fancy name for a fatty chain of atoms that can attach itself to nutrients and transport them round the body. Cholesterol works just like the washing up liquid you use to dissolve grease and oils from your dinner plates. Washing up liquid is a very clever molecule made up from a section that binds to fats, and a section that dissolves in water. The portion that binds to fats is called hydrophobic because it doesn't like water (but it loves fat) and the portion that dissolves in water is called hydrophilic (it loves water; hydro just means water, as in hydro-electric or in a British spa town, just 'Hydro'). Cholesterol is named after sterol which is derived from stearic acid. And stearic acid is the starting point for soap and detergent.

When you add washing up liquid to your dishwater, it dissolves in the water, thanks to that hydrophilic part, and the fat-busting hydrophobic part reaches out and attaches itself to the fat and grease, making them soluble and lifting the grease from your plate.

Cholesterol does something a bit similar in your body, attaching nutrients and delivering and releasing them to the cells. It does a wonderful job, but the problem is that although you get very little cholesterol-like 'lipids' from your food, it is nevertheless very important that you eat the right diet.

There are good cholesterols and bad cholesterols and it is a case of getting the right balance between them. There are literally thousands of different cholesterol lipids in your body, but they are grouped into high-density lipids (HDL) and low-density lipids (LDL). There are also ultra-low density lipids called triglycerides.

When you do a cholesterol test, you need to know your levels of HDL cholesterol, LDL cholesterol and triglycerides.

It has been decided that if your total cholesterol is unacceptably high and you have a low HDL, then this is a bad sign for your health. You'll now be prescribed statins. But the wrong ratio of cholesterol lipids is just a symptom of something else going wrong in your body. You're better to tackle these first.

The common causes of raised cholesterol are as follows:

1. **Borderline hypothyroidism.** Indeed, thirty years ago a raised cholesterol level was almost routinely treated with thyroid hormones. Mostly, you are probably deficient in iodine. Try mixing in dried seaweed with your salad, because seaweed is very high in iodine. The Japanese eat a lot of seaweed, and traditionally the Japanese have had a low rate of heart disease until recently when they changed to a Western diet.

2. **Vitamin D3 deficiency.** Cholesterol is the raw material that your body converts to Vitamin D through the action of sunshine on the skin. Your body monitors the level of Vitamin D3 because it is so important to the successful working of your cells, and when it perceives a deficiency in D3 (and this is almost universal in the British and Scandinavian climates), then the liver pushes out more cholesterol so that when ultraviolet radiation does land upon the skin, there is plenty of cholesterol for vitamin D3 to be made. All that extra cholesterol hangs around in your body waiting for you to throw off your clothes and go nude bathing, to soak up some sunshine. Vitamin D3 deficiency itself is a major risk factor for coronary heart disease.

3. **Vitamin B3 deficiency.** A small study of six patients with chronic fatigue syndrome have shown them all to be deficient in vitamin B3 (niacinamide) and it may well be that this deficiency is widespread in the general population. Indeed, before the advent of statins, vitamin B3 was widely used for the treatment of high cholesterol and it is still available on NHS prescription specifically for the treatment of high cholesterol. There are various forms of vitamin B3 and some, such as nicotinic acid, cause flushing of the skin which patients find embarrassing. This was an unacceptable side effect for some sufferers and so its use went out of fashion. However, niacinamide 500mg does not cause flushing, is extremely helpful for some patients with fatigue syndrome, and it certainly lowers cholesterol naturally.

4. **Copper deficiency.** There is an inverse relationship between cholesterol levels and copper - so the higher the copper level in the blood, the lower the level of cholesterol and vice versa. Furthermore, copper absorption is inhibited by zinc. Actually, the best test of copper status (and also zinc and manganese) is to measure levels of superoxide dismutase. This is one of the most important antioxidant enzymes. Superoxide dismutase crops up again later in cancer screening.

5. **Vanadium** deficiency may be implicated in a raised cholesterol, but there are only limited studies available and I would not recommend you go and buy a vanadium supplement because too much of it is a cause of manic

depression. But vanadium-rich foods are OK - foods rich in vanadium include mushrooms, shellfish, parsley, and a few special foods like black pepper and dill seed. Fruit and vegetables are generally low in vanadium. In fact vanadium is a strange element, which has been reported as having some unusual effects when deficient in some animals. For example goats fed a vanadium deficient diet were found to have high abortion rates, and almost half of the kids born were small and died within 3 months. But similar kids born to non-deficient mothers exhibited normal growth and had very low death rates. Presumably the same could apply to humans.

6. **Wrong ratio of omega 3 oils and omega 6 oils.** Eating too many omega 6 oils and not enough omega 3 oils upsets the balance of prostaglandins in your body and causes sticky plaques that gum up your cardiovascular system. More of that later.

There is some evidence that a high dose of vitamin C also reduces cholesterol levels. Clearly nutrients in food are very important, but you probably know that by now.

Here are some simple food choices you should make.

Eat more	Eat less or give up altogether
Garlic, porridge oats	coffee, fried food, white bread, pasta
Oily fish (mackerel, salmon, herring)	nicotine, excess alcohol
Unsalted nuts, seeds, olive oil	saturated/ hydrogenated oil and trans-fats
Blueberries, prunes, strawberries	processed food, biscuits, soft drinks
Fruit and vegetables	processed meats
Beans, pulses, wholegrains	sugar

Plant sterols are natural plant fats that are very similar to cholesterol and these foods are being suggested as beneficial additions to your diet, where they reduce the amount of animal cholesterol that is absorbed through your intestines from the meat in your diet. Sterols are present in pulses, peas, vegetables, nuts, seeds and vegetable oil. This is hardly ground breaking advice, however, as you should be including these in your diet anyway, instead of getting them from designer margarine.

There is now a huge market for plant sterols in spreads and processed foods but there is no substitute for a proper diet.

I discuss cholesterol more fully in 'Do you have High Cholesterol?

Do you have EXCESS EAR WAX?

You may be deficient in ESSENTIAL FATTY ACIDS

Essential Fatty Acids, or EFA's are - well, as the name suggests - essential. Excess ear wax is a classic symptom of deficiency in fatty acids, unless you actually have a troublesome ear infection.

Deficiency of EFA's can also cause dandruff.

Most people are deficient in EFA's to some degree or other. Our modern diet is lacking in the type of fats that are good for us, because the diet has been replaced with cheap oils and trans-fats that are indigestible and have the wrong EFA content.

EFA's are also damaged by processing in the manufacture of cooking oils, margarines, shortenings, partially hydrogenated vegetable oils, trans fatty acids, and are also damaged by sautéing, frying, and deep-frying in food preparation. We need to get our EFA's from food, not fat and oil.

Essential fatty acids include linoleic acid and arachidonic acid, which are omega-6 fatty acids, and linolenic acid, eicosapentaenoic acid, and docosahexaenoic acid, which are omega-3 fatty acids. In the body, arachidonic acid can be made from linoleic acid, and eicosapentaenoic and docosahexaenoic acids can be made from linolenic acid.

EFA's are needed for many physiologic processes, including maintaining the integrity of the skin and the structure of cell membranes and synthesizing prostaglandins and leukotrienes. Eicosapentaenoic acid and docosahexaenoic acid are important components of the brain and retina. See the Cholesterol section for more information.

Does your child have BEHAVIOURAL AND LEARNING PROBLEMS?

If you have excess ear wax, the chances are you have a diet low in EFA's. And if you have a diet low in EFA's then your children will probably have an even lower intake of EFA's than you. And children with low blood levels of essential omega-3 fatty acids, have a greater tendency to have problems with behaviour, learning and health consistent with attention deficit hyperactivity disorder (ADHD).

Or maybe they just take no notice of you because they can't hear you. They're so stuffed up with ear wax they appear to be deaf to your ranting and raving!!

Do you have tinnitus (ringing in the ears) or other hearing problems?

You might have a dietary deficiency or a blood disorder.

Tinnitus is the medical term for ringing in the ears, but tinnitus is rarely due to an actual sound, such as blood rushing through an enlarged vein—a problem that requires medical treatment. More commonly the problem is due to nerve irritation from an unknown source or an underlying ear problem often induced by noise damage.

Symptoms may include hearing buzzing, roaring, ringing, whistling, or hissing sounds. These sounds may be intermittent, continuous, or pulsing. Tinnitus might interfere with normal activities and sleep, and there may be an associated decrease in the ability to hear conversation or other sounds in the environment. Often, tinnitus produces a feeling of disassociation and confusion.

Ménière's disease is a condition characterized by tinnitus, vertigo, and hearing loss. Menieres disease is often associated with an inner ear infection, but the cause of the problem has not really been fully established, and there are many metabolic abnormalities, including elevations of serum cholesterol and/or triglycerides and abnormal regulation of blood sugar, that have been associated with the disease. In one trial, people with Ménière's disease who replaced refined carbohydrates in their diet with foods high in fibre and complex carbohydrates frequently experienced an improvement or disappearance of their tinnitus.

Here are some of the factors thought to be associated with Menieres disease and tinnitus.

- Iron deficiency
- Magnesium deficiency
- Vitamin A deficiency
- Vitamin B12 deficiency
- Vitamin D deficiency
- Zinc deficiency
- Excessive fat or excessive sugar in the diet
- Poor circulation of blood in the ears due to poor blood viscosity.

A number of sources suggest that nutritional supplements may be helpful. Zinc supplements have been used to treat people who had both tinnitus and hearing loss (usually age-related). Of those who had initially low blood levels of zinc, about 25% experienced an improvement in tinnitus after taking zinc (90-150 mg per day for three to six months). Two controlled clinical trials found no benefit from zinc supplementation in people with tinnitus. However, participants in these studies were not zinc deficient, so these results were not surprising. Research suggests that zinc supplementation is only helpful for tinnitus in people who are zinc deficient.

Decreased hearing ability associated with low vitamin A levels was found in a group of patients suffering from alcoholic liver disease. Animal studies have demonstrated degenerative changes in the ganglion cells on a vitamin A-deficient diet.

Some improvement in tinnitus and associated complaints were observed in 12 patients with low vitamin B12 levels following vitamin B12 replacement therapy.

In children with hearing losses, fluctuations in hearing ability appeared to vary according to their level of fat intake. Dietary changes led to a drop in cholesterol levels and a return to near normal hearing.

A number of papers have reported a 5 to 15 decibel improvement in the pure-tone threshold in patients with hearing loss supplemented with a combination of vitamins A and E.

Treatment of vitamin D deficiency in patients with hearing problems should prevent progressive hearing loss, which may be partially reversible, says one study.

In another study, Zinc supplements were given to tinnitus sufferers with low blood zinc levels, resulting in a significant improvement in symptoms in 52% of cases, especially in cases of continuous tinnitus. And 259 tinnitus sufferers were given either the medicinal herb Ginkgo biloba extract or almitrine-raubasine or nicergoline. Ginkgo biloba was found to be a particularly effective treatment for tinnitus.

Magnesium protects hearing too. In a trial 300 young, healthy individuals with normal hearing, undergoing military training with exposure to high noise levels, were given either magnesium aspartate or placebo. Thresholds for noise-induced permanent hearing loss were significantly higher in the magnesium group. Magnesium supplementation was therefore found to be protective against damage to hearing caused by exposure to noise. No-one in this study explained how these bizarre studies come about in the first place. Menieres disease is usually permanent but there is certainly no harm in trying some of these supplements.

URINE

Does your baby's urine smell of maple syrup?

If so, you should seek medical attention.

Maple Syrup Urine Disease (MSUD) is an extremely rare inherited metabolic disorder characterized by a distinctive sweet odour of the urine and sweat. It is a serious disorder that, unless treated promptly and correctly, can be life threatening. Therapy must be started at the earliest possible age to achieve the best results. MSUD is manageable, just as diabetes is manageable, but care and attention must be given to diet and to the treatment of even minor illnesses.

Symptoms develop because the body is unable to break down (metabolise) three of the essential amino acids, leucine, isoleucine, and valine. These produce a distinctive smell. They are essential because they are used by the body to build proteins, and they are three of 11 amino acids that must be obtained as part of the daily diet since the body cannot synthesize them. These three amino aids share a common characteristic of chemical structure and are thus known as the branched chain amino acids (BCAA's). An affected newborn will have abnormally high concentrations of acidic metabolic by-products of the BCAA's in the blood and other tissues (metabolic acidosis) that, if left untreated, may lead to seizures or coma, and may be life-threatening.

Does your urine smell funny?

Urine smells explained

We are told that Hippocrates, the father of all doctors used to taste his patient's urine (the mother of all medicines). Apparently sweetness identified diabetes and rancidity identified a urinary infection, but with practice Hippocrates no doubt became quite expert at diagnosing other disease this way too. One wonders, with all his obsession on bodily waste whether he was an ex Crete and not a native Roman after all.

The Body Language of Health

It is true that the smell of urine varies depending on your state of health, and a strong smell is indicative of the rancidity that Hippocrates noted when there is an infection lurking deep in your plumbing system.

Now, I wouldn't recommend that you routinely collect and taste your urine, although there is not likely to be any harmful effect from drinking small amounts of urine. Actually, it is more likely that you can only accurately determine the taste of someone else's urine, but can't diagnose your own, for the same reason I explained earlier that when you lick your own fingers they will only taste salty if they have more salt on them than the rest of your body.

But it is a jolly good idea to get to know your urine smells, and become attuned to any significant changes because that could signify the early symptoms of a problem.

We do need to be careful, however, because some foods will affect urine smell and colour. For example Asparagus produces a strange smell to your urine, due to two chemicals, methylthioacrylate and methylthiopropionate that are in the asparagus. Some other foods are likely to have an effect too. Colour can be affected by vegetables and spices too, for example Turmeric turns the urine bright yellow. That is why piccalilli makes your pee turn fluorescent yellow.

A strange smell to your urine can be associated with an underlying medical condition. If you're concerned about the odor of your urine, talk to your doctor. Here are a few guidelines:

Ammonia smell	Not enough fluids, dehydration
Foul smell	Bacterial infection of kidneys or bladder
Sweet smell	Uncontrolled diabetes
Musty smell	Liver disease; phenylketonuria, a rare, inherited metabolic condition
Maple syrup smell	Maple syrup urine disease, a rare, inherited metabolic disorder

Pear drops smell (sometimes also detected on the breath) is likely to be due to ketones that develop when you are breaking down fats, for example when exercising too hard or dieting too drastically. It is a frequent side effect of the Atkins diet.

More than 100 different clinical tests can be done on urine. A routine urinalysis usually includes the following tests:

- **Colour.** Many factors affect urine colour, including fluid balance, diet, medications, and disease. The intensity of the colour generally indicates the concentration of the urine; pale or colourless urine indicates that it is dilute, and deep yellow urine indicates that it is concentrated. Vitamin B supplements can turn urine bright yellow. Reddish brown urine may be caused by certain medications; by blackberries, beets, or rhubarb in the diet; or by the presence of blood in the urine.
- **Clarity.** Urine is normally clear. This test determines the cloudiness of urine, also called opacity or turbidity. Bacteria, blood, sperm, crystals, or mucus can make urine appear cloudy.
- **Odour.** Urine usually does not smell very strong, but has a slightly "nutty" (aromatic) odour. Some diseases can cause a change in the normal odour of urine. For example, an infection with *E. coli* bacteria can cause a foul odour, while diabetes or starvation can cause a sweet, fruity odour.
- **Specific gravity.** This measures the amount of substances dissolved in the urine. It also indicates how well the kidneys are able to adjust the amount of water in urine. The higher the specific gravity, the more minerals are dissolved in the urine. When you drink a lot of liquid, your kidneys should produce increased amounts of dilute urine with low specific gravity. When you drink very little liquid, your kidneys should make only small amounts of concentrated urine with high specific gravity.
- **pH.** The pH is a measure of how acidic or alkaline (basic) the urine is. A urine pH of 4 or less is strongly acidic, pH7 is neutral (neither acidic nor alkaline), and pH9 or more is strongly alkaline. Sometimes the pH of urine may be adjusted by certain types of treatment. For example, efforts may be made to keep urine either acidic or alkaline to prevent formation of certain types of kidney stones.
- **Protein.** Protein is normally not detected in the urine. Sometimes a small amount of protein is released into the urine when a person stands up (this condition is called postural proteinuria). Fever, strenuous exercise, normal pregnancy, and some diseases, especially kidney disease, may also cause protein in the urine.
- **Glucose.** Glucose is the type of sugar usually found in blood, but normally there is very little or no glucose in urine. However, when the blood sugar level is very high, as in uncontrolled diabetes, it spills over into the urine. Glucose can also be found in urine when the kidneys are damaged or diseased.
- **Nitrites.** Bacteria that cause a urinary tract infection (UTI) produce an enzyme that converts urinary nitrates to nitrites. The presence of nitrites in urine indicates a UTI.
- **Leukocytes (WBC esterase).** Leukocyte esterase detects leukocytes (white blood cells) in the urine. The presence of while blood cells in the urine may indicate a urinary tract infection.
- **Ketones.** When fat is broken down for energy, the body produces by-products called ketones and releases them into the urine. Large amounts of ketones in the urine may signal a dangerous condition known as diabetic ketoacidosis. A diet low in

sugars and starches (carbohydrates), starvation, or prolonged vomiting may also cause ketones in the urine because the body takes its nutrition from your fat.

- **Microscopic analysis.** In this test, urine is spun in a centrifuge so the solid materials settle out. This sediment is spread on a slide and examined under a microscope. Types of materials that may be found include:
- **Red or white blood cells.** Normally blood cells are not found in urine, but inflammation, disease, or injury to the kidneys, urethras, bladder, or urethra can cause blood in urine. Strenuous exercise (such as running a marathon) can also cause blood in urine. White blood cells are often a sign of infection, cancer, or kidney disease.
- **Casts.** Some types of kidney disease can cause plugs of material (called casts) to form in tiny tubes in the kidneys. The casts can then get flushed out into the urine. Casts can be made of different types of material, such as red or white blood cells, waxy or fatty substances, or protein. The type of cast can provide clues about the type of kidney disease that may be present.
- **Crystals.** Healthy people often have only a few crystals in their urine. However, a large number of crystals, or the presence of certain types of crystals, may indicate kidney stones or a problem with how the body is metabolising food.
- **Bacteria, yeast cells, or parasites.** Normally there are no bacteria, yeast cells, or parasites in urine. Their presence can indicate an infection.

Urine normally has a stronger smell first thing in the morning, as at this time it is usually rather concentrated. There can be a distinctive fruity smell of by-products from certain foods that you may have eaten the night before. Asparagus is a typical example of a substance that is passed through the kidneys into the urine that gives a powerful aroma, but even medication such as penicillin may do this too. In addition there are many other substances such as nitrates and phosphates in the urine that can colour it and give it a distinctive odour. The more dilute your urine is and the blander your diet, the less you will notice these smells.

Some drugs such as Sertraline are sometimes capable of causing urinary symptoms, particularly difficulty urinating, and should only be taken with great caution if there is any degree of kidney or prostate impairment.

Most urinary infections respond well to drinking 3 litres of water every day with cranberry juice or lemon barley water. The latter is particularly good for any kind of kidney infection and it will help remove kidney stones as well.

Dogs have been very successful in sniffing out bladder cancer from a urine sample. There have been anecdotal reports of dogs spotting cancer in their owners, but now researchers say they have proved this phenomenon scientifically. In 1989, researchers wrote a letter to the Lancet medical journal about how a woman claimed to have sought medical help as a direct result of her dog's unusual interest in a skin lesion that turned out to be a skin cancer. Such areas are thought to produce distinctive odours which a dog's nose can distinguish. Apparently, spaniels seem to develop the most discriminating noses for this sort of thing.

Dogs are also very good at detecting bladder cancer by sniffing a sample of the patient's urine. They don't have to drink it. Someone should have suggested this more palatable method of diagnosis to Hippocrates.

Do you have unusual stools?

Stools explained

Bars have them, toads have them, and milkmaids have three legged varieties. Indecisive people are torn between two of them. But we're not talking here about unusual seating arrangements, we're back to shit again.

My style of humour might be hard to digest, but everything you eat and drink has to escape through the urinary system or the bowel, so it is not surprising that what comes out reflects what went in. And what they say about the computer, GI-GO (garbage in, garbage out) is never more true that in the human body.

Because your intestines are a repository for vast populations of bacteria, around half of the volume of faeces is dead bacteria. The rest is bog standard fibre, from your food, mixed with bile that was used in the digestive process, and that is what produces the characteristic brown colour found in the excrement of all mammals.

If your digestive system is working well, your bowels should be stimulated daily or every other day, often after breakfast or some other meal. The faecal load should be of reasonable volume and the faecal matter should be shaped into undulating soft fecal turd that escapes the anal cavity with tapered ends. If the quantity of fibre is correct, these should just float in the water in the toilet, like an iceberg with about nine tenths of the volume below the waterline.

They shouldn't be so big they could sink the Titanic, nor so small that they break up into little floating mines in the water. If you can only produce rabbit droppings, that is a sign of dehydration and probably a poor digestion. Time you said 'What's up Doc?'

The waste in your colon should be evacuated within 18 to 36 hours, which is the time it takes for food to travel from mouth to anus through the 20 feet (6 metres) of the small intestine in an average person. This is called the 'fecal dump time'

To work out your evacuation time, you can do 'hands on' scientific experimentation. Cook a good helping of sweetcorn and eat it with your dinner. Then wait. Remember to inspect your stools when you go to the toilet. The indigestible sweetcorn husks will make an appearance in your stools when they have passed through the body. The time it takes is your dump time, that's why scientists say they are going 'for a dump'.

It is not good for the intestines for food to stay in the bowel too long because it degrades and causes build up of toxic material; that can cause all sorts of problems.

Bristol Stool Scales

The Bristol Stool Form Scale or simply 'Bristol Stool Chart' is an unlikely name for a classification of the form and size of stools as they appear in a toilet. It was developed by K W Heaton at the University of Bristol and was first published in the British Medical Journal in 1990. The form of the stool depends on the time it spends in the colon and the classification puts them into seven distinct groups depending on their consistency and shape. The ideal stool has sometimes been called 'The Goldilocks Stool'.

This is because it is not too hard and not too soft but is "just right". All shipshape and Bristol fashion, you might say. Actually Bristol has been an important English seaport for more than a thousand years. The city is actually several miles from the sea and stands on the river Avon estuary. Bristol's harbour has one of the most variable tidal flows anywhere in the world and the water level can vary by more than 30 feet between tides. Ships that were moored there were beached at each low tide, so they had to be of especially sturdy construction and the goods in their holds needed to be securely stowed. That's where the saying came from. Nothing to do with 'Bristols' incidentally, that refers to cockney rhyming slang associated with Bristol City.

The shape and form represent the amount of moisture and fibre in the stool, and if you have a look at 'Bristol stool scales' on the internet you can find some interesting *motion pictures.*

SENSES

Do you sneeze in bright sunlight?

You probably have a deficiency in METHIONINE

Methionine is an essential amino acid that is effective in liver detoxification and in the breakdown of fats. It is also a powerful antioxidant and helps protect the body from toxins and destructive free radicals. Methionine helps in some cases of schizophrenia by decreasing the blood level of histamine which can cause the brain to relay incorrect messages. It is also helpful in the treatment of depression. Histamine, of course is involved in sneezing and allergies, for which you take antihistamines.

Good sources of Methionine

Methionine is not synthesized in the body. It must be obtained from food or supplements. Food sources include

- Beans, soya beans, onions, garlic
- Fish and meat
- Eggs
- Seeds
- Yoghurt

Methionine supplies sulphur and other compounds required by the body for normal metabolism and growth. Methionine belongs to a group of compounds called lipotropics, or chemicals that help the liver process fats (lipids).

People with AIDS have low levels of methionine. Some researchers suggest this may explain some aspects of the disease process, especially the deterioration that occurs in the nervous system that can cause symptoms such as dementia. A preliminary study has suggested that high doses of methionine may improve memory recall in people with AIDS-related nervous system degeneration.

There are eight key essential amino acids, each with vital actions to perform in your body that are not to be sneezed at. Here is a quick review of them.

Phenylalanine is used to build insulin and helps to regulate blood sugar levels. It also contributes to the fibrous texture of skin and keeps it flexible. It is found in chicken, fish, soya, eggs, and milk and dairy products, especially chocolate.

Tryptophan maintains mental function and mental clarity, and it also relieves depression through increasing serotonin levels. It also aids good sleep. It is found in eggs, beef, nuts, turkey, cheese, cottage cheese and especially bananas.

Leucine, isoleucine and valine are related products that are needed for muscle building and healing wounds. This group is found in nuts and seeds.

Lysine is essential for absorption of calcium from foods, and it is valuable in maintaining our immune system, especially in treating herpes and other persistent viruses like HIV. It is also needed to maintain good skin. It works with methionine to produce another amino acid, called carnitine which helps carry fatty acids to cells as fuel – hence carnitine is a vital ingredient in weight management and is sometimes taken as a supplement. Lysine is found in all meats, dairy, oily fish and shellfish, eggs, mung beans, chickpeas and hazelnuts.

Methionine we have already discussed. It is a known allergy-fighter, and is also essential for regulating metabolism, and it produces serotonin, the mood relaxing neurotransmitter. Methionine is found in meat and dairy products, sunflower seeds and avocados. Some say that methionine deficiency is a cause of hay fever because of its link with histamine, so it could be involved in allergies too.

Threonine is best known for its immune boosting powers, and it also plays a vital role in dealing with inflammatory conditions like arthritis, eczema and irritable bowel disease. It is found in wheatgerm, oats, ricotta and cottage cheese.

Do you have Poor Sensory Systems?

You may be deficient in VITAMIN B12, B1 and MAGNESIUM

Vitamin B12 deficiency symptoms, like those of many other treatable health conditions, can be virtually identical to age dementia symptoms, senile dementia symptoms and Alzheimer's symptoms. As many as 20% of people over age 65 have low

Vitamin B12 levels and deficiency may even cause needless worry about dementia. Correcting the deficiency can help older people resume full and normal lives.

Vitamin B12 deficiency symptoms include:

- Loss of appetite
- Diarrhoea
- Numbness and tingling of hands and feet
- Paleness
- Shortness of breath
- Fatigue
- Weakness
- Sore mouth and tongue
- Confusion or change in mental status in severe or advanced cases. This is sometimes confused with dementia. More importantly, even a moderate deficiency of this important vitamin and its counterpart, folic acid, may ultimate contribute to the onset of Alzheimer's disease or other related dementias.

You need vitamin B12 to make red blood cells and keep the nervous system healthy. It is also needed to absorb folic acid and it helps to release energy. It is absorbed through your intestines from a variety of foods, but mainly meat, fish and dairy products. It can be stored in the body in small amounts, and around 80% of this is stored in the liver. It may take three or four years for the symptoms of deficiency to develop because your liver store is considerable and lasts a long time.

Vitamin B12 cannot be absorbed on its own. It has to combine with another substance called 'intrinsic factor' which is produced by your stomach lining.

Vitamin B12 deficiency therefore usually develops for one of the following reasons:

- Your stomach cannot produce enough intrinsic factor
- Your intestine cannot absorb enough vitamin B12
- You do not eat enough food containing vitamin B12 (this may easily happen to people following a Vegan diet)

Vitamin B1

Vitamin B_1 (thiamine) deficiency may result from a deficiency in the diet. People whose diet consists mainly of polished (refined) white rice are at risk of vitamin B_1

deficiency, because polishing removes almost all of the vitamins. Alcoholics, who often substitute alcohol for food, are at high risk of developing this deficiency.

Early symptoms are vague. They include fatigue, irritability, memory impairment, loss of appetite, sleep disturbances, abdominal discomfort, and weight loss. Doesn't this sound like symptoms of alcoholism? Eventually, a severe vitamin B_1 deficiency (beriberi) may develop, characterized by nerve, heart, and brain abnormalities.

Brain abnormalities due to vitamin B_1 deficiency occur primarily in alcoholics. Brain abnormalities actually may develop when a chronic vitamin B_1 deficiency is suddenly worsened by a rapid, substantial decrease in the vitamin B_1 level (which can be caused by an alcoholic binge) or by a sudden increase in vitamin B_1 requirements (which may occur when an undernourished alcoholic is fed intravenously).

Brain abnormalities may develop in two stages: an early stage called Korsakoff's syndrome and a later stage called Wernicke's encephalopathy. Together, these stages are called the Wernicke-Korsakoff syndrome which causes memory loss, and Wernicke's encephalopathy which causes mental confusion, difficulty walking, and eye problems (including nystagmus and paralysis of the eyes). If Wernicke's encephalopathy is not promptly treated, symptoms may worsen, resulting in coma and even death.

Magnesium

Magnesium is an essential mineral in the human body. It is needed for bone, protein, and fatty acid formation, making new cells, activating B vitamins, relaxing muscles, clotting blood, and forming adenosine triphosphate (ATP; the energy the body runs on). The secretion and action of insulin also require magnesium.

Magnesium also acts in a way related to calcium channel blocker drugs. This effect may be responsible for the fact that under certain circumstances magnesium has been found to potentially improve vision in people with glaucoma. Similarly, this action might account for magnesium's ability to lower blood pressure.

Since magnesium has so many different actions in the body, the exact reasons for some of its clinical effects are difficult to determine. For example, in preliminary research magnesium has reduced hyperactivity in children. Other research suggests that some children with attention deficit-hyperactivity disorder (ADHD) have lowered levels of magnesium. In a preliminary but controlled trial, 50 ADHD children with low magnesium (as determined by red blood cell, hair, and serum levels of magnesium) were given 200 mg of magnesium per day for six months. Compared with 25 other magnesium-deficient ADHD children, those given magnesium supplementation had a significant decrease in hyperactive behaviour.

Magnesium levels have been reported to be low in those with chronic fatigue syndrome (CFS), and magnesium injections have been reported to improve symptoms. Oral magnesium supplementation has also improved symptoms in those people with CFS who had low magnesium levels in another report, although magnesium injections were sometimes necessary. However, other research reports no evidence of magnesium deficiency in people with CFS. The reason for this discrepancy remains unclear. People with CFS considering magnesium supplementation should have their magnesium status checked beforehand by a doctor. Only people with magnesium deficiency appear to benefit from this therapy so perhaps this explains patchy results.

People with diabetes tend to have lower magnesium levels compared with those who have normal glucose tolerance. Supplementation with magnesium overcomes this problem so it may help some diabetics improve glucose tolerance.

Surprisingly, magnesium may be beneficial for bladder problems in women, especially common disturbances in bladder control and the sense of "urgency." A double-blind trial found that women who took magnesium twice daily for four weeks had better bladder control and fewer incontinence symptoms than women who took a placebo. All that double-blindfolding must have played havoc with finding the lavatory in a hurry, though.

Magnesium supplementation may reduce dehydration of red blood cells in sickle cell anaemia patients. Administration of magnesium to sickle cell anaemia patients was found to reverse some of the characteristic red blood cell abnormalities and to dramatically reduce the number of painful days for these patients after six months treatment. This preliminary trial was not a blind trial, however, so a placebo effect could not be ruled out.

You will find many references to zinc deficiency and loss of taste and smell elsewhere in this book.

HAIR

Do you have premature grey hair?

You may be deficient in PARA-AMINO BENZOIC ACID

Para-amino benzoic acid or PABA is one of the nutrients the body uses to make B vitamins, especially vitamin B5 which has itself been linked with slowing down the rate of both greying and hair loss. Before you rush out and buy a PABA supplement you need to appreciate that the trials which indicated this welcome benefit only worked when prematurely greying hair was the result of either stress or a nutritional deficiency that the PABA could correct. Simple age-related greying will not respond well to this treatment if you are not deficient.

In fact, PABA was initially being assessed for the treatment of a condition called Vitiligo where patches of skin turn chalky white. This unfortunate pigment loss condition has been made famous by Michael Jackson. Vitiligo is associated with autoimmune and inflammatory diseases, commonly thyroid overexpression and underexpression. Jackson's doctors also testified that he has lupus, a chronic autoimmune disease that is potentially debilitating and sometimes fatal as the immune system attacks the body's cells and tissue, resulting in inflammation and tissue damage. This may be why his facial features have changed so much, as he has always declared that he never had significant cosmetic surgery. If you succumb to debilitating disease in your life, just hope you're not famous as well. The press love to pick the famous to pieces, don't they?

Some people with Vitiligo also have prematurely grey hair and what the researchers found was that a very small percentage of patients responded really well to a combined dose of PABA and magnesium. A side effect was that not only their skin but also their hair colour returned to normal. Maybe worth Michael Jackson trying this, after all we don't really know whether he dyes his hair or not, do we?

Good sources of Para-Amino Benzoic acid :

* Liver, kidney
* Brewer's yeast, molasses
* Whole grains
* Mushrooms, spinach
* PABA is made by intestinal bacteria. (It seems we evolved to eat soil).

The Body Language of Health

Schizophrenia and PABA

Dr. Carl Pfeiffer reports that large doses of PABA, 2 grams per day, have been used with good results in schizophrenia. He speculates that PABA may prevent certain amines from forming hallucinogens. There is a chemical found in quantity in the bodies of schizophrenics that is an indole called adrenochrome. Adrenochrome (which is oxidized adrenalin) has an almost LSD-like effect on the body. That might well explain the behaviour of schizophrenics. PABA might therefore be a useful compound to help people come off other amines, such as amphetamine and Ecstasy.

Niacin (Vitamin B3) serves to reduce the body's production of this toxic material. In fact there is reference on the web to Vitamin B3 having produced remarkable stabilisation of schizophrenia. Probably not surprising, because Niacin and PABA are both part of the Vitamin B group of compounds.

Can we put two and two together to make four, and suggest that premature grey hair might indicate risks of psychosis or schizophrenia? Well, probably. I know several people who fit into this category. Does this explain Michael Jackson's unusual habits?

Another puzzle that someone else can perhaps solve is that for some reason schizophrenia and rheumatoid arthritis seldom occur in the same person. There are many links like this which medical science has not found interesting, but surely there are links that can point us to a simple nutritional cure. Perhaps medicine is not interested because nutritional cures can't be turned into vastly profitable, expensive wonder drugs.

I told you earlier that we are throwing our ability to synthesise niacin into the genetic dustbin. You might ask, does it matter?

Firstly, let us remind ourselves what this substance is. Niacin is also known as nicotinic acid or vitamin B3. It is a water-soluble vitamin whose derivatives such as coenzymes NADH, NAD and NADP play essential roles in energy metabolism in cells and DNA repair.

Without niacin, cells that accumulate a large amount of DNA damage, or no longer effectively repair damage incurred to their DNA, can either become dormant and be useless to the body, can commit suicide in a process called apoptosis, or can start unregulated cell division. We have another name for this. Cancer.

Niacin is therefore pretty important.

The Body Language of Health

A deficiency of niacin causes a horrible disease called pellagra. It got its name from northern Italy in the early 1700's because pelle agra means literally 'rough skin'. It is even thought that sufferers were so disfigured that this outbreak set off the legend about vampires in the region. Pellagra causes dermatitis and skin lesions, extreme sensitivity to sunlight, insomnia and dementia. Maybe that sounds like Count Dracula? Pellagra kills within about four years, but consuming niacin effects a rapid cure.

Humans can synthesise niacin from Tryptophan. That, you will remember is an essential amino acid that is a constituent of meat, eggs and fish. But pellagra develops in people who get most of their food from a diet of maize, like those peasants in Italy in the early 1700's, because this diet is also deficient in tryptophan. Unfortunately if the legend is true, what Count Dracula needed was some read meat (or a drink of blood??) but instead someone misheard and administered the wrong sort of stake.

Pellagra can still be common today among people who live in rural South America where corn is a staple diet. The symptoms usually appear during spring, increase in the summer due to greater sun exposure, and return annually. It is also one of several diseases of malnutrition still common in Africa, and was endemic in the poorer states of southern USA. like Mississippi and Alabama as well as among the inmates of jails and orphanages. It was also common amongst prisoners of Soviet labor camps, such as the infamous Gulag. Pellagra is also occasionally found in cases of chronic alcoholism.

The story about pellagra and its discovery by US Surgeon General Joseph Goldberger in 1915 is a fascinating one, but pellagra only occurs in the absence of niacin and tryptophan. You may ask yourself why should pellagra be an issue when we can get hold of tryptophan if not niacin. Surely it will be a thing of the past when we can make vitamin B3 (niacin) from tryptophan?

Yes we can, but the synthesis is extremely inefficient; 60 parts of tryptophan are required to make one part of niacin. And it looks as though mankind is losing the ability to perform this synthesis because of his meat eating habits over the last ten thousand years or more. You remember, we decided earlier that man originated as a vegetarian? His teeth pattern, his digestive system and his inability to manufacture vitamin C put him firmly with the guinea pigs. It seems we are now losing the ability to make niacin too.

That will be fine unless a future world disaster forces us back into a foraging existence in which niacin becomes a very scarce commodity. We would be destined to become pellagra-disfigured extras in a Hammer horror film starring The Count himself. It is this sort of long term genetic change that could be the downfall of the human race if conditions on Earth change significantly.

Are you experiencing hair loss?

If you do, you may be deficient in BIOTIN

Biotin is a water-soluble vitamin, generally classified as a B-complex vitamin. Biotin is required by all organisms but can only be synthesized by bacteria, yeasts, moulds, algae, and a few plant species.

Although chronic biotin deficiency is very rare, the human requirement for dietary biotin has been demonstrated in two different situations: prolonged intravenous feeding without biotin supplementation and consumption of raw egg white for a prolonged period.

Avidin is a protein found in egg white, which binds biotin and prevents its absorption. Cooking egg white denatures avidin, so it cannot then prevent the absorption of dietary biotin. If you are experiencing hair loss, lay off the raw eggs.

Baldies may also be deficient in Essential Fatty Acids and in Zinc, to a latter extent, since these are also associated with excessive hair loss.

Male pattern baldness and health

Male pattern baldness (MPB) is different, and progressive. I have only heard that apricot kernel extract has been beneficial in restoring hair growth, but again only in certain people. There is little you can do about this but by way of compensation, studies have found that women are genuinely attracted to balding men.

MPB is caused by testosterone and its derivative, *dihydrotestosterone* (DHT) that acts on the skin, sometimes producing acne, and on the hair follicles, putting hair on the chest but often taking it off the scalp. The classic MPB sufferer has a balding head but lots of facial and body hair. DHT also stimulates the growth of prostate cells, producing normal growth in adolescence but contributing to benign prostatic hyperplasia (BPH) in many older men. So if you are bald with an excess of chest hair, this suggests that you need to take care of your prostate.

Perhaps this is rather good advice, according to scientists in Australia. They evaluated 1,446 men who were diagnosed with moderate to high-grade prostate cancer before age 70 and compared them with 1,390 men of the same age who were free of the disease. They found that men with bald spots at the top of their heads

The Body Language of Health

(*vertex baldness*) were one and a half times more likely to have prostate cancer than those without bald spots. The association was particularly strong for men who were diagnosed with high-grade prostate cancer at 60–69 years of age. In contrast, there was no link between a receding hairline (*frontal baldness*) and cancer.

An American study also found that men with bald spots were more likely to develop coronary artery disease than men with full heads of hair. Mild vertex baldness was linked to a 23% increase, moderate baldness to a 32% rise, and severe baldness to a 36% increase in risk. As in the Australian study of prostate cancer, frontal baldness was not associated with risk.

So MPB chaps need to look after their prostate and heart. There is strong evidence that lycopene, the plant chemical found in tomato products lowers risk of prostate cancer. One important study showed that men who ate 10 or more servings of tomato based foods per week had more than a 30% lower risk of prostate cancer. Since lycopene is fat soluble, it helps to have your tomatoes with a little fat such as olive oil. Maybe that's the real secret as to why Italian food is so healthy. You'll also find lycopene in other red foods like pink grapefruit and watermelon.

A high-fat diet, especially high saturated fat, may increase risk so it makes sense to choose the leanest cuts of meat, remove skin from poultry, use lower-fat diary products and keep your meat portions small. Replace some of your meat meals with fish. The omega-3 fatty acids found in fish such as salmon, mackerel, herring, sardines and trout, have been linked to lowered cancer risk. And a recent study suggests that a diet rich in omega-3 fats not only protects against heart disease but might help to inhibit the spread of disease in men with early prostate cancer.

Eating more cruciferous vegetables such as broccoli, cabbage, cauliflower, kale, pak choy and turnip also provides protection. These contain selenium.

Selenium, an essential trace mineral and important antioxidant, is being studied for its role in lowering risk of prostate cancer. In one major study, selenium significantly reduced the incidence of lung, prostate and colorectal cancers in participants who received 200 mcg selenium for 4.5 years. The best sources of selenium are Brazil nuts, seafood, some meats and fish, as well as bread, wheat bran, wheat germ, oats and brown rice. Eating more whole grains continues to be an important health strategy.

Vitamin D found in fortified foods including cows milk, margarine, fortified plant-based beverages, some fortified orange juice, some fortified yoghurt as well as fatty fish also appears to play a protective role.

BODY

Do you have Asthma?

Make sure you have enough VITAMIN D3

Researchers in asthma say that Vitamin D could be used to prevent thousands of life-threatening asthma attacks in the event that steroid treatments do not take effect, after research showed that vitamin D3 could substantially improve a patient's responsiveness to steroid treatments.

Conversely, if you are an asthmatic, how about taking a high dose of Vitamin D3 or a supplement of D vitamins and seeing if your asthma is more manageable?

At this stage I would normally expand on asthma but I couldn't do better than to refer you to Dr Morrow-Brown's superb website at www.allergiesexplained.com which has some fascinating stories and excellent pictures. Dr Morrow-Brown was responsible for Becotide inhalers which revolutionised the treatment of asthmatic conditions, so all sufferers owe him tremendous thanks. Please pass on details of his website to your friends as well because this site deserves better recognition and has my support.

Do you have a pot-belly?

Your risk of heart disease is increased by 40%

A twelve-year study of over a hundred thousand men and women has reinforced the suspicion of strong links between your waist size and the risk of heart attacks. This mammoth study by American researcher Dr Carlos Iribarren found that belly size was more of an indicator than body mass indicator (BMI) because abdominal fat is more metabolically active than fat stored elsewhere in the body. He found that the risk of heart attacks increased by up to 44% for men and women with a pot-belly.

Women should not get complacent because the belly-size-to-heart-disease relationship was said to apply to them too. But this might come as some comfort for British women, who tend to store fat on their buttocks rather than on their belly.

The Body Language of Health

Presumably then the pot-belly trait is more prevalent for women in USA, since this was an American study, but this advice is a lesson for us all.

So what is a pot-belly? Well, in Britain we tend to call it a 'beer belly' instead, and it is thought to be associated with lack of muscle tone due to consumption of large volumes of Britain's favourite tipple. Some people erroneously also think it is due to an enlarged liver through drinking excess.

Sorry, but a 'beer belly' or whatever you like to call it is just plain and simple fat that likes to be laid down round the belly especially in men, and it has very little to do with beer, apart from the fact that beer is loaded with sugar and the alcohol also increases your appetite, so you drink far more calories than you burn off.

Exercising the stomach (that is, with exercise, not food) does nothing to remove fat from this region. The only thing that works is burning calories, in other words burning up more energy in exercise than you consume in food.

Hippocrates got it right a couple of thousand years ago when he promoted a highly physical lifestyle to keep muscle tone active into old age. His philosophy was 'that which is used develops, and that which is not wastes away'. In modern terminology doctors would say that any part of the body which is not used undergoes atrophy, and any part which is used a lot undergoes hypertrophy.

If you have a pot-belly, it is a good idea to make a concerted effort to reduce it by taking more exercise, because the mere act of exercising also reduces the appetite. The alternative, of suffering with heart disease in later life is not worth contemplating. Why not set yourself a target and when you reach it you can give yourself your own trophy. And if you beat your target by a mile (well, a few inches anyway), you could reward yourself with a hyper-trophy.

Women with large hips risk gallstones

British women don't get away with it either. Those women who have larger waist and hip measurements can face almost double the risk of developing gallstones and a requirement of subsequent surgery to remove them, according to research published in the tantalising online journal 'Gut'.

Writing in the Times, Sam Lister reports that the research, conducted at the University of Kentucky Medical Centre, involved the monitoring of over 42,000 women aged between 39 and 66 between 1986 and 2000. In that period 3,197 of the women required surgery to remove gallstones. It was found that those women with waistlines of 92cm (36in) or above, were twice as likely to require surgery to remove gallstones than those whose waistlines were 66cm or less.

Additionally, women with a higher waist-to-hip ratio, of around 0.86, had a 40% higher risk of developing gallstones compared with those whose ratio was 0.70 or less. Gallstones occur in roughly 10% of older adults, and are more common in women than in men.

Are you pregnant?

You are probably deficient in everything

Pregnancy is good for some women, they seem to radiate an aura of well-being, but for others it is a nine month uphill struggle.

Put pregnancy + deficiency as search words on the internet and you will find literally millions of entries. Using these as a yardstick for the number of deficiencies that exist, I found that iron (anaemia) comes top, followed by folic acid, then vitamin D then Vitamin B. After that are individual stories covering just about everything, but with a predominance of zinc, magnesium and biotin.

That's not surprising is it? Your baby makes huge demands on your body and has such a voracious appetite that it takes your mineral and vitamin supplies for its own. This is a big enough demand on your body, but now it seems a mother's burden is even greater than we thought.

"Women who do not eat properly in the run-up to *falling pregnant* could be risking the future health of their children", says Professor David Barker, of the MRC Epidemiology Unit at the University of Southampton. He believes that the nutrition the foetus receives in its first few days is vitally important.

"If mums-to-be do not eat the right things in the build up to getting pregnant', he says, 'There could be damaging long-term effects'. Starting to eat properly once a woman finds out she is pregnant may be too late".

The Body Language of Health

"Research monitoring the eating habits of 12,000 women in Southampton aged 20 to 34 suggested that 40% were eating an unhealthy diet", he said. He suggested that vulnerability to chronic disorders such as diabetes were set in the womb.

Other studies have suggested that the quantity a baby eats in its first few weeks after birth may influence future risk of diabetes.

Professor Barker presented his findings at a conference in Lyon. He said: "Much of what is important in pregnancy happens really early - life in the womb establishes the risk for coronary heart disease in later life". You are what your mother ate, it seems.

"We're not suggesting anything revolutionary at all in terms of diet but the point is that many young women are not anywhere near getting it right."

He suggested that prior to conception, women needed to eat a diet rich in fruit, vegetables and dairy produce - and not to eat too much meat in relation to carbohydrates. He said that at least two portions of carbohydrates should be eaten for every portion of meat, and blasted the fashionable Atkins diet, which focuses on high-fat and high-protein foods.

We already know that a deficiency of folic acid can cause a series of neural tube defects in the baby and that is why new mothers are given folic acid supplements, but we also know that by the time a woman finds she is pregnant it is actually too late to be taking a supplement. So if you are of childbearing age, are fertile and are sexually active you should be taking a folic acid supplement anyway or eating lots of food that contains folic acid. Once you become pregnant, it is too late.

We also know that genetic imprinting prepares the child for the sort of life led by the mother. And of course we know that the mother is also forming her daughter's eggs while she is in the womb, so she is responsible for her grand-daughters as well. This is quite a responsibility!!

So, as you can imagine, diet is vitally important to the mother and especially to the child. So what should a mother be eating? The UK government has issued several pretty good booklets on healthy eating while pregnant. Here is a summary of their various recommendations.

When pregnant, or trying to become pregnant, ideally you should:

The Body Language of Health

- Eat a healthy balanced diet.
- Include foods rich in calcium, folate, and iron.
- Avoid certain foods and drinks which can be harmful to the pregnancy.
- Watch your weight gain and aim to lose weight before becoming pregnant if you are obese.
- Cut right back on drinking if you drink alcohol.
- Take folic acid supplements.

Eat a healthy balanced diet

A healthy diet for pregnancy is much the same as for everyone! Briefly, it is as follows.

Eat plenty of starch-based foods (complex carbohydrates)

The bulk of most meals should be starch-based foods (such as bread, cereals, potatoes, rice, and pasta), together with fruit and vegetables. Some people wrongly think that starch-based foods are 'fattening'. In fact, they contain about half the calories than the same weight of fat.

Eat at least five portions of a variety of fruit and vegetables each day

One portion is: one large fruit such as an apple, pear, banana, etc, OR two smaller fruits such as plums, satsumas, etc, OR one cup of small fruits such as grapes, OR two large tablespoons of fruit salad, stewed or canned fruit, OR one tablespoon of dried fruit, OR one glass of fresh fruit juice (150ml), OR a normal portion of any vegetable, OR one dessert bowl of salad.

Eat protein foods in moderation

Meat, fish. pulses, chicken, and similar foods are high in protein. You need some protein to keep healthy, but most people eat more protein than is needed.

Eat plenty of fibre.
This helps prevent constipation and is found in wholegrain bread, pasta, rice, pulses and fruit and vegetables

The Body Language of Health

Don't eat too much fat

For example: try not to fry much food. It is better to grill, bake, poach, barbecue, or boil food. If you do fry, use unsaturated oil such as corn, sunflower or olive oil. Drain off the oil before eating. Choose lean cuts of meat. Use low fat spreads. Have low-fat milk, cheeses, yoghurts, and other dairy foods rather than full-fat varieties.

Don't have too many sugary foods and drinks

These are high in calories, and too much may cause weight gain.

Try not to eat too much salt

Use small amounts of salt with cooking, and don't add more salt at the table. foods rich in protein such as lean meat and chicken, fish (aim for at least two servings of fish a week, including one of oily fish), eggs and pulses (such as beans and lentils). These foods are also good sources of iron (see 'Do I need extra iron?' below)

Healthy snacks to have instead include malt loaf; currant buns without icing; sandwiches or pitta bread filled with cottage cheese, chicken or lean ham; low-fat yoghurts; vegetable and bean soups; and fruit including fresh, tinned in juice or dried fruit such as raisins or apricots.

Include foods with plenty of iron, calcium and folic acid
A growing baby needs these nutrients right from the start of the pregnancy.

- **Iron** is mainly in red meat, pulses, dried fruit, bread, green vegetables and fortified cereals.
- **Calcium** is found mainly in dairy products such as milk, cheese, and yoghurt. (Low-fat milk, cheeses and yoghurts usually contain just as much calcium as the full-fat varieties.)
- **Folic acid** is mainly in green vegetables, brown rice, fortified bread and breakfast cereals.

Avoid foods and drinks which can be harmful to the pregnancy

Don't eat anything with a lot of vitamin A

You need a small amount of vitamin A to keep healthy. However, large amounts can harm an unborn baby. So, avoid:

- liver and liver products such as liver pâté and cod liver oil supplements.
- vitamin tablets or supplements which contain vitamin A.

Don't eat food which may have high levels of listeria

Listeria is a bacterium (germ) which does not usually cause problems in people who are not pregnant. However, pregnant women are more likely to become infected with listeria, and it sometimes causes miscarriage, stillbirth, or infections in the baby after birth. Foods which are most at risk of carrying listeria are:

- undercooked meats and eggs. For example, this may occur in some pre-cooked meats and pre-prepared meals. Make sure all meat foods are cooked until piping hot. Eggs should be cooked until both the white and yolk are solid.
- soft cheeses such as brie. (Hard cheeses and processed cottage cheese are safe.)
- pâtés.
- shellfish and raw fish.
- unpasteurised milk. Note: goat's milk is often unpasteurised, and goat's milk products such as cheeses are often made from unpasteurised milk.

Don't eat fish from sources which may contain a lot of mercury

A high level of mercury can damage the developing nervous system of an unborn baby. So:

- Do not eat shark, merlin, or swordfish.
- Limit the amount of tuna that you eat. You should eat no more than two medium sized cans (drained weight = 140 gm per can), or one fresh tuna steak per week. (This would be about six tuna sandwiches, or three tuna salads per week.)

Don't have too much caffeine

You should limit the amount of caffeine to no more than 300 mg per day. Having a lot of caffeine increases the risk of having a baby with low birth weight, and increases the risk of miscarriage. The main sources of caffeine are coffee, tea, chocolate, cola. Caffeine is also added to some 'energy' drinks and to some cough and cold remedies. As a rough guide:

- One cup of brewed coffee has about 100 mg caffeine.
- One cup of instant coffee has about 75 mg caffeine.
- One cup of tea has about 50 mg caffeine.
- One 50g chocolate bar has about 50 mg caffeine.
- One can of cola has up to 40 mg caffeine.
- One can of 'energy' drink may contain up to 80 mg caffeine.
- Check the label on medicines for quantities of caffeine.

So, you do not have to stop your favourite drinks, but you may need to limit their amount. For example, you will reach the 300 mg limit for one day if you eat two bars of chocolate, drink two cups of tea, and have a cup of brewed coffee.

Consider if you should eat peanuts

If you have an atopic disease such as asthma, eczema, or hay fever, or if a close family member has one of these conditions, then you may wish to avoid eating peanuts when you are pregnant. This may reduce the risk of your child developing peanut allergy in later life (which can be a serious and life-threatening allergy).

This advice about peanuts in pregnancy is precautionary and further research is needed to clarify this issue.

Watch your weight

When you are pregnant, don't 'eat for two' and overeat. Too much weight gain will increase your risk of developing problems with the pregnancy, and extra weight is difficult to lose after the birth. The best way to avoid weight gain is simply to eat a healthy balanced diet detailed above.

If you are already obese or overweight, ideally you should try to lose some weight before becoming pregnant. This is to reduce the risk of pregnancy complications which are more common in obese women. See other government leaflets called 'Weight Reduction - How to Lose Weight' and 'Obesity and Overweight'.

Cut right back on drinking if you drink alcohol

If you have one or two drinks of alcohol (one or two units), once or twice a week, it is unlikely to harm your unborn baby. However, the amount of alcohol that is safe in pregnancy is not definitely known. So, many women have little or no alcohol when they are pregnant. It is known that if you drink heavily you have an increased risk of miscarriage, and may cause serious harm to the baby's growth and brain development.

A unit of alcohol is 10ml (1cl) by volume (8g by weight) of pure alcohol. This is about equal to:

- A half-pint of normal strength beer, cider, or lager.
- A pub measure of spirits (25ml), or of fortified wine such as sherry (50ml).
- A small glass (125ml) of wine containing 8% alcohol by volume.

Note: using the above 'rough guide' it is easy to underestimate how much alcohol that you drink. This is because many beers are now strong, and wines are often served in 175ml glasses. Many wines are also stronger than standard (some contain 12-14% alcohol by volume).

If you find it difficult to cut down or stop drinking alcohol, then seek advice and help from your practice nurse or GP. (note that women usually weigh much less than men and have a higher bone/fat to muscle ratio which significantly increases the proportion of alcohol in the body compared to men – Ed)

Take folic acid supplements

You should take folic acid tablets for at least the first 12 weeks of pregnancy - even if you are healthy and have a good diet. Folic acid is a vitamin which occurs naturally in certain foods. However, you need a good supply of folic acid when you are pregnant. If you take folic acid tablets in early pregnancy you reduce the risk of having a baby born with a spinal cord problem such as spina bifida. You can buy folic acid tablets from pharmacies.

- **You should start taking folic acid tablets before becoming pregnant** (from the time you plan to become pregnant). If the pregnancy is unplanned then start taking folic acid tablets as soon as you know that you are pregnant.
- For most women the dose is 400 micrograms (0.4 mg) a day.
- If your risk of having a child with a spinal cord problem is increased then the dose is higher (5 mg a day - you need a prescription for this higher dose). That is, if:
  - you have had a previously affected pregnancy.
  - your partner, or a first-degree relative, have a spinal cord defect.

- ○ you have coeliac disease (as your intake of folate may be affected by this condition).
- ○ you are taking medication for epilepsy.
- ○ you have sickle cell anaemia or thalassaemia.

What to avoid

There are certain foods that you should avoid when you're pregnant, because they might make you ill or harm your baby:

Some types of cheese

Avoid cheeses such as Camembert, Brie or chevre (a type of goats' cheese), or others that have a similar rind. You should also avoid blue cheeses.

These cheeses are made with mould and they can contain listeria, a type of bacteria that could harm your unborn baby.

Pate

Avoid all types of pate, including vegetable. This is because pate can contain listeria.

Raw or partially cooked eggs

Avoid eating raw eggs and food containing raw or partially-cooked eggs. Only eat eggs cooked enough for both the white and yolk to be solid. This is to avoid the risk of salmonella, which causes a type of food poisoning.

Raw or undercooked meat

Make sure you only eat meat that has been well cooked. This is especially important with poultry and products made from minced meat, such as sausages and burgers. Make sure these are cooked until they are piping hot all the way through and no pink meat is left. Always wash your hands after handling raw meat, and keep it separate from foods that are ready to eat. This is because raw meat contains bacteria that can cause food poisoning.

Liver products and supplements containing vitamin A

Make sure you don't have too much vitamin A. This means you should avoid eating liver and liver products such as pate and avoid taking supplements containing vitamin A or fish liver oils (which contain high levels of vitamin A). You need some vitamin A, but having too much means that levels could build up and may harm your unborn baby. Ask your GP or midwife if you want more information.

The Body Language of Health

Some types of fish

You can eat most types of fish when you're pregnant. But there are a few types you should avoid and some others where you should limit the amount you eat.

Avoid eating any shark, swordfish and marlin. Limit the amount of tuna you eat to no more than two tuna steaks a week (weighing about 140g cooked or 170g raw) or four medium-size cans of tuna a week (with a drained weight of about 140g per can). This is because of the levels of mercury in these fish. At high levels, mercury can harm a baby's developing nervous system.

Have no more than two portions of oily fish a week. Oily fish includes fresh tuna (not canned tuna, which does not count as oily fish), mackerel, sardines and trout.

But remember that eating fish is good for your health and the development of your baby, so you should still aim to eat at least two portions of fish a week, including one portion of oily fish.

Undercooked ready meals

Avoid eating ready meals that are undercooked. Make sure you heat them until they are piping hot all the way through.

Raw shellfish

Avoid raw shellfish when you're pregnant. This is because raw shellfish can sometimes contain harmful bacteria and viruses that could cause food poisoning. And food poisoning can be particularly unpleasant when you're pregnant.

Gardening and changing cat litter

Always wear gloves when you're gardening or changing cat litter, and wash your hands afterwards. This is to avoid toxoplasmosis, an infection caused by a parasite found in meat, cat faeces and soil. The infection can be harmful to unborn babies.

You can eat:

- Live or bio yoghurt
- Probiotic drinks
- Fromage frais
- Creme fraiche

- Soured cream
- Spicy food

Mayonnaise, ice cream, salad dressing - as long as they haven't been made using raw egg. Generally, mayonnaise, ice cream and salad dressing you buy in shops will have been made with pasteurised egg, which means it's safe to eat. But it's better to avoid home-made versions if they contain raw egg. If you're not sure about any of these foods when you're eating out, ask catering staff for more information.

So, how about that, I bet you were thinking I wrote the above summary, but no, it was the advice of Big Brother. For general advice I reckon that is pretty concise and well written. My only complaint is that the magical Merlin quoted early in the Government's advice had changed to marlin on their health website. And I am not sure about the peanuts thing. Recent research has shown that the peanut allergy problem has been grossly overstated, due to the inefficiencies of allergy testing.

Of course this is government advice, so no-one will take any notice. Therefore maybe I am doing everybody a great service by including it in the Body Language book. Still not as good a plot as 'Sword and the Stone' though, is it, despite it's Merlin connection? But I reckon it is sound advice for everyone, actually, pregnant or not.

Do you have vertical creases on your forehead?

You may have a duodenal ulcer.

Many of us end up with a permanent frown as our forehead takes on deeper and deeper wrinkles. But if your wrinkles run vertically on your forehead, these vertical creases appear to be a reliable Body Language sign that you may have a duodenal ulcer.

If you have digestive problems or ever feel abdominal pain, you should see your doctor straight away. Your doctor should carry out a test for a micro-organism called Helicobacter pylori (abbreviated to H pylori by the medics) that lives in your stomach and is responsible for many stomach ailments like ulcers, and gastritis. It can also occasionally develop into stomach cancer, so it should be taken seriously.

H pylori is pretty much the only bacterium that can survive the stomach's very acidic environment. It has developed a spiral shape (hence the 'helico' name) to tunnel itself into the mucous lining of the stomach. The term 'pylori' comes from Greek pylorus meaning 'gatekeeper' hence the name for the pyloric valve which leads from the stomach into the duodenum.

H pylori was isolated and cultured by German scientists as early as 1875, but its significance then, and in many research applications since was not realised. It took the combined talents of physician Dr Robin Warren and his maverick colleague Dr Barry Marshall to reveal the true significance of H pylori in the 1980's. Marshall went through medical school in Western Australia being told that everything about medicine had already been discovered, simply because that is how medicine is taught. But in practice as a physician he often found that people had gastric problems of some sort or other that no-one could do anything about.

At the same time, Warren routinely found an unusual bacterium in samples of stomach lining from areas of inflammation. He discussed this with his colleagues so much that they tired of his bug-fixation because everyone thought that no bacteria could survive the stomach acid.

When Marshall was looking round for a bacteria-based research project to work on, it was suggested he contact Warren who by now was well known as a bit of a bugger amongst his colleagues.

The pair spent several months trying to cultivate H pylori and only succeeded when the petri dishes were left over an Easter break without being washed because they were short staffed. They postulated that these bacterial growths could be the cause of stomach irritation in patients with H pylori infections.

Even with their research findings, they found the medical establishment sceptical to the idea that ulcers were caused by bacteria, because everybody thought that ulcers were caused by spicy food, stress, and irregular eating patterns. It took a brave (some would say, foolish) decision by Marshall to consume a dish of H pylori culture to see what would happen, to prove it caused disease.

About a week later, Marshall started vomiting blood and suffering painful gastritis, which is now recognised as being classical symptoms of chronic H pylori infection. He then showed it could be treated effectively and quickly with antibiotics, not with antacid preparations. In fact under these circumstances antacids and indigestion potions simply make life more comfortable for the bacterium so they spread more easily into other folds of the stomach.

The Body Language of Health

Even so, it took him ten years of lecturing and publishing technical papers to convince the medical world that H pylori was responsible for many digestive ailments. Warren and Marshall's discovery has contributed to renewed interest in the idea that many chronic diseases that can flare up may be caused by persistent unrecognised infections that can be easily treated.

Even today the medical profession is slow to accept that many digestive problems are associated with H pylori, but their cautious approach with antibiotics just might prove to be prudent after all. It has been suggested that about two thirds of the world's population are already infected by this bacteria but it causes them no problems. It is estimated that about 70% of cases are asymptomatic, i.e. they have no visible ill effects. And although the rate of infection has been decreasing in developed countries probably because of better hygiene and increased use of antibiotics, acid reflux and cancer of the oesophagus has increased. But this could simply be due to the influence of numerous other factors such as the quality of food.

Helicobacter pylori can be tested for using rapid tests which look for the body's antibodies to H pylori infections. These are very simple and just use a spot of finger prick blood. Doctors use a rather more complicated method which requires a laboratory.

How do we all get infected by H. pylori? Interestingly, H pylori is carried on the feet of houseflies and they spread the bacteria to our food when they land on it. So the key is to clear refuse promptly and avoid flies in the house. Saving money on fortnightly bin collections may prove to be rubbish if it increases medical bills thousands of times over due to outbreaks of gastric ulcers.

So how does a duodenal ulcer cause vertical lines on your forehead? No-one is sure, but quite independently I have found the ancient art of Chinese face reading confirms these vertical lines as a Body Language sign, along with many others that have been around for thousands of years. The Chinese say horizontal lines indicate stomach and spleen problems, and a dot or pimple in the middle of the forehead indicates the power of the pituitary gland. Eyebrows that disappear towards the outer edge indicate poor thyroid functioning, while two vertical lines above the nose where the eyebrows end signify gallbladder problems.

My own explanation centres on the advice from researchers which says that sufferers of peptic ulcers more often than not tend to be thin, morose individuals who often worry about finances and work. Maybe this attitude gives them a tendency to develop a worried look typified by a deeply furrowed brow. Worrying tends to increase stomach acidity, and irregular eating habits cause the stomach to shrink, producing folds of skin in which H pylori can multiply in luxury and produce areas of irritation. So this could be why people who worry a lot are said to be susceptible to ulcers.

It also comes back to our evolutionary roots. Humans were designed to be browsers eating periodically throughout the day, not carnivores who gorge on one meal a day, if they are lucky. Skipping meals is likely to give H pylori the opportunity it needs to be aggravating. So eat little and often, and for goodness sake don't worry. Literally.

Do you have haemorrhoids (or piles)?

You may have a deficiency of fibre in your diet.

Haemorrhoids, also known as piles, are rather like varicose veins in the canal of the anus. Here, just under the mucous membrane (inner lining), is a considerable network of veins extending upwards for an inch or so from the level of the skin to just above the anal canal, where it joins the rectum. When the veins of this network become swollen with blood, haemorrhoids develop.

The vein swelling can affect the part of the network just above the anal canal, where it is less well supported by the muscular ring or sphincter, and this causes internal haemorrhoids. Or it may affect the veins at the lower end of the canal, just under the skin, causing external haemorrhoids. Some unfortunate people have both, not being content with a few haemorrhoids they have to have piles of them.

Haemorrhoids are a common problem and affect around 50% of people at some time in their life. Although uncomfortable and embarrassing, it is not normally a serious condition unless they bleed sufficiently to cause anaemia.

The common symptoms of haemorrhoids are:

- Itching around the anus
- Signs of blood (bright red) on toilet paper after a bowel motion
- Soreness and discomfort during and immediately after a bowel motion
- A visible swelling around the anus
- A feeling that your bowels have not been completely emptied

Sometimes haemorrhoids inside the anal canal protrude outside the anus. These are known as prolapsed or prolapsing haemorrhoids. At first, the haemorrhoid may go back in by itself, but later you might need to push it back in yourself using your finger.

Protruding haemorrhoids can lead to skin irritation and discomfort and there is usually mucus discharge from the irritated mucous membrane. Internal haemorrhoids can become inflamed and swollen, but are rarely very painful, unless associated with an anal fissure.

Haemorrhoids are generally thought to be caused by constipation. If you have constipation over a period of time and often have to strain to pass hard stools, this can damage the lining of the anal canal. If this happens often enough, the veins may lose their normal support and protection. Some people are thought to have veins especially liable to this kind of injury. This is probably just a matter of chance anatomical variation. But we are led to believe that haemorrhoids are a modern phenomenon, due to a diet poor in fibre, and a lifestyle lacking in hard physical exercise, causing many of us to exceed our optimum weight.

We have it on good authority that haemorrhoids are not caused by sitting on cold hard surfaces, prolonged standing or sedentary work. Not sure about sitting on a horse for most of your life, though. I have often wondered if cowboys in films walk like that because their legs have developed a bandy shape or whether they just have a sore bum. The hell they have.

The veins around the anus drain into larger veins that carry the blood through the liver and up to the heart. This part of the system of large veins has no valves in it, and the whole weight of the blood bears down on the lowest veins in the system, that tend to stretch. Anything restricting the free upward flow of blood through these veins leads to an increase in pressure in them. This is why haemorrhoids are so common in pregnancy, especially in older mothers.

Do you have a low fibre diet?

Dietary fibre is the undigested remains of plant materials, particularly indigestible plant carbohydrates (i.e. the non-starch polysaccharides). Fibre is found only in foods derived from plants, and all plant food provides at least some fibre; how much depends on whether it has been processed. Unpeeled fruit and vegetables and whole meal or whole-grain cereal foods (which still contain the outer layers of the grain) will provide the most. For example, brown rice can contain seven times more fibre than white rice. The exact balance of the various components of dietary fibre (cellulose, hemicelluloses, pectin and lignin) varies between foods.

Soluble and insoluble fibre

Dietary fibre can be soluble or insoluble. Soluble fibre dissolves in the gut, to form a viscous gel that slows down the release of some nutrients, particularly the sugar glucose, into the bloodstream; it is therefore good for diabetics. It can also reduce the risk of heart disease, by reducing blood cholesterol levels. Soluble fibre is present in fruit, vegetables, pulses (e.g. kidney beans, baked beans, lentils) and foods containing oats, barley or rye. That's why porridge for breakfast is great at reducing cholesterol.

Insoluble fibre has a sponge-like effect in the gut, soaking up water and swelling in size. This effect produces a feeling of fullness and adds bulk to the gut contents, making waste matter heavier and speeding it through the large intestine, and thus reducing the risk of constipation, and possibly even reducing the risk of cancers of the digestive system.

Personally I am a big fan of oats, and not just because of my Scottish ancestry. Oats provide fibre and are an excellent carrier to cleans the digestive system. In some countries with primitive healthcare porridge containing herbs is used as a chelating agent, to remove toxic metals from the body after cases of poisoning. Porridge also reduces cholesterol levels in the body. Although there is a modern tendency to supply everyone with a lifetime's supply of statins to reduce cholesterol, this could be achieved quite effectively if we all had porridge for breakfast. Oats do not have the gruelling side effects of statins either. I make the bread in our household and usually mix white flour, wholemeal or spelt flour, oats, linseed or omega 3 seeds, yeast, sea salt and olive oil. Brilliant. Oh, but I did say there were no recipes in this book.

Cereal and grain products (e.g. bread, flour, breakfast cereals, rice, pasta), especially wholemeal varieties, and fibrous vegetables (e.g. carrots and celery) are primary sources of insoluble fibre.

Fibre is good for us

Fibre is something most people should eat more of. The overall nutritional balance of our diets could be improved just by eating a few more high-fibre foods. However, fibre in an isolated form as a supplement (such as bran) is not the answer because bran can actually reduce the absorption of minerals from our food. Fibre is thought to be far more beneficial if it is consumed as an integral part of food, rather than as bran supplements or fibre-containing drinks.

Sources of dietary fibre

- Wholemeal bread,
- Whole-wheat pasta,
- Dried apricots,
- Baked beans,
- Jacket potato, including the skin
- Breakfast cereal.
- Porridge

Do you get white spots on your shoes?

If you do, you may be Diabetic

When someone is diabetic, they excrete sugar in their urine. Hippocrates used to taste the urine of his patients and could readily identify a diabetic this way by the sweet taste of the sugar in the urine.

But shoes do not get diabetes, so where do the white spots come from?

Well, when men urinate they usually get splashing as the urine stream hits the toilet bowl or urinal. And when the urine splashes dry on their shoes the sugar content crystallises out and causes the spots to turn white.

So white spots on your shoes could indicate that you're diabetic. Or maybe you've just emulsioned a ceiling. There is another alternative scenario. Possibly you stood too close to someone else who was urinating. That's the trouble with these modern high-density public urinals.

Diabetes is a chronic disease that affects the way your body utilises sugar. A healthy body will digest food and convert it into glucose, a sugar that fuels the cells of the body. A hormone called insulin is essential to this process. Insulin is needed in order for the body to have the energy it needs to grow and stay healthy. People with diabetes are unable to produce, or efficiently use, insulin. It is a very serious condition and can be life-threatening. However, with early diagnosis and good management, people can live a normal life with diabetes.

What are the causes?

Diabetes can come in two forms: type 1 diabetes, which is usually diagnosed in children and teenagers, and type 2 diabetes which is usually diagnosed in adults. The causes of both types of diabetes are still unknown, however, type 1 is thought to have genetic causes while type 2 is more strongly linked to lifestyle factors such as obesity, lack of exercise and poor diet. In particular, chromium deficiency is commonly linked to diabetes type 2.

How common is this condition?

In 2000, 171 million people worldwide suffered from diabetes. This is expected to be 366 million by 2030 - mainly due to a huge rise in diabetes in the numbers in African and Asian countries that are now introducing Western foods into their lifestyle.

The commonest symptoms are as follows:

- Frequent urination
- Excessive thirst/hunger
- Excessive tiredness
- Blurred vision
- Dalmation shoes

Your body relies on you to supply it with the right amount of quality food, but the food suppliers want you to buy only their product, so there is a conflict straight away. They tempt you with abnormal amounts of sugar, salt, flavour enhancers, colourants and added flavourings. So your taste buds are fooled into thinking that you are getting a good diet while your body has other ideas. That is believed to be the main reason obesity levels are at an all time high. Our stomach still hasn't received the nutrients it needs, so it tells the brain to tell the mouth to keep on eating.

Ideally we need to be telling food manufacturers to stop providing us with an unnatural diet, but the food chain is big business and the governments won't cut out their gravy train of taxation. We need to act ourselves.

The Body Language of Health

Your body breaks down most of the food you eat and uses it to gain energy and extract nutrients. If you lack certain nutrients in your diet, your body processes will not be able to function properly. Likewise, if you exceed the appropriate sugar levels in your body, you will risk getting diabetes. You should choose a wholesome diet without junk food and take supplements, because otherwise the food you eat is unlikely to provide you with all the nutrients you need. Three very important nutrients that your body needs to carry out this function are chromium, vanadium and vitamin A.

The Chromium link

The Diabetes UK website advises the following:

Chromium forms a substance in the body known as the glucose tolerance factor. People with a deficiency of chromium can therefore develop problems with glucose tolerance.

Good dietary sources of chromium are Brewers yeast, meat, cheese, vegetables, whole grains, nuts, wine and beer. So if you are taking a balanced diet you are very unlikely to be low in chromium. (However, as we have found, most people don't get a balanced diet and nutritionists advise that most of us are deficient in something-Ed)

At present Diabetes UK suggests that chromium is given as a supplement, where a chromium deficiency has been diagnosed. Otherwise it is recommended that people with diabetes try to follow a healthy, balanced diet to ensure adequate intake of all essential nutrients.

It crossed my mind when reading their advice about a good diet, that this perfectly describes a ploughman's lunch washed down with a pint of beer. But beer is loaded with sugar and the alcohol is converted to sugar as well, so for Diabetes UK to include beer on their list is bad advice. Unfortunately Diabetes UK focuses on type 1 diabetes whereas by far the biggest group of sufferers have type 2 diabetes, for whom any sugar at all may be difficult for the body to cope with. There seems to be very little good advice for sufferers of type 2 diabetes out there. So I have produced my own.

Steps to healthy eating to control Type 2 diabetes

Again, the internet quotes various advice for type 1 diabetics, but for the vast millions of people who are diabetic type 2 the advice is wrong.

The Body Language of Health

If you have type 2 diabetes, the following steps will help you to control your blood glucose levels as well as regulate your weight. These steps are good advice whether you are diabetes type 2 or not, as they will help prevent the disease as well.

Eat regular meals based around vegetables. Limit your intake of starchy carbohydrate foods such as bread, pasta, chapattis, potatoes, rice and cereals. This will help you to control your blood glucose levels. Whenever possible, choose wholegrain varieties of carbohydrate that are high in fibre, like wholemeal bread and wholemeal cereals to help maintain the health of your digestive system and prevent problems such as constipation.

Cut down on the fat you eat, particularly saturated (animal) fats, as this type of fat is linked to heart disease. Choose monounsaturated fats, e.g. olive oil. Eating less fat and fatty foods will also help you to lose weight. Grill, steam or oven bake instead of frying or cooking with oil or other fats. Don't use or consume any trans-fats or other 'manufactured' oils or fats. Eat plenty of fish. Avoid Statins at all cost.

Eat more fruit and vegetables — aim for at least five portions a day to provide you with vitamins and fibre as well as to help you balance your overall diet. A portion is, for example, a piece of fruit or a serving of a vegetable. Sugar in fruit is OK because it is locked in plant cells and is released into the body slowly. Try raw vegetables, roast vegetables, or a vegetable curry but without sugar if it is out of a tin or packet.

Cut out sugar and sugary foods — your body does not require sugar, you get more than enough energy from the other foods. Manufacturers have wrongly classified sugar as a food and it isn't at all. Eating sugar is as bad for your body as it is to put rocket fuel in your car engine. Read the ingredients in all processed food carefully because most are loaded with sugar. Use sugar sparingly as an ingredient in foods and in baking if you have to. Only use sugar-free or diet squashes and fizzy drinks, as sugary drinks cause blood glucose levels to rocket. Be aware that most junk food is loaded with sugar. Cheap supermarket ice cream is about 20% sugar and the rest is nasty omega 6 oil. How dare they make and sell such rubbish? How can you buy it?

Avoid alcohol or drink in moderation only — that's two units of alcohol per day for a woman and three units per day for a man. For example, a small glass of wine or half a pint of normal-strength beer is approximately one unit. Never drink on an empty stomach, as alcohol can make hypoglycaemia (low blood glucose levels) more likely to occur.

If you are overweight, losing weight will help you control your diabetes and will also reduce your risk of heart disease, high blood pressure and stroke. Take care with any dieting. Aim to lose weight slowly over time (1-2 lbs per week) rather than crash dieting. Even if you don't manage to get your ideal weight, losing a small amount and keeping it off will help with your blood glucose control and improve your overall health.

Exercise is the key. Try a mixture of walking, dancing, gardening, swimming, aerobics, weight training, exercise machines, and plenty of sex (if you can still manage it after all that exercise). Burning off calories with gentle consistent exercise is the best way to balance your sugar and avoid diabetes; sex will take your mind off food.

Snacks are not a problem, try nuts, sticks of vegetables or root veg crisps, fruit, crackers, hummus, cottage cheese, unsweetened yoghurt, and various nut, seed and fruit mix from your local health shop. Or try a little bag of unsweetened muesli occasionally. But avoid things cooked in trans-fats and Omega 6 oils like sunflower oil.

Don't be tempted by 'diabetic' foods or drinks. They are expensive, unnecessary and have no added benefit for people with diabetes.

Are you overweight or obese?

If so, you may be searching for that vital nutritional element missing in your diet

Bet you thought I had the usual criticism for you if to happen to be a Bunter. Eat less pies, Fatty. But my thinking is taking a different approach, because experts now agree that the Western World is overfed and undernourished. We eat to gather the nutritional elements we need, and when our food fails to deliver them, we eat some more because our body is still not satisfied and is still searching for those missing ingredients.

We don't trigger the 'I'm full' switch because we haven't eaten what we really need. So we get fatter and fatter, and in doing so, make even more demands on our body.

Many food companies employ experts to make their food more addictive so they make more profit. They add anything that's cheap and addictive, usually sugar, salt, lactic acid, artificial flavourings and colours. America has 200 million tons of lactic acid to dispose of from the manufacture of dairy produce like cheese, so manufacturers put it into everything we consume. Even crisps are sprinkled with lactic acid. In a recent survey, 97% of the food we eat in the western world was found to be artificially treated to make it more palatable. Coupled with the poor nutrition of the soil, it is not surprising we are undernourished.

In April 2006 in the UK research showed that nearly 2 million schoolchildren were overweight and 700,000 were obese because of a poor diet and lack of exercise, according to research by the International Obesity Taskforce. Experts have said that across the UK 160,000 school-age children are displaying signs they could develop heart disease, while 150,000 have high blood pressure and unhealthy cholesterol levels. Researchers reviewed data from 39 studies and discovered that there were signs of type 2 diabetes, which normally only occurs in adults, in up to 4,000 children.

The research also revealed that 58,000 children in the UK have impaired glucose tolerance, which is an early sign that they are at an increased risk of developing diabetes. The report said that the number of overweight children across the EU is set to top 26 million within four years, with 6.4 million of them being classed as clinically obese.

And now, we are imposing the Western nutrition on the third world through clever marketing, into a population which already has dire nutritional imbalances through malnutrition. That's a disaster waiting to happen.

So how do you tackle obesity?

The first thing to do is find out what your fundamental needs are and then supply them. Review the Body language signs and symptoms and find those that relate to you. Each one lists foods that you should focus on.

The internet and the popular press are bulging at the seams with advice on weight. Ignore it. You don't need special diets, slimming foods etc. You need good wholesome food. Here is my advice. Throughout the research for Body Language I have come across 'superfoods' and they are all the old basics - not expensive, easy to prepare and tasty. Here they are – include an abundance of these and you'll not go far wrong.

Eggs are the perfect food. They contain absolutely everything needed to sustain life in one convenient package. All the protein, minerals etc. And cheap, easy to cook and versatile. The famous cricket umpire, 'Dicky' Bird used to make sure he only ate fried eggs and chips when on tour in foreign climates, and he took his own eggs with him. This enabled him to monitor a cricketer's performance without getting the runs himself. Howzat for a play on words?

Choose liberal helpings of the following:

- Carrots and all other green, red or orange vegetables.
- Nuts
- Cheese in moderation
- Brightly coloured fruit
- Chicken, preferably free range, and game birds
- Oily fish
- Lean meat in moderation
- Water / mineral water

Be careful with chicken, most suppliers now feed their chickens beef fat to make them so plump in 4 weeks that there's more fat in a chicken portion than in a burger. But game birds have recently been voted pleasant creatures as they have lean meat and a high level of selenium which is an anti-cancer element.

Think you can't stick to this diet? Well, you can eat as much as you want, and even if you hate the stuff it is a fact that if someone eats something 20 times they will then love it. Apparently it's an in built conditioning factor that helps us survive on things like earthworms, rats, or grasshoppers, which happens to be the diet of millions of people in the world every day.

Maybe this is your diet. I have eaten some strange food in foreign countries, especially in China where people still starve to death so I should think myself lucky really. My diet has included raw shrimps, boiled donkey penis and raw jellyfish (a surreal experience as it is jelly-like and tastes vaguely of riverwater but is strangely fantastically crunchy as you bite through that transparent muscle).

Do you have pernicious anaemia?

You may be deficient in Vitamin B12 and Cobalt

Pernicious anaemia is a specific type of anaemia that occurs when your stomach and gut cannot absorb Vitamin B12. It is characterized by abnormally large red blood cells, gastrointestinal disturbances, and lesions of the spinal cord. Because B12 is based on cobalt, pernicious anaemia can often be due to insufficient cobalt in your diet.

The Body Language of Health

Pernicious anaemia is also known as megaloblastic anaemia and is different in several ways from every other kind of anaemia. This name is really no longer appropriate. It was given at a time when the cause and treatment of the disease were unknown and the outcome was usually death. Nowadays the condition is easily and effectively treated. Early diagnosis is, however, still vital.

Pernicious anaemia is most common in older people. It affects about 1 in 8,000 people over the age of 60. It is more common in women than in men and is more prevalent in people with fairer colouring. There is some evidence that pernicious anaemia may be genetic although its mode of inheritance is poorly documented.

Good sources of Vitamin B12

- Dairy produce
- Eggs
- Yeast extract
- Seaweed
- Spirulina algae
- Liver

Pernicious anaemia was first described in 1855 by the English physician Thomas Addison. The name "pernicious anaemia" was coined in 1872 by the German physician Anton Biermer. The later studies of George H. Whipple on the benefits of feeding liver in anaemia followed by those of George R. Minot and Wm. P. Murphy on the beneficial effects of feeding liver specifically in pernicious anaemia. This led to the cure of pernicious anaemia and resulted in all three experts receiving the Nobel Prize in 1934.

This was good old fashioned science. Murphy bled dogs to make them anaemic then fed them various substances to see if anything would make them healthy again. He found that feeding liver made them better then set about finding what was so special in the liver that gave such a miraculous and rapid cure.

In nature, B12 is solely produced by bacteria found in animals, but the B12 molecule is complicated and includes a vital atom of cobalt, without which Vitamin B12 cannot be produced. So a deficiency of cobalt is deadly serious. While vegetarians should get enough B12 through dairy products or eggs, it can sometimes be lacking in those following a vegan diet. Several studies of vegans on raw food diets show that raw food offers no special protection against B12 deficiency.

The usual way to determine Vitamin B12 deficiency is to carry out a Schilling test. In the first part of the test the patient is given Vitamin B12 containing radioactive cobalt. Urine is then collected for 24 hours. If it contains at least 10% radioactive Vitamin B12 the patient has normal B12 levels and has excreted the excess. If the result is less than 5% radioactive B12 the patient has a deficiency and has absorbed the new supply. The test is redone using additional cofactor to see if the patient has a problem absorbing B12, which could be due to coeliac disease, Whipple's disease or a liver problem. Despite its name, this test is very expensive to carry out.

Are you taking Antibiotics?

You are at risk of a Yeast Infection

The problem with antibiotics seems to be that they are so universally prescribed that it is rare to find an individual who has gone through life without them. And most people you talk to say that they feel odd when they are taking them, and their food tastes strange.

The problem is not just confined to taking medication though, because 80% of all the antibiotics made are used on animals, so we consume a dose of antibiotics every time we eat animal products.

This section should have been straight forward to research, but it was difficult for one reason. There are some extremely committed anti-antibioticists out there who would have you think that every aliment you are ever going to contract is caused by....... well I imagine you can guess. Still not sure about the term anti-antibioticists though, treated mathematically the anti-anti cancel out and we are left with ... something that sounds rather like bioterrorists actually. Ironic therefore that these people are so fanatical they appear to treat the manufacturers of antibiotics as bioterrorists themselves.

Wading through this data has revealed two overwhelming facts. The first is that when your body has genuinely been invaded by some serious bacteria, (and there are some Trojans out there) you need one thing and nothing else will do. And that one thing is antibiotics.

The Body Language of Health

The second thing is that when your body can cope with an infection, there is just one thing you should keep away from, and that's antibiotics too. They are useless on viruses anyway, and that is where almost all of our coughs and colds originate.

So, I have focussed on three questions which I think are important. When should you take antibiotics?; when should you refrain?; and what should you do when you've already taken them?

Actually, I had my own Eureka moment while I was researching this section, and it made me raise my eyebrows. (maybe this is a Body Language sign for 'interesting discovery!'). As a schoolboy I had learnt about Alexander Fleming and his chance discovery in 1928 of a petri dish culture in which mould had produced a substance (penicillin) that repelled bacteria which were thriving elsewhere on the culture medium. More of that later.

What I suddenly realised in my Eureka moment is that penicillin mould is a *mould; a fungus.* And its natural tendency is to drive out bacteria to make a home for its mouldy old friends instead. Take antibiotics and you have made perfect conditions for yeast proliferation. Obvious actually, but for some reason I had never quite thought of it in those terms, and I wondered if others had failed to make the same connection. It's a bit like enjoying the shooting star display to start with, only to find that tomorrow you will be living with a Triffid. Invading your body!!!

A bit like employing and arming Saddam Hussein to get him to take care of Iran for you, isn't it, then realising you have set up a tyrant? Or like giving a home to Sally to eat your grass, not realising she would find roses and rhododendrons much more interesting.

As a typical human you have three to four pounds of beneficial bacteria and yeast cells living within your intestines. These microbes compete for nutrients from the food you eat. Usually, the strength in numbers of beneficial bacteria keeps the ever-present yeast in check.

However, every time you take a course of antibiotics, you kill the beneficial bacteria within your intestines. When you do so, you upset the delicate balance of your intestinal flora. Yeasts grow unchecked into large colonies and take over, in a condition called dysbiosis.

In the 1980's I did some property developing and ended up treating timber and damp. I developed my skills in timber fungal attack to the extent that I would often receive commissions to survey large, old properties, sometimes from Elizabethan times, and report on the fungal infestations that I observed. Occasionally I would be stunned by the extent of fungal growth. I remember one old property consisting of four storeys plus a cellar. Wet rot had started in the corner of the cellar and had allowed dry rot to get hold. There were mycelia, the very fine strands of fungus feeding roots, all over the cellar, and they had penetrated behind the plaster and extended right up the walls to the fourth storey where they had broken out into big fruiting bodies releasing trillions of spores. This network of myceliae was so complex and intricate yet so delicate at the same time that I could not help admiring the driving force within such a simple organism that had grown as big as an oak, held up by the house.

Yeasts are opportunistic Triffids. They will encase your bread and cheese in mycelia and devour it as soon as conditions are favourable, and they won't stop even if the loaf is four storeys high.

This means that, as the antibiotic drives out your intestinal bacteria, yeasts will thrive, especially when their dietary needs are met with a supply of sugar in your diet. Yeasts can use their myceliae, or hyphae, to literally poke holes through the lining of your intestinal wall. This results in a syndrome called leaky gut. Yeasts are not the only possible cause of this syndrome. Some scientists have linked non-steroidal, anti-inflammatory drugs (NSAIDS) such as naproxen and ibuprofen to the problem as well. Given their ability to alter intestinal terrain, antibiotics are very likely to contribute to leaky gut syndrome.

I can imagine the yeast overgrowth associated with leaky gut syndrome to be similar to the properties I surveyed, with yeast cells becoming a parasite within the gut. Some experts inform that is why yeast infections have been linked to various ailments such as ME or 'yuppie flu' and many allergies and underlying aliments that simply make you feel under par. I have already mentioned, for example, that those people I know with asthma seem to have athlete's foot, which is another type of yeast infection, suggesting a possible link here because it stimulates your immune system.

There is some evidence that parasitic yeasts can also cause you to change what you eat in that they encourage you to binge on carbohydrates, perhaps because they mop up sugars in your diet, leaving you feeling sugar deficient. This may be why food tastes strange when you are on antibiotics. So, it should come as no surprise that massive weight gain counts as one of the telltale signs of antibiotic damage and subsequent yeast overgrowth. Now, that's real Bio-terrorism.

My good friend Simon Galloway has recommended a clever test to see if you have a Candida yeast infection. And like all the best tests, it is simple and logical.

The Body Language of Health

First thing in the morning, before you put anything in your mouth, get a clear glass and fill it with water. But don't drink it. Work up a bit of saliva in your mouth and spit it out into the glass. Chances are it will sit there floating on top or else it will ball up and sink. Put the glass down where it won't be disturbed (or drunk by someone at the breakfast table) and observes it every quarter of an hour for an hour or so.

Is the saliva still floating after an hour? You're OK. Are there cloudy specks suspended in the water, has the saliva dropped to the bottom of the glass? These are indicators of other things but not Candida. Is saliva still floating on top with strings (like legs) travelled down into the water? You have a Candida infection. Brilliant.

Huge though it is, human consumption is not the biggest use of antibiotics. Far more, in fact 80% of all the antibiotics that are made are fed to livestock on a daily basis, with the intention of protecting them against bacteria. This practice not only possibly contributes to antibiotic resistance in humans, but many experts believe that it is animal weight gain, and not disease prevention, that is the real reason antibiotics are so widely used. Remember we said in people, yeast infection causes weight gain? Fat cattle sell for more than thin cattle. That's all very well, but imagine the antibiotics present in beef, pork, chicken, milk and all the processed foods containing dairy produce that we then eat. No-one knows what that is doing to our health.

So, when should you take antibiotics? Most definitely when you have as serious bacterial infection that will not clear up with your body's natural defences. Antibiotics are necessary in these circumstances, even though many scientists will agree that, great though antibiotics are, very many more lives have been saved in the world through simple improvements in basic hygiene.

When should you refrain from taking antibiotics? The answer is whenever they will not benefit your health. Colds, coughs (other than streptococcus infections) and numerous ailments for which antibiotics are dished out at the moment that will not benefit from antibiotics. One of the most common diagnoses given at a doctor's office in America is the upper respiratory infection (URI). It accounts for up to 70 percent of all antibiotics dispensed and virtually all are unnecessary. Taking them when not needed will not only render you prone to a yeast infection. They will build up bacterial immunity to the drug making it less effective when you really do need it.

What should you do when you've already taken them? Well, we only take antibiotics when we are sick, when our immune system is weakened or fighting another invader. But antibiotics destroy the friendly bacteria in our intestines, such as Lactobacillus acidophilus, Bifidus and Bulgaricus. Triffids are even more likely to get a hold, so we should take probiotic supplements of these friendly bacteria. They protect us against pathogens such as Salmonella, yeast, cholera, Escheria coli (E coli), Pseudomonas, Clostridium, Klebsiella, and by Candida yeast, the Triffid of the fungi family.

In order to make some informed decisions, you could also consider the following general advice.

1. Take an ounce of prevention. Exercise, eat intelligently and take a few supplements. Avoid alcohol, smoking, and recreational drugs. Get more rest. Relax with a video - watch 'Day of the Triffids' (that advice was mine).

2. Ask questions if you visit your doctor when you have an infection. If your doctor diagnoses you with an upper respiratory infection, sore throat (in which the strep test is negative), bronchitis, sinusitis, or ear infection, and you wonder if you really need an antibiotic, make a point of asking them about it. Most doctors are pleasantly surprised that one of their patients would take the trouble to be knowledgeable about their condition and consider trying to recuperate without antibiotics. Ask if you can treat your condition symptomatically and come back or call in a couple of days if you are not better. Try one of my natural Immune Boost patches that include allicin and zinc.

Most people do get better without drugs and a lot of people tend to underestimate their body's healing abilities. Remember that the illnesses that 'do the rounds' are vital to your immune system, they are doing you a favour by keeping the system running smoothly and alert to any invaders, though it doesn't seem that way at the time. Trust the decision of your doctor because they are always in a better position than you are to make the decision whether or not to prescribe drugs.

3. Take an objective look at yourself and your life-style. If you keep coming down with the same thing, do some research and a little thinking. Review this book, make changes and get in shape. The point is that a myriad of factors contribute to "wellness."

There are a few things you can do to help your body when you are on a course of antibiotics.

1. Take an antioxidant supplement. Vitamin C would be ideal, with plenty of water. But beware, sweetened orange is the WORST thing you could drink.

2. Keep your bowels moving. If antibiotics kill off your friendly, intestinal bacteria, once you cease taking antibiotics you'll run a higher risk of infection by other, more hostile bacteria. These bacteria will be quick to find and exploit pockets of debris that could be collecting and putrefying in

your intestines if you happen to become constipated. So, be sure to keep your digestive tract as clear as possible until you can repopulate it with friendly bacteria. Eat plenty of high fibre food. Heard of 'feed a cold'?

3. Replace the good bacteria in your intestines. Supplement with an acidophilus supplement for a few weeks following any course of antibiotics. Do not take these simultaneously with your antibiotic, or you will simply end up with a lot of very dead, albeit still friendly bacteria in your intestines. At the very most, take acidophilus supplements either in between antibiotic doses or after you have completely finished your prescription.Look back at why you became ill to begin with. Diet plays at least as much a role as actual exposure to germs as to whether we get sick -- when we are healthy and eating correctly, our bodies are remarkably resistant to infection.

4. One, last note: Please ignore advertisements that recommend guzzling orange juice for the vitamin C it contains. A big dose of sugar is what you'd actually be getting. I have heard several people say that once they felt they were coming down with something, they immediately began downing glass after glass of orange juice, only to get even sicker. They concluded that they must not have caught the illness in time, which couldn't have been any further from the truth. The fact is, they probably simply fuelled the fire of their infections with lots of sugar, all because they trusted a manufacturer's advertisement to educate them about proper healing strategies. Sugar is Trifid fertilizer. Your body is 70 percent water - and that is exactly what it needs! Water.

Back to Professor Alexander Fleming, a bacteriologist working in 1928 at St Mary's Hospital in London who accidentally discovered Penicillin. It was the first of the antibiotics but he failed to stabilize the substance because the germ-destroying qualities lasted for only a few days. The next major breakthrough was achieved when stabilization was achieved by Australian-born pathologist Howard Florey and the German-born Ernst Chain, a chemist, working at Oxford University in 1940. The war gave them sixty five million casualties and their product appeared just in time.

The invention of antibiotic has proved to be the "miracle drug" but indiscriminate use has led to resistant strains such as the British super bug MRSA. (methicillin resistant Staph. aureus). Many microbiologists will tell you that, great though antibiotics have been, it was improvement in basic hygiene that gave the greatest rewards to health. And antibiotics are being targeted more and more now as the bringers of long term ill health and poor food quality due to indiscriminate use throughout farming.

The Body Language of Health

Some experts believe the increasing use of antibiotics to treat disease might also be responsible for the rising rates of asthma and allergies. By upsetting the body's normal balance of gut microbes, antibiotics may prevent our immune system from distinguishing between harmless chemicals and real attacks.

"The microbial gut flora is an arm of the immune system," says Gary Huffnagle at the University of Michigan in Ann Arbour. His research group has provided the first experimental evidence in mice that upsetting the gut flora can provoke an allergic response.

Asthma has increased by around 160 per cent globally in the last 20 years. Currently about a quarter of schoolchildren in the US and a third of those in the UK have the condition, but pinning down the causes of the rise has proved difficult. Some researchers have blamed modern dust-free homes, while others have pointed to diet.

Antibiotics have been implicated as the cause by some epidemiological studies. For example, the rise in allergies and asthma has tracked widespread antibiotic use. Furthermore, research in Berlin, Germany, has found that both antibiotic treatment and asthma were low in the east compared to the west when the wall came down. As antibiotic use has increased in the east though, so has asthma. This study is particularly valuable because the politically divided populations were genetically very similar and enjoyed much the same menu.

There is also a highly significant association between Crohn's disease and prior antibiotic use in this data. This is unlikely to be explained by reporting bias because all prescriptions are recorded without any intention of using that data for this type of epidemiological study. If this association is real then it is thought that antibiotics may explain about a quarter of all Crohn's disease.

INTEGRATED MEDICINE

Geologists, naturopaths, and forward thinking doctors are telling us that most of us are chronically deficient of some nutrient or other. Why? Because our modern diet is far from ideal, and intensive farming has depleted many essential trace elements from the soil, so even the healthiest diet is still lacking in some essential nutrient or other.

Dr Julian Kenyon, an eminent expert in 'life threatening diseases' (in Britain a doctor is no longer allowed to advertise their expertise in cancer diagnosis so the title has been watered down to 'life-threatening disease') started the British Society for

The Body Language of Health

Integrated Medicine because he realised that medicine was more than waiting until the condition became serious and then treating the symptoms with drugs.

His Royal Highness Prince Charles is also a great believer in an integrated approach, though this has not always gone down well with the establishment who believe the National Health Service should be providing drugs not alternative healthcare activities like nutrition. He set up the Prince's Foundation for Integrated Health because he believes that good health is not just about freedom from illness. It also requires mental and physical well being. He believes that many approaches to healthcare – from mainstream medical science through to traditional healing arts – can help us stay healthy, get better, and ease our pain.

Recently I got involved in The Princes Trust and realised they help over forty thousand individuals in one of four categories each year. These groups are unemployed young people, young people underachieving in education, young people leaving care, and young offenders and ex-offenders. I decided that The Prince's charities were high on the list of organisations that I would support with the profits from this book if it became successful.

Often, it takes someone from outside the establishment to look in and spot the obvious shortcomings. Maybe that is what Prince Charles has done. And I do believe that my background as a forensic scientist has enabled me to look objectively at health and its signs and symptoms without a blinkered approach. All I am suggesting is we try to balance out our minerals and vitamins with targeted nutrition, and with supplements provided we use caution and don't go overboard. At worst, we will better understand our bodies and the inevitable shortcomings of a poor quality modern diet and should be trying to eat a more balanced diet. At best we can treat our minor deficiencies before they turn serious.

So why has no-one identified these general nutritional needs before?

The probable answer is that this chronic shortage of one nutrient or other takes a long time to show because your body uses up the last smidgen of these nutrients before deficiencies start to reveal themselves in serious effects. This delay in cause and effect has fooled a lot of previous scientists into thinking the two were not linked. That is probably why it took many years to realise the cause of pellagra, for example, while millions of people suffered terribly, all because their diet based around maize lacked niacin. But many of today's population are suffering similar problems, the difference is the symptoms are underlying sub-optimal symptoms and poor nutrition is to blame.

The Body Language of Health

In the Western world, medicine is mainly curative, not preventive, i.e. we are treated with drugs/chemicals when we become ill. Healthcare and nutrition seem to be disconnected in modern medicine, even though this relationship has been known since Hippocrates' times two thousand years ago.

Modern diets are little better. We have developed a society where products are mainly judged on quantity not quality. Products sell because they are cheaper, so manufacturers are constantly pressurised into reducing price at the expense of quality. That is why fast food has developed into the less-than-a-dollar burger. Palm oils, hydrogenated oils, lactose, lupin flour, and many other ingredients are used to bulk out manufactured products that have become an unnatural diet to man.

Many doctors seem to underestimate the influence of nutrient depletion because they don't study much nutrition at medical college, and of course food and pharmaceutical companies won't tell them. As we have already found out, doctors are 'indoctrinated' to believe that everything about medicine has already been discovered.

But just as simple basic hygiene has had far more reaching impact than all the antibiotics put together, I believe that basic nutrition has the potential to make much more impact on health than we realise. A good wholesome diet has the potential to do away with that complicated health system which merely deals with the modern ailments that a poor or inappropriate diet causes.

After all, it has served modern man for 130,000 years and almost two million years before that while the human race was developing. So it's not surprising it is totally ingrained into our very bodies. That is why we function best on a cave man diet. We have evolved to eat the natural foods all around us.

If you notice any of the symptoms I describe in this book early on, that's good. Until Body Language came along, minor symptoms often remained hidden -- or their causes went undiscovered -- until life-threatening consequences appeared. Depleted levels of vital body nutrients also lead to lowered immune system function, in turn causing a host of other maladies. Now, at least, you can target your deficiency with the right food.

Common Drugs can result in Common Problems

Modern drugs like antibiotics are a marvel of modern living. Drugs modify your body and many of them are vital, but a few can also cause imbalances that may be in themselves rather serious. Here are a few of the interactions between drugs and other factors I have collected, but you should be aware these are difficult to verify.

Aspirin, acid-blockers, and cholesterol-lowering drugs can put you at risk for anaemia by depleting the body of iron, the signs of which include weakness and hair loss. If your doctor identifies that you are anaemic, they may offer iron supplementation yet still not identify your medication as the source of the problem.

A lot of drugs also interfere with nutrient absorption or with nutrient metabolism, storage, transport or use by cells. Because the initial signs of nutritional deficiency are subtle, cells and organs may become prone to disease conditions before the need for supplementation or change of medication is recognized. Drugs that interfere with calcium absorption, for instance, can lead to osteoporosis.

Antibiotic use is a good example of a drug affecting our well-being, because they kill helpful bacteria. Women taking antibiotics consequently often develop an overgrowth of Candida, including vaginal yeast infections, and doctors then prescribe even more medications to combat the yeast. This cycle can lead to immune system disturbance if overused. Antibiotics also deplete B vitamins that are necessary for hundreds of biological processes, including proper nervous system functioning -- suggesting, yet another array of pharmaceutical interventions.

Hormone replacement therapy (HRT) is another category of nutrient-depleting drugs. Vitamin C, zinc, and magnesium can be depleted, causing lowered resistance to colds and stress; magnesium depletion also interferes with absorption of calcium. Low levels of vitamin B6, B12, and folic acid associated with HRT or oral contraceptives also have a high correlation with elevated homocysteine levels, which result in arterial plaque build-up. When the heart has to work harder to adapt to plaque-narrowed arteries, blood pressure rises. And you risk developing heart disease.

Medications that lower blood pressure cause escalating problems of their own. Some reduce the levels of coenzyme Q10, a powerful antioxidant that is essential for cell energy and repairing free-radical damage to the heart muscle. Deficiencies can put you at risk of heart disease. Pretty ironic for a cardiovascular medicine.

Blood pressure medications further deplete vitamin B6 (already depleted by oestrogen replacement), thereby interfering with neurotransmitters that regulate mood, sleep, and appetite--all disturbances that can cause depression. To treat depression, doctors often prescribe antidepressants that would be unnecessary if the causes of depression were recognized. Some antidepressant drugs also deplete Vitamin B2, and can even trigger suicide attempts.

The Body Language of Health

Many medications can contribute to making the body too acidic, a condition in which opportunistic diseases can take hold and in which cancer cells can thrive. The typical Western diet, rich in meat, dairy products, sugar, alcohol, and processed foods, already tends to make the body acidic; medications may compound the problem.

Correcting the Problem

In Europe, one third of cancer sufferers now also take alternative medication along with their drugs. Currently the EU Directive on Supplements and the FDA supplements list in America is aiming to severely limit the use of supplements and herbs, despite the fact that our bodies have evolved with these as our natural medicine.

Many health problems can be alleviated through methods other than prescription drugs. If you choose to try alternatives, be certain to consult with a health professional before stopping any current prescription medication, and continue to take nutritional supplements to counteract the existing deficiencies. Your best advice will probably come from a practitioner of integrated medicine, which is an area that is bound to expand in future unless the pharmaceutical companies succeed in killing off herbs and supplements. If that happens, you will be able to diagnose all these Body Language signs and symptoms but you won't be able to do a darned thing about them.

Do you have Thyroid Swelling?

You may be deficient in IODINE

Iodine deficiency is one of the world's most prevalent causes of brain damage. Yet it could so easily be prevented, by providing the third world with cheap iodised salt.

Iodine deficiency disorders jeopardize children's mental health – often their very lives. They start before birth. Serious iodine deficiency during pregnancy may result in stillbirths, abortions and congenital abnormalities such as cretinism, a grave, irreversible form of mental retardation that affects people living in iodine-deficient areas of Africa and Asia. Iodine deficiency also causes babies to be born without thumbs. However, of far greater global and economic significance is iodine deficiency's less visible but more pervasive level of mental impairment that lowers intellectual power at home, at school and at work.

Good sources of Iodine

- Seaweed
- White fish
- Iodised table salt

Iodine deficiency disorder affects over 740 million people, 13% of the world's population, and 30% of the remainder are at risk.

• Iodine deficiency disorder preys upon poor, pregnant women and preschool children, posing serious public health problems in 130 developing countries.

• Iodine-deficient people may be giving up 15 IQ points. Iodine deficient candidates for Mensa can only join Densa instead. (You can do the U.S. 'Densa Test' on the web).

• Nearly 50 million people suffer from some degree of Iodine deficiency disorder-related brain damage

You can find more information on Iodine and 'Derbyshire Neck' elsewhere.

Do you have Catarrh, Sinusitis, or have you had tonsils or adenoids removed?

You may be intolerant to cows milk

Hippocrates first reported adverse reactions to cow's milk around 370 B.C. Since then the prevalence & awareness of intolerance has increased steadily but today many (some would say most) allergies are still caused by milk. My good friend, Dr Harry Morrow-Brown, one of the world's leading authorities on allergies, says this is not surprising. Cows milk is for baby cows, not humans.

Most people in the world cannot really digest milk. Ironically, this white 'liquid meat' is only tolerated by white western Europeans because they retained the right enzyme to digest it. Lactose intolerance is the inability for the body to digest the sugar lactose that is in milk. This is usually because there is insufficient level of the enzyme lactase in the gut to digest the sugar when you consume milk. This ability to produce lactase is inherited but the ability can disappear due to illness. As western Europeans colonised the new world, such as America, they took their lactase metabolism with them.

We are all born with the enzymes to digest milk because we need them to digest our mother's milk. But there comes a time when the enzymes disappear, because that is nature's way of forcing us to wean ourselves off milk and on to solid food. Europeans, though, hold on to some enzyme production and it would allow us to continue breast feeding almost indefinitely if cultural rules allowed it. Much of the following, therefore, refers to people of European origins.

As you get older the amount of lactase produced by your body reduces, making the intake of milk a bigger problem as you age. Those communities who do not use milk as part of their adult diet will have very little lactase in their bodies and then any large intake of milk will cause problems. African and Asian communities often suffer from lactose intolerance because they are unable to digest raw cows milk. You can always tell when a society have lactase deficiency because they can only digest milk once it has been cooked or when it has been fermented and turned into cheese.

The inability to digest lactose can cause a number of symptoms that are listed below. Lactose intolerance is not life threatening in the way that a milk allergy might be, but it can cause problems when associated with other illnesses such as Crohn's disease, Irritable Bowel Syndrome and Colitis.

Milk is made up of an emulsion of water, protein, lactose, minerals, fats and a variety of other substances. There are over 30 different proteins in milk, and these are broadly categorised as members of the casein or whey group of proteins. When milk ferments, naturally or aided by chemicals in the dairy, the milk changes into a solid fraction (curd) and a watery fraction (whey). The solid fraction contains the proteins belonging to the casein group, in which there are 4 main proteins. The liquid portion contains most of the other proteins, and these belong mainly to the whey group of proteins. So how can fermenting make milk more digestible?

What types of adverse reactions are possible?

Adverse reactions can be allergic (in this case, milk allergy), intolerance-based (in this case, lactose intolerance), or due to constituents that are less a matter of individual sensitivity. We now already know that some proteins cause allergies. Different mechanisms cause different adverse reactions but unfortunately the symptoms may be quite different from each other or they can be confusingly similar. Your body is able to mount a variety of defence mechanisms against proteins it regards as foreign or harmful. Experts don't really understand why food proteins are regarded as harmful by the body, or how these adverse reactions occur. For example, some milk-sensitive individuals produce immunoglobulin E (IgE) antibodies to milk proteins, but others develop a milk protein "intolerance," which results from the body mounting a non-IgE immune response to milk protein.

Milk allergy refers specifically to adverse reactions involving IgE antibodies to one or more protein fractions of milk, either the casein group or the whey protein group. Proteins belonging to the casein group are heat-stable, that is, they cannot be broken down using heat. Therefore individuals who are allergic to casein proteins cannot tolerate any cow's milk, including boiled milk.

In most instances, whey proteins can be broken down by heat, so individuals who are allergic to whole milk but not to boiled milk will be allergic to whey proteins.

You might think from this that you can decide for yourself what sort of intolerance you have, simply by trying boiled milk. But it is usually not quite that simple because the majority of IgE-mediated reactions to milk involve both the casein and whey fractions, which means that most milk-allergic individuals cannot tolerate boiled milk anyway. Allergy to milk may occur in anyone but the group of people most commonly affected by milk allergy are young children. But to complicate matters even more, people can suddenly develop a milk allergy at any age. We don't know why that is.

One of the problems with milk is that it contains a lot of growth hormones that the cow produces to stimulate growth in the calf. We don't need those. Ever wondered why Danish and Dutch men and women are so tall? They consume more dairy products than virtually anyone else on the planet.

Some countries such as USA feed their cows with a hormone called recombinant bovine growth hormone or rBGH, a synthetic hormone that virtually doubles milk production. Europe is against rBGH use but we are now importing milk from many other countries so cheaply that virtually the only way foreign farmers can guarantee cheap supply is through the use of rBGH. When we drink this we consume rBGH ourselves plus another hormone produced by the cow, growth factor-1 or IGF-1. A study by Harvard of 15,000 men published in the journal Science found that those men with elevated IGF-1 in their blood were four times more likely to get prostate cancer.

We should be careful of studies like this, because prostate cancer is not easy to monitor, but there is no doubt that milk and allergies go together.

Do you experience poor healing?

You may be deficient in ZINC

The first signs of zinc deficiency are impairment of taste, a poor immune response and skin problems. Other symptoms of zinc deficiency can include hair loss, diarrhoea, fatigue, delayed wound healing, and decreased growth rate and mental development in infants. It is thought that zinc supplementation can help skin conditions such as acne and eczema, prostate problems, anorexia nervosa, alcoholics and those suffering from trauma or post-surgery.

Impaired wound healing is a classic symptom of zinc deficiency, but it can also indicate deficiency in essential fatty acids.

The other signs and symptoms of zinc deficiency include anorexia, growth retardation, delayed sexual maturation, hypogonadism and hypospermia, alopecia, immune disorders, dermatitis, night blindness and impaired taste (hypogeusia). The first signs of zinc deficiency in marginally nourished children are sub optimal growth, anorexia, and impaired taste.

The most serious manifestations of zinc deficiency were reported in Iranian dwarfs. These adolescent boys, who consumed large amounts of clay, were retarded in growth and sexual development and had anaemia, hypogonadism, hepatosplenomegaly, rough skin, and mental lethargy. Clay eating, incidentally, is a clever trick that our ancestors learnt in times of famine. Because our need for minerals is so great, our stomachs have the capability of extracting them from many sources. In the absence of food, we can eat clay and extract the mineral nutrients from the clay as it passes through our digestive system. Not as potty as it sounds.

After treatment with a well-balanced diet containing adequate amounts of zinc for one year pubic hair appeared, sexual organs increased in size, linear growth was resumed, and the skin became normal. The anaemia responded to iron supplements too.

Zinc deficiency develops in some patients with cirrhosis because the ability to retain zinc is lost.

Clinical assessment of mild zinc deficiency is difficult because many of the signs and symptoms are non-specific. Nonetheless, if a malnourished person has a borderline-low plasma zinc level, is subsisting on a high fibre and phytate diet containing whole-grain bread (which reduces zinc absorption), and has reduced taste sensitivity, poor immunity (low lymphocyte level), and reduced gonadal hormone function, then zinc deficiency should be suspected, and treatment with zinc supplements should be tried.

Maternal zinc deficiency may cause anencephaly in the foetus. Secondary deficiency occurs in liver disease, in malabsorption states, and during prolonged breast feeding. Night blindness and mental lethargy may also be involved.

Good sources of Zinc

- lean meat
- seafood - especially oysters
- Eggs
- soybeans
- peanuts
- wheat germ
- cheese

Do you have Premenstrual Syndrome (PMT, PMS)?

You may be deficient in MAGNESIUM, ZINC and ESSENTIAL FATTY ACIDS

Premenstrual Syndrome (PMS) is a disorder characterized by a set of hormonal changes that trigger disruptive symptoms in a significant number of women for up to two weeks prior to menstruation. Of the estimated 40 million suffers in USA, more than 5 million require medical treatment for marked mood and behavioural changes. Often symptoms tend to taper off with menstruation and women remain symptom-free until the two weeks or so prior to the next menstrual period. These regularly recurring symptoms are typical of Premenstrual Syndrome.

Men find PMT difficult to fathom, because astonishingly more than 150 symptoms have been attributed to PMS. After complaints of feeling "out-of-control", anxious, depressed and having uncontrollable crying spells, the most common complaints are headache and fatigue. But symptoms may vary from month to month and there may even be symptom-free months. Fortunately, women seem to suffer from one or other at any time but not all the symptoms at once. Characteristically symptoms may be both physical and emotional. They may include physical symptoms such as headache, migraine, fluid retention, fatigue, constipation, painful joints, backache, abdominal cramping, heart palpitations and weight gain. Emotional and behavioural changes may include anxiety, depression, irritability, panic attacks, tension, lack of co-ordination, decreased work or social performance and altered libido. But not all at once, thankfully.

PMS sufferers have frequently been found to have deficiencies of zinc and magnesium. It is therefore worth increasing the diet of the foods rich in these elements, or even trying a supplement. Essential fatty acids have also been found to have a beneficial effect in reducing the symptoms. You will find lots of sections in this book referring to sources of these ingredients.

Do you have Cervical Dysplasia?

You may be deficient in BETA CAROTENE and FOLIC ACID

Cervical dysplasia is a term used to describe the appearance of abnormal cells on the surface of the cervix, the lowest part of the uterus. These changes in cervical tissue are classified as mild, moderate, or severe. While dysplasia itself does not cause health problems, it is usually considered to suggest a pre-cancerous condition. Left untreated, dysplasia sometimes progresses to an early form of cancer known as cervical carcinoma in situ, and eventually to invasive cervical cancer.

At one stage of my career I worked on a device for sampling and testing for chlamydia in vaginal mucous. Cervical smear samples are taken from the area round the Os, the medical name for the opening into the uterus. Point of care Chlamydia tests are based on a sample of mucous from the Os, and I worked on a wand containing a brush device that women could use themselves to collect a suitable sample. On reflection, a good name for this wand would have been The Wizard of Os.

Several population-based studies have suggested that eating a diet rich in nutrients from fruits and vegetables may protect against the development of cervical dysplasia. The precise cause of cervical dysplasia is not known, but studies have found a strong association between cervical dysplasia and infection with human papilloma virus (HPV) responsible for warts, however additional factors such as smoking and high levels of free radicals are likely to aggravate the condition. HPV screening is now possible to establish whether you are at risk as an HPV carrier, warts and all.

Beta-carotene

Some research suggests that individuals deficient in beta-carotene may be more likely to develop cancerous or pre-cancerous cervical lesions, but this relationship remains clinically unproven. Other studies indicate that oral supplementation with beta-carotene may promote a regression, or decline in the signs of cervical dysplasia. Despite these promising results, the benefit of using beta-carotene supplements to prevent the development of cervical dysplasia or cervical cancer has been disappointing, probably because the study includes those who are not particularly deficient in beta carotene, and does not say whether participants were HPV carriers.

Even so, there are 600 or so carotenoids that are important for health and they are all believed to be associated with anti-cancer properties. Carotenoids are found in yellow, red, and deep green vegetables and fruits. Don't rely on beta carotene colourant in many foods and drinks because it is synthetically manufactured and doesn't have the diversity of natural carotenes that you find in coloured fruits and vegetables.

Beta-carotene is converted in the body to vitamin A. The breakdown of beta-carotene occurs in the walls of the small intestine (intestinal mucosa) and is catalysed by the enzyme beta-carotene dioxygenase. The retinol formed is stored in the liver as retinyl esters. This is why cod liver oil may be taken as a vitamin A supplement, though too much is toxic.

Beta-carotene, on the other hand, is a safe source of vitamin A. The efficiency of conversion of beta-carotene to retinol depends on the level in the diet. If you eat more beta-carotene, less is converted, and the rest is stored in fat reserves in the body. That is why too much beta-carotene can make you turn orange.

Past studies have shown that broccoli, Brussels sprouts and green cabbage decrease the risk of cancer through the high concentration of glucosinolates which your body metabolises to anti-cancer isothiocyanates. Scientists at the University of Warwick have recently found that the usual British standard method of boiling vegetables severely damages the anti-cancer properties associated with Brassicas.

Boiling had a serious effect on these compounds, and after 30 minutes boiling broccoli lost 77%, Brussels sprouts lost 58%, cauliflower 75%, and green cabbage 65%. Even boiling for five minutes caused significant loss.

However, steaming for 20 minutes, microwave cooking for 3 minutes or stir frying for 5 minutes had no significant effect on the glucosinolates. So to get the maximum benefit from your five-portions-a-day vegetables boiling is out. Stir fry, steam or microwave them. Even better, eat them raw in a salad. They will taste better and be better for you, and you will be spared that awful stench of boiling brassicas that drive away your dinner guests without you even realising it.

Folic acid (Vitamin B9)

Like beta-carotene, some evidence suggests that folate (also known as vitamin B9) deficiencies may contribute to the development of cancerous or precancerous lesions in the cervix. Researchers also theorize that folate consumed in the diet may improve the cellular changes seen in cervical dysplasia by lowering homocysteine (a substance believed to contribute to the severity of cervical dysplasia) levels. The benefit of using dietary folate to prevent or treat cervical dysplasia has not been clinically proven because surprisingly no-one seems that interested. Not so good if you are a sufferer of course.

Other dietary nutrients that may protect against the development of cervical cancer include:

- Vitamin C
- Selenium
- Vitamin E
- Vitamin A

In addition, some of the risk factors for cervical dysplasia may cause certain nutritional deficiencies at the same time, so perhaps it is the deficiency rather than the 'risk factor' that produces the risk. For example, smoking may contribute to a deficiency in vitamin C, and long-term use of birth control pills may diminish folate levels. Maybe that is why smoking and the Pill are seen as risky. Research has yet to prove whether taking vitamin C and folate supplements can help prevent or treat cervical dysplasia or cervical cancer. At the same time, it seems prudent to eat a diet rich in fruits and vegetables which contain vitamin C, folate, and beta-carotene, as these nutrients have been shown to have many other health benefits as well.

So why are these nutrients good at preventing cervical dysplasia? Probably because they are the anti-cancer nutrients. They are not just the ticket for cervical dysplasia, they are valuable for combating all types of cancer.

Do you have Arthritis?

You probably have a BORON and SULPHUR deficiency

Many years ago I was introduced to an eminent Russian scientist who had developed an innovative cancer screening system. But it was another invention of his that caught my attention because it showed how fast the body clock was running. Some people seem to wear out quicker than others, and he seemed to be able to identify the longevity of people using his biochemical markers for the body clock. He detected a compound called somatotropin, which is a growth hormone linked to the rate at which we utilise energy.

Unfortunately I was not able to use this technique because of the difficulties in getting research projects through the British Ethics committee, especially since this was around the time of the Alderhey Hospital tissue biopsy problem where samples had been retained for research without raising the correct paperwork. Clinical trials became very difficult to justify.

So I had to stick to traditional literature based research to start with. While investigating Russian patents, which are granted on a totally different system to the one we use in the West, I came upon their water research topics.

Russians take great store in the quality of their water and have electronic systems to produce 'clustering' of the water molecules which gives the water special properties. I was somewhat sceptical of the process, but it did generate my interest in water. My Derbyshire home is close to several local spa towns, Matlock Bath, Buxton and Ashbourne. There are many more in Britain dating from Roman times.

So that is a convoluted route to explain my interest in water and the minerals it contains, but sometimes science is like that. Anyway, I began to wonder what it is in healing springs that give the water such incredible healing powers. Buxton and Matlock in particular are noted for their powers to heal arthritis.

The answer seems to be that these waters are mineral-rich. And in the best spa waters there is boron in the water, and usually significant amounts of sulphur. I found that boron has been extensively quoted as essential to prevent arthritis, even sometimes effecting a miracle cure once it is added to the diet. Even so, boron is still not widely recognised as a beneficial element for joint quality.

The Body Language of Health

In Australia, arthritis affects less than 1% of the population, and very few animals get arthritis, maybe because there is more boron in the soil, and more boron in the water than in the Western world.

In Israel there is even less arthritis, and guess what, the soil is rich in boron.

Arthritis and its close relative osteoporosis affect about 30% of all people today. These are 'jointly' responsible for more long-term hospital cases that any other single cause. Yet the boron solution has been known for over twenty years, but the impending EU regulations are even seeking to ban boron in supplements.

What is Sulphur?

We all need a lot of sulphur in our body. Our skin, hair and nails all have a high sulphur content - in fact if you have ever been unfortunate enough to burn your hair or skin, the nasty smell that follows is largely the sulphur content burning!

The Ancient Greeks were aware of the health values of sulphur, and used sulphur fumes from hot springs and sulphur-rich onion or garlic to treat many different conditions. Although sulphur is the fourth most plentiful mineral in the body, and can be found in almost every cell, it is only in recent times that we have begun to rediscover the importance of sulphur. Recent interest in sulphur has been stimulated by its veterinary use in the form of methylsulphonylmethane (MSM) on horses. MSM is a naturally occurring organic sulphur compound found in all living plant and animal tissues. MSM is easily destroyed by food processing, and this, in combination with the fact that sulphur is continually excreted by the body, points to the need to include MSM or other forms of sulphur in the diet all the time.

MSM is responsible for the flexible bond between cells, including those that make up the skin. It acts to block undesirable chemical and physical cross-linking or bonding of collagen which is associated with tough, ageing skin. Approximately half of the total body sulphur is concentrated in the body's muscles, skin, and bones. It is present in keratin, the tough substance in the skin, and nails and hair. Sulphur is necessary for making collagen, the primary constituent of cartilage and connective tissue, but it is also responsible for the conformation of body proteins through the formation of disulfide bonds, which hold connective tissue together. MSM does this in conjunction with vitamins and amino acids, and the process is going on 24 hours a day. The body never stops making new cells, and this calls for an unceasing supply of MSM and all other essential nutrients. This is good news for a racehorse, especially one supplied with an ample supply of MSM.

The Body Language of Health

Tests conducted with laboratory animals indicated that wound healing occurred faster with a group receiving MSM, but even faster with both MSM and vitamin C supplementation. Common signs of sulphur deficiency include slow wound healing, scar tissue formation, brittle hair or nails, gastrointestinal problems, arthritis, acne, depression, and lots more. The body is in a constant state of repair, but if we do not have all the necessary 'parts' the body will produce weak, dysfunctional cells.

Organic sulphur is a vital ingredient in the formation of keratin, collagen and elastin (it has disulphide bonds) which give flexibility, tone and strength to muscles, bones, joints, internal membranes, skin, hair and nails.

Good sources of Boron

- Fruit
- Vegetables
- Meat

Good sources of Sulphur

- Grains
- Legumes,
- Fresh unprocessed vegetables like garlic, onions, cabbage, broccoli and Brussels sprouts.
- MSM is also found in meat, fish, poultry, eggs and milk (milk for example contains between 2 and 6 parts per million)
- Onions and garlic are especially rich in sulphur.

When we fart, the gas emitted is nitrogen, carbon dioxide, methane, hydrogen sulphide, and mercaptans which also contain sulphur. We need lots of sulphur to make smelly farts. In fact you can tell the sulphur content of the food by the smell factor of the fart. For example, eggs, onions, cauliflower. But not all at once please.

In contrast, baked beans produce lots of wind but little smell, because the gas is methane, made by fermenting of the sugars in the beans, not from hydrogen sulphide gas production.

Methane is one of the more powerful greenhouse gases, and most of it comes from rotting rubbish and from the bottoms of animals and baked bean fanatics. Cows and sheep are responsible for one third of the methane that passes into the atmosphere in Europe, so I would imagine New Zealand to be a major contributor to global warming, simply because there are one hundred sheep for every inhabitant in New Zealand. One sheep produces 25 litres a day, while a cow can produce around 280 litres a day. That's why some farmers actually fuel their cars by fermenting cow shit. You could literally tow a trailer full of horses and run the car off their fart gas. You could say the more horses you tow, the higher the horsepower of the engine.

In comparison to animals, humans are modest polluters. At any time there is about 200 millilitres, or a cup full, of gas in your gut, and you will typically expel around half a litre each day, although some people produce up to two litres. But even for these windy beggars one cow equals 140 people, in fact one cow emits about the same as one car. But less than ten per cent of human trumping-gas is methane, because unlike cows and sheep we don't eat and digest raw plant material such as grass.

Men fart around 14 to 25 times a day, but women only fart about 7 to 15 times a day. However, in case you women are feeling righteous, women's farts are said to rate higher than men's on the old stinkometer.

Scientists believe that holding in bowel gases for social reasons can be a contributing factor in certain bowel diseases such as diverticulitis. Apparently in Holland in the 1990's there was a campaign by the National Liver and Intestine Foundation to break wind as often as possible. Maybe that is why Holland has so many windmills. Presumably neighbouring Germany who received the prevailing westerly wind thought this was 'nicht so gut'. The message seems to be don't hold it in and poison yourself. Just let it out and poison others.

If we hold in a fart, intestinal pressure forces the gases into the bloodstream and out through the lungs instead. There is scientific evidence that in such social situations our breath contains a greater proportion of the very light, inflammable gas, hydrogen. Being lighter than air, it will increase the pitch of the voice proportionate to the amount the breath contains. In practice it is so slight there will be little variation, but it says a lot for the digestive system of Mickey Mouse. Maybe the Bee Gees name is short for Bowel Gases. A touch of the Saturday Night Fever perhaps?

Incidentally, the smell associated with faeces is a chemical called Skatole. It is an especially fetid smell that apparently is a vital ingredient in some food flavourings, for example, ice cream.

Some fungi have learnt to mimic the smell of farts to attract flies in order that they become attached to the sticky surface, when they are digested and become food for the fungi. Conversely some men I know have developed a smell that attracts flies, but they're hardly fun guys.

Whether you suffer from arthritis now, or might suffer in the future, you should include boron and sulphur in your diet. Even if you are crippled with arthritis right now, I have seen evidence that these minerals will help, after all we get a new set of bones as we age and your new ones could be a lot better.

And what of my Russian friend? He still has his somatotropin 'life expectancy' test and I am still trying to find a way to get it introduced. And his Cancer test is now being trialled in America and I wish him every success with it. Hopefully I did my bit in encouraging him to pursue it. And I would like to thank him for introducing me to the possibilities of relief from arthritis.

Do you have Measles?

If you do, you may have a deficiency in VITAMIN A

It may be fairly obvious by now that there are clear links between diet, deficiencies and physical attributes like blemish-free skin. But there are also important interactions between micronutrient deficiencies and infectious diseases.

I remember when I had measles in about 1960 I had to be kept in a darkened room, because that is what parents did with their children when measles struck in those days. My father even painted the light bulb so that it just produced a faint glow. But I never connected eye damage with measles and the link between them - Vitamin A.

Vitamin A deficiency and measles act synergistically to exacerbate the severity of measles and precipitate vitamin A blindness and even death or severe disability. I was a lucky one, I survived the ordeal with no long term effects other than lifelong immunity to the disease.

So if measles and Vitamin A are synergic, (synergic just means that the combined effects are far greater than the individual effects of each one on its own) it stands to reason that taking vitamin A will help to cure you. And this has been proven in trials. Vitamin A supplementation during acute measles significantly reduces risks of morbidity and mortality.

This is because Vitamin A helps regulate the immune system. The immune system helps prevent or fight off infections by making white blood cells that destroy harmful bacteria and viruses. Vitamin A may help lymphocytes, a type of white blood cell that fights infections, function more effectively.

Vitamin A deficiency is also closely linked to eye damage, hence the wisdom of my parents darkening my bedroom when I had measles all those years ago. They did it by putting up thick curtains at the window, and painting a light bulb so that it dimly illuminated the bedroom. These silly old fashioned precautions were not so silly after all.

Globally, 3 million children suffer clinical Vitamin A deficiency, exhibiting the signs and symptoms of eye damage. However, the full magnitude of Vitamin A deficiency often remains hidden: an estimated 140-250 million children under five years of age are at risk of sub-clinical Vitamin A deficiency, mainly in Asia and Africa. Though showing none of the ocular signs or symptoms these children suffer a dramatically increased risk of death and illness, particularly from measles and diarrhoea, as a consequence of Vitamin A deficiency.

Long known to be a principle cause of childhood blindness (250,000-500,000 children lose their sight each year), Vitamin A deficiency is now recognized as a major contributing factor in an estimated 1-3 million child deaths each year.

The simple provision of high-dose vitamin A supplements every 4-6 months not only protects against blindness but also has been repeatedly shown to have a dramatic and multiple impact on the health of young children.

- Overall, all-cause mortality is reduced by 23%
- Measles mortality is reduced by 50%
- Diarrhoeal mortality is reduced by 33%
- 85% coverage can result in a 90% reduction in the prevalence of severe opthalmia

Vitamin A and Malaria: A recent study in Papua New Guinea found that when young children were given vitamin A supplements three times a year they had 30% fewer malaria attacks and the number of malaria parasites in their blood dropped by 36%.

Vitamin A and HIV/AIDS: Trials are currently on-going to determine if vitamin A supplementation can reduce the mother-to-child transmission of HIV during breast feeding.

Every year, some 12 million children in developing countries die before they reach their fifth birthday, many during the first year of life. Seven out of ten of these deaths are due to acute respiratory disease infections (mostly pneumonia), diarrhoea, measles, malaria or malnutrition - or more commonly some combination of these conditions. These same children are often most at risk of vitamin A deficiency, a known contributing factor to these causes of death and disease. Vitamin A deficiency can be prevented by including foods rich in vitamin A or beta-carotene as a regular component of the diet; liver, meat, eggs and dairy products are examples. Foods rich in beta-carotene include red peppers, carrots, pumpkins, as well as those just mentioned. Margarine is rich in beta-carotene, because this chemical is used as a colouring agent in margarine production. In Africa, Indonesia, and the Philippines, vitamin A deficiency is prevented by public health programs that supply children with injections of the vitamin whenever money is available.

Good sources of Vitamin A

- Eggs
- Milk
- Liver
- Fresh colourful vegetables
- Carrots are an especially rich source

Do you have Persistent Diarrhoea leading to fatigue?

You may have a deficiency in MAGNESIUM and POTASSIUM

Diarrhoea causes us to lose lots of magnesium and potassium. We're talking here about diarrhoea after a stomach upset. If you have persistent diarrhoea for any unknown causes you should refer the problem to your doctor without delay.

Our bodies can also lose large amounts of magnesium through the kidneys. People who take diuretics or drink too much alcohol and caffeine, which increase urine excretion, are exposed to potential magnesium deficiency. Diabetics who have to use insulin also tend to excrete more magnesium via the kidneys and are at risk of magnesium deficiency.

Any condition that increases magnesium loss through the kidneys or bowels, such as prolonged bouts of diarrhoea, kidney disease, and epilepsy, can cause magnesium deficiency.

Symptoms of magnesium deficiency

Magnesium plays an important role in health, disease prevention, and possibly in boosting athletic performance. Because South Africa has many regions where the magnesium content of the soil and drinking water is very low, experts believe there are many people in that country who either suffer from a sub-clinical, or an outright magnesium deficiency.

Magnesium is another one of those co-factors like copper which help enzymes in the human body function properly.

In particular magnesium helps to activate enzymes that split and transfer phosphate groups which are involved in the production of a substance called adenine triphosphate or ATP. This is one of the most important compounds in the body's energy system and a lack of magnesium can lead to inefficient energy production. This is probably why athletes can benefit from increasing their magnesium intake.

The latest research suggests that the real culprit in causing high blood pressure is a diet low in calcium, potassium and magnesium intake, not in the level of salt you take.

Potassium

Patients with diarrhoea often develop potassium depletion owing to large faecal losses of this element. These losses are greatest in infants and can be especially dangerous in malnourished children, who are frequently potassium-deficient even before diarrhoea starts. More serious symptoms of potassium losses are:

- General muscular weakness;
- Cardiac arrhythmias;
- Paralytic ileum, especially when drugs such as opiates are also taken.

Some other effects can lead to excessive losses of potassium from the body:

- Prolonged use of stimulant laxatives, such as those that contain senna, can cause excessive loss of potassium.

- Cisplatin, a chemotherapy medication, may cause excessive loss of potassium.
- Steroidal anti-inflammatory medications, including prednisone and cortisone, increase the loss of potassium in the urine.
- Neomycin, an antibacterial drug, decreases blood levels of potassium by reducing the absorption of dietary potassium and/or increasing urinary excretion of potassium.
- Theophylline and aminophylline, medications used in the treatment of asthma, may promote potassium deficiency.
- Tobramycin, an antibiotic that is administered intravenously, can cause potassium depletion.
- Diuretics, or "water pills", flush fluid out of the body, and are often prescribed for the treatment of high blood pressure. While certain diuretics limit potassium loss, others decrease potassium levels. Because potassium can be helpful in maintaining normal blood pressure, these diuretics may make it even more difficult to treat high blood pressure.

Do you have muscle cramps?

If you do, you may be deficient in MAGNESIUM

Many people experience cramps when they sleep, and this can sometimes be associated with excruciating pain. It can lead to bedroom athletics in the middle of the night as the sufferer does the long jump out of bed followed by the hurdles and the hop, skip and jump triathlon. Real athletes, on the other hand, tend to develop muscle cramps when they are exercising.

Many factors produce painful muscles contractions; the following are common causes:

- A mineral deficiency involving potassium, calcium, magnesium and/or sodium.
- Dehydration, which can occur in athletes when they exercise hard in hot conditions and do not drink sufficient liquid.
- Excessive intake of fluid (drinking 2-3 litres or more of water in addition to your daily fluid intake) - this can flush these minerals out of your body.
- Lack of fitness - well-trained muscles are less likely to suffer from muscle cramps. Although this mainly applies to athletes, people who are not fit and get too little exercise often develop cramps because their muscles are so poorly used.

- Wearing tight constrictive clothing, especially in bed. Try to wear comfortable, loosely fitting clothes at all times (be comfortable, rather than stylish if you are plagued by cramps), as constriction of the blood supply to muscles can cause them to contract painfully.

Calcium

Most people are not aware of the fact that calcium is essential for the normal contraction of muscle tissues, including those of the heart. Patients with extremely low blood calcium levels can develop a condition called tetani where the muscles fibres contract continuously. When this happens, heart failure can occur.

Such severe calcium deficiencies are rare, except in cases of anorexia and other eating disorders, but sub-optimal calcium intakes are relatively common, especially in teenagers and young women who go on poorly balanced ill-conceived diets.

Magnesium

People eating a western diet that lacks fresh fruit, vegetables, legumes and unprocessed grains and cereals, may well have inadequate intakes of magnesium. If you suffer from muscle cramps, you can try increasing your intakes of the foods listed above (especially green, leafy vegetables such as spinach, cabbage, lettuce, broccoli) or take a calcium and magnesium supplement (taking these two minerals together improves their mutual absorption).

Potassium

Potassium is one of the most abundant minerals available in common foods and most people should not develop a deficiency. However, eating monotonous diets to lose weight, concentrating on fast foods with little nutrition, or avoiding fruits, vegetables, grains and cereals, can cause a potassium deficiency. Drinking too much water can also deplete your potassium reserves.

The easiest way of ensuring that you have abundant potassium is to eat five or more servings of fruit and/or vegetables a day, especially bananas. If you think you lack potassium, buy a variety of fresh or frozen vegetables and boil them lightly in chicken stock to make a delicious, fat-free soup that is loaded with potassium. If you have a juicer, make an apple and banana or grape and carrot drink to boost your potassium intake. Bear in mind that if you boil vegetables the potassium will end up in the water, so use the water in soup or stock, or boil it down to a low volume and use it to make gravy.

Potassium supplements should preferably only be taken if your potassium levels have been checked by a medical doctor and have been found to be low. Supplements should only be taken under the supervision of your doctor, because a number of medications can influence the potassium levels in the body - for example, the so-called 'potassium-sparing diuretics' help to reduce loss of potassium from the body. If you take a potassium supplement, you could develop hyperkalaemia (excess potassium in the blood), which is also harmful. So you are better to eat fruit and vegetables and whole grains to top up on potassium, than take supplements. In fact this message is common throughout Body Language. If you could buy the right food like the old fashioned varieties described by David Thomas, you wouldn't need supplements.

Sodium

Most people on a western diet, which is based on processed foods, won't develop a sodium deficiency because their food will be laced with salt, sodium chloride. However, drinking too much water, sweating a lot, and certain imbalances in kidney function can lead to sodium depletion, which in turn can cause cramps.

If you do a lot of exercise in hot weather or if you are an athlete training hard, you need to make sure that you are getting enough sodium in your diet. In fact people who develop cramps should always consider that they might have a sodium deficiency.

Do you suffer from hypertension (high blood pressure)?

If you do, you may be deficient in MAGNESIUM

I have not got sick yet - sick of quoting magnesium. And if I did, you could bet a dose of magnesium could cure it. Magnesium comes up time and time again so it just shows you how important it is to our bodies. Just look at magnesium entries in the index.

An observational study examined the effect of various nutritional factors on incidence of high blood pressure in over 30,000 US male health professionals. After four years of follow-up, it was found that a lower risk of hypertension was associated with dietary patterns that provided more magnesium, potassium, and dietary fibre.

The Body Language of Health

New scientific evidence from clinical trials was so significant that the Joint National Committee on Prevention, Detection, Evaluation, and Treatment of High Blood Pressure stated that diets that provide plenty of magnesium are positive lifestyle modifications for individuals with hypertension. The group recommended magnesium as a beneficial eating plan for people with hypertension and for those with "pre-hypertension" who are looking to prevent high blood pressure.

At last, some healthcare professional are starting to realise that blood pressure tablets are wrongly targeted for many people, and can cause undesirable side effects.

Magnesium and diabetes

In recent years, rates of type 2 diabetes have rocketed along with the rising rates of obesity.

Magnesium plays an important role in carbohydrate metabolism. It may influence the release and activity of insulin, the hormone that helps control blood glucose levels. Low blood levels of magnesium are frequently seen in individuals with type 2 diabetes.

Low magnesium may worsen insulin intolerance, a condition that usually precedes diabetes and invariably leads to type 2 diabetes. The kidneys will excrete magnesium during periods of severe hyperglycaemia (significantly elevated blood glucose). In older adults, correcting magnesium depletion may improve insulin response and action.

One health study followed over 170,000 health professionals through diet questionnaires. Over time, the risk for developing type 2 diabetes was greater in men and women with a lower magnesium intake.

Most of the body's magnesium occurs in bone; very little is present in the blood. Magnesium is necessary for the formation of bone and teeth and for normal nerve and muscle function. Many enzymes in the body depend on magnesium to function normally. The body takes in magnesium from the diet and excretes it in urine and stool.

Hypomagnesaemia

In hypomagnesaemia, the level of magnesium in the blood is too low. The most common causes of hypomagnesaemia are decreased dietary intake (due to starvation, dieting, poor nutrition, eating disorders) and decreased intestinal absorption (malabsorption).

The Body Language of Health

Hypomagnesaemia occurs frequently in people who consume large amounts of alcohol and in people who have protracted diarrhoea. High levels of aldosterone, antidiuretic hormone, or thyroid hormones can cause hypomagnesaemia by increasing the excretion of magnesium by the kidneys. Diuretics, antifungal drugs or chemotherapy can also cause hypomagnesaemia.

Symptoms of hypomagnesaemia include nausea, vomiting, sleepiness, weakness, personality changes, muscle spasms, tremors, and loss of appetite. The diagnosis is made by carrying out a magnesium analysis of the blood.

A good way of boosting you magnesium levels is to take milk of magnesia.

Hypermagnesaemia

In hypermagnesaemia, the level of magnesium in the blood is too high. Hypermagnesaemia usually develops only in people with kidney failure who are given magnesium salts or who take drugs that contain magnesium (such as some antacids or laxatives).

Symptoms of hypermagnesaemia include weakness, low blood pressure, and impaired breathing. When hypermagnesaemia is severe, the heart can stop beating. So go steady on that milk of magnesia. Like all the advice in this book, take everything in moderation, and go to your doctor if symptoms persist.

People with severe hypermagnesaemia are given intravenous calcium gluconate. Intravenous diuretics can increase the kidneys' excretion of magnesium, but if the kidneys are not functioning well, dialysis is usually needed.

Magnesium supplements can improve energy production within the heart, improve delivery of oxygen to the heart, reduce demand on the heart, inhibit the formation of blood clots, and improve heart rate. Magnesium supplementation has been used in many of these applications for over 50 years, and was invaluable in the days before sophisticated cardiovascular treatments.

Magnesium is also effective with Chronic Fatigue Syndrome. People with CFS have low red blood cell magnesium levels. A recent study in the United Kingdom conducted a double-blind experiment with CFS patients and magnesium supplements. The researchers concluded that 80% of the patients receiving magnesium reported "significantly improved energy levels, better emotional state, and less pain."

Page 294

The Body Language of Health

On a daily average, more than 9 million Western people are exposed to noise levels above 85 decibels, the level where the risk for permanent hearing loss increases exponentially. Since magnesium is essential in regulating cellular membrane permeability and neuromuscular excitability, researchers decided to test the hypothesis that noise-induced hearing loss and magnesium are related. The researchers were right! They discovered that magnesium supplementation is highly effective in preventing noise-induced hearing loss.

Magnesium plays important roles in the structure and the function of many parts of the human body. The adult human body contains about 25 grams of magnesium. Over 60% of all the magnesium in the body is found in the skeleton, about 27% is found in muscle, while 6 to 7% is found in other cells, and less than 1% is found outside of cells

Severe magnesium deficiency can result in low levels of calcium in the blood (hypocalcaemia). Magnesium deficiency is also associated with low levels of potassium in the blood (hypokalemia).

Good sources of magnesium

- Brown rice, soya beans, nuts, pulses
- Wholemeal flour, green vegetables
- Fish, milk.

Do you suffer from osteoporosis?

You are deficient in MAGNESIUM and BORON and probably have the WRONG DIET

Experts say go to the gym regularly, eat lots of dairy produce and red meat, and your bones will stay healthy. Right?

Wrong.

The Body Language of Health

Osteoporosis is a modern disease brought about by this very advice that experts are still quoting you. The above diet is high in acidic foods and low in fruits and vegetables. Remember our cave-man diet with very little meat and no dairy produce? That is how to keep bones healthy. Correct Nutrition is the key to preventing osteoporosis.

The idea that meat and dairy produce could be good for your bones originated in the 1920's when doctors noticed that patients with kidney failure (in those days dialysis was not available) had unusually delicate skeletons. When doctors gave them bicarbonate to relieve acid stomach (another symptom of kidney failure) they noticed their patient's bones gradually got stronger. So they thought milk was good for the skeleton because it is also rich in calcium (though not as good as lots of green leafy vegetables!!).

But cows milk is designed for baby cows, not humans. Dairy produce is cheap and is added to almost every convenience food, but it is not good for human skeletons. All these years the experts who have told women to drink lots of milk have been having precisely the opposite effect to the one they were trying to promote.

Why is this? The reason is to do with something called pH, the symbol for acidity and alkalinity. Water is neutral when it has a pH of 7.0. Numbers below this are acidic, and above this are alkaline. Anything that lowers the pH makes the body more acidic and anything that raises the pH makes the body more alkaline.

Your body works best at a pH of 7.4 and we have complicated mechanisms in the body to maintain that balance. One of the ways the body does this is to use its calcium reserves from your bones to mop up any excess acidity. This is rather like putting acid rain onto calcium carbonate, or limestone. The alkalinity of the limestone neutralises the acid and the calcium dissolves. As the water slowly evaporates in caves it precipitates calcium out again as stalagtites and stalagmites.

When your body's balance is tipped towards the acid side from dairy produce, sugar, carbohydrate (pasta, bread etc) and meat, the body has to rob alkaline calcium carbonate from its skeleton to keep that balance of pH 7.4 Therefore you would expect populations on a Western diet containing these acid-producing foods to have high incidences of osteoporosis, and this is exactly what epidemiologists have found. But if your diet is restricted to a simple cave man diet, your body stays neutral. So a cave man diet is best yet again.

But bones are not just made up of calcium. Many other trace elements are equally important including magnesium, zinc, selenium, boron, chromium and many others. We

The Body Language of Health

also know essential fatty acids are important for your bone health, and so are vitamins C, D, K and the vitamin B group. In order to make healthy bones, we need the whole spectrum of vitamins, minerals, essential fatty acids and trace elements. These are also available from fruit and vegetables that form the cave man diet.

You should also not be taking a calcium supplement routinely. By taking just calcium it is possible to unbalance other trace elements and worsen the risk of osteoporosis. Remember too, that drinking milk and eating cheese is the worst thing you can do. Here is a summary of what is best.

- Eat plenty of fruit and vegetables
- Reduce or cut out dairy products altogether
- Reduce your intake of meat to a minimum
- Cut out highly acidic foods and food ingredients, such as refined white sugar, refined white flour, high-fructose corn syrup, soft drinks, cola, biscuits, chocolate, sweets, and sugary desserts.
- Make sure you have a daily dose of trace elements especially magnesium and boron by choosing foods rich in them or using a mineral supplement containing all elements including boron.
- Eat foods that are rich in sulphur and minerals. An old Chinese remedy for brittle bones or arthritis is to drink broth made from chicken bones.

There are two vitamins which are particularly important. The first is vitamin D. Absorption of calcium from the gut is a vitamin D dependent process. It is not so much a question of how much calcium is in the diet, but how much can be absorbed from the gut. Once absorbed, does it go to the right place? Without vitamin D calcium could be deposited in the wrong place such as arteries or gall bladder and kidney (stones). It is impossible to get adequate vitamin D through sunshine during a British winter. The daily requirement is one quarter of that time necessary to tan or turn pink on arms and face. Either use a sun lamp, or take a winter holiday in the sun. Alternatively take a vitamin D3 supplement.

The second important vitamin is vitamin K. This is highly protective against osteoporosis because it strongly stimulates bone production. Vitamin K is found in green leafy vegetables, eggs, and meat. Antibiotics can reduce vitamin K by 50% since bacterial fermentation of foods in the gut is an important source of vitamin K. Antibiotics kill the gut flora, and stop you receiving this supply of vitamin K so be sure to take extra K-rich foods. Note that vitamin K is antagonistic to warfarin and should not be taken as a supplement with warfarin anti-coagulant heart treatments.

The Body Language of Health

Experts do not recommend prescribed female sex hormones to prevent osteoporosis because any benefit is temporary and bone is rapidly lost again when the hormones are stopped. Female sex hormones are associated with increased risk of oestrogen dependent cancers, thrombosis, mental disorders and chronic fatigue. HRT treatment affects the balance of calcium in the body and it is occasionally found that calcium deposits in healthy breast tissue, sometimes requiring surgery to avoid a high risk of future breast cancer.

You might be wondering why you have not heard this advice before. Perhaps it is because osteoporosis is a highly lucrative disease - more than 17 billion dollars were spent treating osteoporosis in America in 2001 alone. But osteoporosis is nothing more than brittle bones, or a loss of bone mass or bone density. There's really nothing complicated about it.

Osteoporosis is really caused by only three things. They are: 1) inappropriate diet, 2) inadequate physical exercise, and 3) lack of exposure to natural sunlight. It's really not that complex.

When it comes to diet and osteoporosis, most people think that a lack of calcium is the number one dietary concern. But this isn't true -- calcium is only a minor factor when it comes to preventing and treating osteoporosis.

Do this annual home test to measure osteoporosis

The annual home osteoporosis test couldn't be simpler. It is done by measuring your total height standing barefoot with your heels, back, shoulders and head square against a wall. Have a friend place a level horizontal on top of your head to place a pencil mark on the wall. Mark that line with the date. Then check your height against this annually. Every birthday, or every new year's day is ideal, because you will remember to do it.

Osteoporosis will appear as a reduction in height from the lifetime maximum height. Only osteoporosis will make you shrink with time. Maintaining a full lifetime maximum height with no height loss whatsoever at 65 years of age is common in healthy individuals, and this should be your goal. Serious osteoporosis exists when a person of 5' - 10" (1778 mm) tall has lost 1.0" (25 mm) in height or a person of 5' - 3" (1600 mm) tall has lost 0.75" (19 mm) in height. Lesser or greater degrees of osteoporosis are compared to these typical readings.

It's that simple.

Do you wear a bra?

If you do you should beware of internet literature

The internet has numerous sites which claim that women who wear a bra are more likely to get breast cancer than those women who don't wear a bra.

What??? I suggest you read that statement once more. Women who wear a bra are more likely to get breast cancer than those women who don't wear a bra. Is this the answer to a major killer of women in the western world? Let's investigate the tantalising link between a bra and cancer. There is another message here. Be careful what you read on the internet!

The theory behind this story is that the elastic in a bra restricts blood flow in the breasts and this can increase the likelihood of developing cancer. As an observer of cleavage at parties (yes you're right, that is my favourite part of the body), I can confirm that breasts that are supported by a brassiere don't wiggle about as much as those that are unfettered, and apparently wiggling is good for the circulation. Who's circulation I am not sure, the scientists responsible for this titillating bit of information didn't say.

Taken at face value this business of not wearing a bra affecting breast cancer could sound feasible. The elastic surrounds the ribcage like a tourniquet which must surely have some effect on circulation, especially round the lymph nodes under the arms.

The story goes that this elastic can restrict the lymphatic fluid flow in your breasts. Normally the lymph fluid helps to remove waste materials and other toxins away from the breasts, but brassieres might inhibit this action, so toxins could start to accumulate in the breast, and that could help cancer to develop.

Bra wearing might also be connected to breast cancer in other ways. You may already be aware that men who wear tight underpants tend to have a low sperm count and it improves when they wear loose briefs, or wear no underpants at all. Travelling pantless is more common than you would think among the youth of today, ladies, so it's not just Scots in a traditional kilt who wear nothing underneath. (There's an old saying 'What's worn under the kilt, Jock?' 'Nothing laddie, it's all in fine worrking orrder!')

The Body Language of Health

This improvement in sperm quality might be because 'free and easy' could be sexually stimulating, but scientists tell us that sperm production is seriously affected by temperature. Males apparently evolved before high street designer stores appeared on the scene, and are equipped to produce sperm under au naturelle conditions with everything dangling in free space. When testicles are nestling snug and secure next to the skin encased in cotton the higher temperature takes its toll on the sperm factory. Sperm, it seems, like their air conditioning turned to the 'brass monkeys' setting and the thermally insulating properties of their donor's underpants gets them all hot and sticky, which is bad for business.

Now, seeing a woman without a bra usually gets most men all hot and sticky too, but for women, wearing a bra slightly increases the temperature of the breast tissue, and as a result, women who wear bras tend to have higher levels of the hormone prolactin in their tissue. This is said to influence breast cancer formation.

But more significantly, medical researchers have noticed that "Westernised" Japanese, Fijians, Maoris, Aborigines and other bra-converted cultures, have developed 'western' levels of breast cancer despite the virtual absence of breast cancer in their native colleagues. But the science may be flawed, because we don't know if the relatively new category of 'bra-converts' changed their lifestyle as well.

Women who don't wear bras might indeed be less likely to develop breast cancer, but this might be nothing to do with the bra itself. You could say the bra is merely lending support to the argument.

The more probable answer is that those women who don't wear a bra are more likely to come from a background where life is more 'natural' and free from cosmetics, dairy produce and food additives, all of which have been associated with breast cancer. So I think this science is flawed, and could just be a storm in a 'T' cup.

If such a size exists.

Imagine that.

I mention this example of Body Language because a lot of 'scientific' information that you come across is not telling the full story, or is flawed logic, and that is particularly true of many aspects of nutrition. You have to take some of it with a pinch of salt.

I don't really know if wearing a bra is an important health issue or not, but certainly you can find a lot of information about it on the internet if you are so inclined and want to keep abreast of the situation. All I do know is that the argument has not been properly investigated by ruling out all the other associated factors, so keep this one close to your chest.

The problem with the internet is that it is so vast, and most of the information available has not been cross-checked, and certainly not peer reviewed like proper scientific papers. So it is sure to contain some information or other from dubious sources that will virtually guarantee you can put in two plus two and come up with five.

I just tried moon + green + cheese as an internet search and came up with seismological evidence for lunar rocks and earth rocks that proves the moon could be made of green cheese after all. Well fancy that.

The website quotes seismic velocities for moon rock compared to those of rocks from various locations. The results were published in *Science* and are shown below:

Seismic Velocities

Lunar rocks	Seismic Velocity (km/sec)
Basalt 10017	1.84
Basalt 10046	1..25
Near surface layer	1.2

Terrestrial rocks	Seismic Velocity (km/sec)
Granite	5.9
Gneiss	4.9
Basalt	5.8
Sandstone	4.9
Marble	6.02
Limestone	5.06 - 5.97

It is clear from this that moon "rock" is considerably less dense to sound waves than any type of rock found on earth. The scientists then decided to examine the seismic velocities of various cheeses from around the world. Some of the results are shown below:

Cheese	Seismic Velocity (km/sec)
Sapsego (Swiss)	2.12
Romano (Italy)	1.74

Cheddar (Vermont)	1.72
Muenster (Wisconsin)	1.57

The seismic velocity of moon "rock" is much closer to cheese than any rock found on earth. The author admits that this is not conclusive proof that the moon is made of cheese, but quotes the words of the scientists: *"Old hypotheses are best after all, and should not be lightly discarded"*

From the author's choice of cheese we can assume he is not British (what, no Wensleydale, Grommit?) but that doesn't make him a lunatic. Just a victim of the freedom of information that the internet gives us.

If you are an academic, here is a plea from the heart. As I researched Body Language most of the academic papers I looked at on the web gave a tantalising synopsis but if I wanted to read the full study I had to pay for the privilege to download the full paper. After trying this a few times I just gave up, because most of what I eventually got was irrelevant. So all your no doubt fascinating stuff remained hidden, and you got a summary of green cheese instead. There is a message here somewhere. If you want your paper to be cited in other works of reference, for goodness sake make it available for free, and for the benefit of science.

Do you have high Cholesterol?

If you do, you don't take enough exercise. You should give up sugar.

Oh, another controversial one. We're told to give up sausages and lard but no-one said anything about sugar until today. Before we start, I want to put your mind at rest with one remarkable statistic.

It has been found that 50% of all men who have a heart attack have normal cholesterol. Does that help you? Well, probably not, because of course the other 50% of men who have a heart attack do have high cholesterol. So if you have high cholesterol you might still be a bit concerned.

But this statistic has really got me worried for another reason. It doesn't mean that cholesterol itself is the cause of heart disease. And if we concentrate on the wrong thing, we miss the real culprit. In fact by concentrating on cholesterol we may be missing the things that we should be doing to prevent heart disease.

This figure shows that cholesterol is not the main factor in heart disease. If it was, a high proportion of heart attack sufferers *would* have a high cholesterol, and they don't. I think that is why the latest statistics have shown that cholesterol-lowering drugs have had no significant effect on the life expectancy from heart disease in Britain.

Statistics like 50/50 are not statistics at all. If someone tried to sell you a machine that predicted the outcome of tossing a coin heads or tails at 50/50 would you buy it? Of course not, a 50/50 outcome is a natural result for a yes/no event. A 50/50 split of heart attacks between high and low cholesterol indicates to me that the level of cholesterol has nothing at all to do with heart disease.

Everyone these days seems to be hooked on lowering cholesterol, but I think they are totally missing the point.

So let's have a look at the facts on cholesterol. It's a bit complicated, but we have already discussed cholesterol once and by this stage of the book you should be in tune with how the body regulates itself so you should be able to grasp this - with no sweat.

Far from being an enemy, cholesterol is essential to your body. It is a carrier which distributes nutrients round the body to the cells. Think of it as a fleet of lorries shipping energy. A bit like the Post Office but this time with a post office in every village and a letter box in the door to every cell in your body, and deliveries arriving on time every moment, day and night.

But the cholesterol in your body is not from food, it is made for you specially in your liver. Dietary cholesterol consumption has almost nothing whatsoever to do with your blood cholesterol level. Numerous excellent medical studies have repeatedly demonstrated that even massive changes in the dietary cholesterol consumption, up or down, have only a very minor effect on total cholesterol levels.

This means that trying to control cholesterol by rigorously avoiding all forms of dietary fat and consuming only low cholesterol foods is misdirected and highly ineffective. In fact, restricting your diet in this way will lead to all sorts of other nutritional deficiencies like the ones we describe elsewhere in this book.

The Body Language of Health

The cholesterol made in your liver travels round the body in the blood stream where the nutrients are absorbed into your cells and gets used. Cholesterol that is not needed is transported back to the liver where it is recycled or simply eliminated.

As a back-up supply, in addition to these deliveries, every cell in your body can also make the cholesterol it needs internally. Every cell in your body has the ability to either receive a lorry load, or make its own. Not only can it receive take-aways, it can do home cooking as well if it has to.

The key to lowering cholesterol is to get your cells to prefer using lorry supplies rather than making its own. **You do this with exercise.** Physical exercise burns up the cholesterol and its energy delivery, and you don't even have to put the empties out on the doorstep afterwards. But of course, we all know that it takes a lot less energy to put a tin of food under the automatic tin opener than get off your backside and chase after your next meal. So we have a problem, because no-one has yet told your liver.

There are two more pieces to the cholesterol puzzle, the first piece has to do with understanding the ratio between the "good cholesterol" and the "bad cholesterol" and the second piece of the puzzle has to do with fully understanding the effect diet has on cholesterol levels.

Let's first of all base our understanding on some medical facts.

- Our cholesterol level goes up in winter and goes down in summer.
- Our cholesterol level increases when we are injured.
- When we have surgery our cholesterol level goes through the roof.
- It increases after dental work, during and after an infection, and when we are stressed.
- It returns to normal when we are healthy and relaxed.

Why does it do this? Because cholesterol is a perfectly normal constituent of our body, in fact it is a healing agent. When we try to artificially regulate it with drugs, we open ourselves to infection, and could damage our cells. When the body needs to heal itself it does this by producing cholesterol and sending it to the site of the damage with a supply of energy for repairs. So depending on our circumstances, it's not surprising that our cholesterol will vary from one day to the next.

Worryingly, our cardiovascular system is our plumbing system and it is constantly under attack from toxins, chemicals, viruses, free radicals and waste because these are all in the blood that passes through them. In a house, we rarely get problems with our plumbing from what is exposed on the outside; it's what passes through the pipes that causes corrosion, erosion and blockages. It's the same with our veins, arteries and heart valves. And like the plumbing in our house, we can't see what is happening inside.

Cholesterol is nature's corrosion inhibitor. Cholesterol patches up any internal defects in the pipes, it lubricates the heart valves, it protects from 'corrosion' caused by free radicals. It delivers nutrition. And it does this in so many clever ways that have only recently been appreciated. And that is where 'good' and 'bad' cholesterol come in, although, again this idea is a lorry load of nonsense.

When our liver gets a message that there is some damage to sort out, it boosts cholesterol of a type that is called low density lipoprotein, or LDL. Because this type of cholesterol is produced by the liver, experts have argued that it must be the baddy and the way to lower cholesterol is to stop the liver producing it.

When the LDL gets to the site of the damage, and has done its job, it turns into a different form of cholesterol, called high-density lipoprotein, or HDL. Because this travels from the site of the injury, back to the liver to be broken down and made into more cholesterol, experts have decided it should be called 'Good Cholesterol'. I have always wondered why experts say that the large molecules in 'hard fat' like lard are bad for us, and the small molecules in oily fats like olive oil are good for us, but then tell us totally the reverse argument by calling low-density LDL as bad, and high-density HDL as good. Now I have researched the matter for myself, I realise why; they are talking out of their hat. Presumably it must be a high-density hat.

Calling LDL bad and HDL good is as silly as calling the ambulance that is coming to collect you a bad ambulance, and the ambulance that is taking you to hospital a good ambulance.

When we have surgery or dental work, or when we injure ourselves, the liver produces more cholesterol, and that is why the cholesterol level rockets in our blood. The same thing happens when we get an infection. So when we have high cholesterol, it is because our body needs it. The last thing we should do is to interfere with this process. When the body is back to normal, cholesterol will stabilise. When we are stressed the body assumes a 'flee or fight' mode that was fine when we were a tasty meal on two legs on the savannah, but useless in modern society. Instead of removing the cholesterol, we need to remove the stress.

The Body Language of Health

When your doctor carries out a cholesterol test and reports it as high, he will prescribes cholesterol reducing drugs, in fact there is sometimes a government initiative in which the doctor gets a bonus whenever he can prescribe statins. So guess how often you get them prescribed.

What you should do is find out why your cholesterol is high. Your doctor should be asking himself, what is wrong with this patient to elevate his cholesterol? But unfortunately doctors have to stick to current policy which in this case attacks the very defence system you are relying on.

You might well ask yourself why don't doctors know any better? Why should I trust the opinions of a forensic scientist? The reason is that practicing doctors get most of their information from the drug companies. Compared to doctors who pioneered much of the medicine we use today, modern doctors don't have the time to review research and evaluate reports. Government targets and statistics gathering see to that. They just go with the instructions the government and the National Institute of Clinical Excellence (NICE) pass to them. Very few know anything about the research into cholesterol, and nor did the lecturers who taught them. Most of my facts come from experts in human nutrition who have nothing to do with the food industry, and their views are well substantiated from numerous clinical trials. And that is NICE...to know.

And don't forget that as a forensic scientist I have based my career looking at fact, not assumption. The facts about cholesterol speak for themselves. Much of the impetus for cholesterol reduction comes from speculation rather than any hard scientific proof. The cholesterol cartel of drug companies, manufacturers of low-fat foods, and others with vested interests have succeeded in infiltrating medical and government regulatory agencies that would normally protect us from this unsubstantiated pressure.

Pharmaceutical companies have become very worried about herbs, vitamin supplements and antioxidants. These are the 'medicines' we have evolved to benefit from. The reason why they are worried is that many of these natural substances have the remarkable ability to mop up natural toxins such as viruses, free-radicals, bacteria etc. in your body. In doing so they help wounds to heal. As the wound heals, the need for the protective cholesterol disappears, so the cholesterol in the form of HDL cholesterol is released. This is why herbs, vitamins, antioxidants and other natural substances increase the HDL cholesterol in the blood for a time. They are protecting their profits.

Why are foods that are rich in cholesterol called 'brain food'?

The Body Language of Health

The richest food source of cholesterol is animal brain at 4,500 mg/100 grams, meaning that 4.5% is cholesterol by weight. Caviar has a very high level, at about 580mg of cholesterol per 100 grams, or 0.58% is cholesterol. But it is only just in front of cod liver oil, which has around 570mg per 100 grams, or 0.57%. That is why cod liver oil is so beneficial to health in all sorts of ways. Quite a lot of cholesterol in there, you will note. And much cheaper than caviar!!

Fresh egg yolk is around 420mg per 100g. Quite a bit again, you'll notice. There is very little cholesterol in egg white. Butter has around 220mg per 100g of cholesterol.

But remember that your cholesterol is actually made in your liver, it is not produced from these foods when you eat them. In fact animal liver has around 0.55%. All these foods do is provide you with plenty of building blocks for your body to make what it needs. There is only a small link between dietary cholesterol and bodily cholesterol.

My grandfather used to say that fish was 'brain food' and I always assumed that was because it was rich in Vitamin D. But I now realise that it is also the cholesterol in fish that is so beneficial to mental capacity. Cod liver oil, as you can see above, is a rich source of cholesterol.

This is because about one quarter of all the cholesterol made in your liver is taken by your brain. Every cell in your body, every structure, and every part of the nervous system needs cholesterol to build and maintain the system. One of the most abundant materials in the brain is a fatty substance called myelin. Every nerve and every fibre is coated in myelin, just like the insulation around an electrical cable. Well, 20% of myelin is cholesterol. When the myelin starts to break down round the nerves, it causes a disease called multiple sclerosis. So if you start interfering with the cholesterol system in your body you put the very structure of the brain into jeopardy.

People with multiple sclerosis should therefore try to make sure they have a good supply of the building blocks for the body to manufacture cholesterol. Plenty of fish, eggs and butter. And, surprise surprise, the richest 'brain food' is .... *animal brain.*

These days there is a big problem in the Western world with the memory of the elderly. We form memory by establishing links in our brain through connections called synapses. Scientists have found that synapse formation and maintenance is almost entirely dependent on a good supply of cholesterol. A special form of cholesterol, called apolipoprotein E is manufactured in the brain for the sole purpose of maintaining synapses. (That's pronounced apo-lip-o-protein, and if you live in Lancashire or Yorkshire you should put the Eeee on the end as well). Without apolipoprotein E we would not be able to remember anything. So that is why the brain soaks up 25% of all the cholesterol we make in our liver.

And that is undoubtedly why cholesterol rich foods have been known for many years as 'brain food'. These are especially vital for the young, who are still forming synapses, and the elderly, who are losing more synapses daily through old age. It is also an especially good reason for the elderly to throw away their statins, sterols, and modified low-cholesterol foods and give up the idea that low cholesterol is good; unless of course you already have heart disease. In fact, I am totally convinced that your cholesterol level is good for you, whatever level it happens to be.

Our brain cells also produce neurotransmitters, and one particular transmitter called acetylcholine is responsible for triggering those synapses associated with memory. And guess what. Acetylcholine is made from ....yes, you guessed right, it is made from cholesterol. Memory loss is one of the most serious side effects from cholesterol-lowering drugs.

You would therefore think that all this gets taken into account when your cholesterol is checked. But the business for cholesterol-reducing drugs is massive – in the UK alone this business is worth £200 billion.

Doctors who practice integrated medicine know about the links between nutrition and health, but they have to tread carefully because conventional medics often call them 'nuts' or 'mavericks' and the medical council can strike them off if they stray too far from normal government's medical policy. So you're prescribed Statins.

We've not quite finished our story. Some people happen to be naturally deficient in cholesterol. Their symptoms tell us something about how important cholesterol is to our body. These unfortunate people are prone to emotional instability and behavioural problems. Low blood cholesterol has often been reported in criminals who commit murder and other violent crimes, in people with aggressive and violent personalities, in people prone to suicide, and people with aggressive social problems and low self-control. It may be no surprise to find that many of these people have what we would now consider to be a poor diet.

Incidentally these people who are cholesterol deficient are no less at risk from heart disease.

Even more worrying, the late Oxford professor, David Horrobin, has warned us all that reducing cholesterol in the population through measures such as statins and sterols on a large scale like the current government targets, could lead to a general shift in more violent behaviour in the public. Most of this would be seen at work and in the family, as retaliation, squabbles, car rage, child abuse, wife beating and general unhappiness. Does that sound a little like modern urban society today?

Those unfortunate people who cannot naturally produce enough cholesterol do need to have more cholesterol in their diet, because, although the cholesterol in our body is not the cholesterol in our food, we do need to be supplied with enough cholesterol in our diet to give us the building blocks our liver needs to produce its own cholesterol.

While our brain takes up 25% of the cholesterol our liver produces, cholesterol is important for other things too. Cholesterol is the building block for the sex hormones. Every steroid in the body is made from cholesterol; testosterone, progesterone, pregnenolone, androsterone, estrone, estradiol, corticosteroids and many others that are produced by the adrenal glands. These hormones carry out many important functions in the body. Our modern busy lives consume a lot of these hormones, leading to people getting 'burnt out' which doctors call adrenal exhaustion. The more enthusiastic we have become about fighting animal fats, the more problems with sexual development and fertility we have encountered. Many of these are related to sex hormonal problems. It is not difficult to understand why.

Our obsession with cholesterol has led to many odd situations in the food industry. We have sterol-fortified margarines, yoghurts, and cereals that lower cholesterol by forming a barrier in the gut that stops fats being absorbed. But this not only prevents vital cholesterol from entering our bodies, it stops other essential nutrients from entering our bloodstream as well. This particular area of business is currently valued at over £14 billion a year. Rather a lot, but of course chicken feed compared to what the statins manufacturers make.

There is another important function for cholesterol that we should be aware of, because this is vital to our well-being too. Cholesterol is used by the liver to produce bile, which is a clever solvent that drains into the stomach to allow us to digest fats. Bile is essential for absorbing and using fat soluble vitamins. We cannot live without these vitamins A, D, K and E. Apart from enabling these vitamins to be used by our body, cholesterol is one of the building blocks of another vitamin, Vitamin D.

Vitamin D is made by our skin from the action of sunlight on cholesterol. Our misguided fears of cholesterol and sun exposure seems to have created an epidemic of Vitamin D deficiency throughout the Western world.

But a deficiency of Vitamin D causes a multitude of problems

The Body Language of Health

- Diabetes (Vitamin D is essential for blood sugar control)
- Heart disease
- Mental illness
- Autoimmune disease (rheumatoid arthritis, lupus, IBD, multiple sclerosis)
- Obesity
- Rickets and osteomalacia
- Muscle weakness and poor coordination
- High blood pressure
- Cancer
- Chronic pain
- Hyperparathyroidism (osteoporosis, kidney stones, depression, chronic fatigue)

So, if cholesterol is not the cause of cardiovascular problems, what is?

For the answer to that you have to look at man's history. Unfortunately for modern man, your body has evolved to keep you safe from predators. One of the consequences is that we have not developed to become couch potatoes. If you eat too much and take too little exercise, cholesterol is not needed as much as it should because the cells are making all the cholesterol they need internally. That means an excess of cholesterol into your blood, which builds up in the blood, tissues, and arteries.

Your body also has that 'fight or flight' instinct that floods your body with cholesterol at times of stress or panic. The idea is that you will be ready for anything, including injury, (that's why you have a flood of cholesterol when you have a fright) but this hardly applies when you are faced with modern stressful situations. Cave man never had to give evidence in court, take exams, drive through city traffic, or forgot to pay the mortgage. Or any of the hundreds of stressful situations you face every day at work, commuting, and at home.

When you exert yourself, your muscles gather cholesterol out of the blood to meet their immediate needs. Then blood cholesterol typically stays well within healthy levels and the important HDL to LDL ratios stay in the healthy range. So exercise is the key to a stable cholesterol level.

But you remember in the heading I say that you should give up sugar. Why is that?

It is because insulin activates an enzyme that causes your cells to make cholesterol internally, which means that high levels of insulin stimulate the continuous production of cholesterol in the cells. And you will recall we said that is the wrong thing to do.

The Body Language of Health

Another enzyme, glucagon does exactly the opposite, it inhibits the enzyme that causes cholesterol production inside your cells, which results in the cell sending messengers to gather the needed cholesterol directly out of the blood, thereby reducing blood cholesterol levels. That is exactly how some of the cholesterol lowering drugs work too, so the pharmaceutical boffins know all this as well.

Too many fatty acids?

But these boffins won't have told you about prostaglandins. They are lipid compounds that are produced by enzyme reactions with fatty acids and they have important functions in all animals. They are technically hormones, although they are rarely classified as such. The name originates from the prostate gland because prostaglandin was first isolated from seminal fluid in 1935 by the Swedish physiologist Ulf von Euler, and independently by M.W. Goldblatt. It was believed to originate from the prostate but it was later shown that many other tissues secrete prostaglandins for various functions. They require a supply of essential fatty acids for their production.

In the body, prostaglandins and EFAs are vital for normal physiology, including:

- producing steroids and synthesizing hormones
- regulating pressure in the eye, joints, and blood vessels
- controlling immune response
- regulating bodily secretions and their viscosity
- dilating or constricting blood vessels
- regulating collateral circulation
- directing endocrine hormones to their target cells
- regulating smooth muscles and autonomic reflexes
- being primary constituents of cell membranes
- regulating the rate of cell division
- maintaining the fluidity and rigidity of cellular membranes
- regulating the inflow and out-flux of substances into and out of cells
- transporting oxygen from red blood cells to the tissues
- maintaining proper kidney function and fluid balance
- keeping saturated fats mobile in the blood stream
- preventing blood cells from clumping together (conglomeration, which is the cause of atherosclerotic plaque, and blood clots, can be a cause of stroke)
- mediating the release of inflammatory substances from cells that may trigger allergic conditions
- regulating nerve transmission and communication

- being the primary energy source for the heart muscle

So, you could say they are good at just about everything except making toast. Prostaglandins are absolutely vital in this story about cholesterol, because although cardiovascular disease is directly caused by high refined sugar diets, prostaglandins switch the method of biosynthesis to one that forms plaques in the cardiovascular system. This is a little complicated but stick with it.

There are three families of prostaglandins, called PGE1, PGE2, and PGE3. (If you're interested, omega 6 fatty acid (DGLA) is converted to PGE1, while arachidonic acid (AA) is converted into PGE2. PGE3 made by the conversion of omega-3 fatty acids).

Both PGE1 and PGE3 are goodies, they're anti-inflammatory agents, protecting against coronary disease by keeping blood platelets slippery and flowing, thus preventing blood clotting. PGE2 is the baddy – it is inflammatory and increases platelet stickiness and blood clotting. This is what causes heart disease.

All three forms must be present to ensure a functioning clotting system. There must be enough PGE2 to ensure healthy clotting, but enough PGE1 and PGE3 to protect against too much stickiness, which can lead to hardening of the arteries, heart attack, and stroke. Likewise, PGE1 appears to act as a diuretic, while PGE2 aids in the retention of water and salts in the kidneys. PGE2 also is required for healthy brain functioning. These three types of prostaglandins therefore serve as a vital system of checks and balances within the body.

However, if arachidonic acid (AA) and its derivative, PGE2, are over-produced or imbalanced with PGE1 and PGE3, they can cause illness or disease. The over-consumption of red meats and the under-consumption of cold-water fish and unprocessed oils can lead to an over-production of inflammation-producing PGE2 and an under-production of anti-inflammatory agents PGE1 and PGE3.

The goal for good health is to consume omega-6 fatty acids in a balance with omega-3 fatty acids. A suggested optimum ratio of omega-6 fatty acids to omega-3 fatty acids that should be consumed is four parts omega-6 to one part omega-3. Ratios of healthy populations range from 2.5:1 in Inuit diets to 6:1 in other traditional diets.

But daily consumption of omega-6 fatty acids by most people is grossly excessive, due to the presence of omega-6 fatty acids in common cooking vegetable oils and processed foods, indeed the ratio of omega-6 to omega-3 fatty acid consumption can often reach a staggering 20:1. That is fatal. To achieve a more desirable ratio, the best approach is to eliminate sources of omega-6 fatty acids, especially those hidden in processed foods, and to increase the amount of omega-3 fatty acids consumed through fish oil or flaxseed supplements. In addition, to convert the omega-6 fatty acids present in oils (such as corn, safflower, or soybean) to GLA requires that the oils be unprocessed and unheated and in the natural form (*cis* form, not *trans* form).

So, all those foods such as potato crisps, and all those 'healthy' products cooked in sunflower oil are out the window because they have been steeped in cooked Omega 6 oil. And that's bad. Don't believe the 'health' rubbish these manufacturers tell you.

In oils that have undergone processing (heating and/or hydrogenation) to prolong shelf life (e.g., many store bought oils) or to form a solid at room temperature (e.g., shortening and margarine), the fatty acid structure has been changed to the *trans* form, and the conversion process of omega-6 fatty acids to GLA will be inhibited. And that is why hydrogenated oils, margarines and so called *trans*-fats are so bad for you.

Interestingly, as soon as the ratio of omega 6 fats to omega 3 fats in food exceeds 4:1 people develop serious health problems. This is especially meaningful since grain-fed beef can have ratios that exceed 20:1 whereby grass-fed beef is down around 3:1. Similar ratios are also found in all grain-fed versus grass-fed livestock products.

Grass-fed animal products are rich in all the fats now proven to be health-enhancing, but low in the fats that have been linked with disease. So it is not the eating of beef that is the problem, it is the eating of cattle fed a rich diet that is the problem. That seems to be sensible. Make the cow artificially fat and when you eat it you'll get fat.

So, if you followed me so far, you'll appreciate that PGE1 and PGE3 are the good guys and PGE2 is the baddie. But even that is not the full story.

That's because the real culprit in the cardiovascular woodpile is ironically what is known by many as 'the white death'. Sugar produces excess insulin secretion, increasing cholesterol biosynthesis and switching immune system from PGE1 and PGE3 to an inflammatory, prothrombotic and plaque-forming PGE2 series instead. Sugar tips the balance towards sticky atherosclerotic plaques that gum up your arteries.

Sugar also overstimulates insulin and that in turn stimulates the production of cholesterol inside the cell, but we have already argued that this is not a good idea. The key to maintaining normal, healthy cholesterol levels is to eat in a way that does not result in excess insulin and in a way that puts glucagon in the metabolic driver's seat in your body. A diet high in carbohydrates, such as sugar, drives the body the wrong way. **And that's why sugar is such a bad idea.**

So cholesterol is like the oil in your engine. It needs to be maintained and looked after. And like a car engine, it needs regular exercise and to be revved up occasionally. And you'd be a dipstick if you ignored it.

Still not convinced? Don't you trust a forensic scientist? Let me quote Dr Natasha Campbell-McBride, a qualified human nutritionist and neurologist from an article in Complimentary and Alternative Medicine March 2007 (6:8, pp38-44).

"New cholesterol lowering drugs, the statins, were introduced in the late 1980's. The most commonly used ones are atorvastatin, fluvastatin, pravastatin and simvastatin. They inhibit the body's ability to produce cholesterol. As these drugs are new, their long-term effect is not known yet.

However, the data so far is not very encouraging; statins appear to result in increased risk of cancer development, breast cancer in particular, in animals and humans. Other side effects include liver damage, nerve damage, short temper, cognitive decline, memory loss and violent behaviour. Taking statins during pregnancy may lead to more serious malformations in the baby than were seen after exposure to thalidomide.

These drugs can cause kidney failure, which has already claimed the lives of several hundred people and resulted in one of the statins, cerivastatin, being withdrawn from the market. Muscle damage can be a very serious side-effect, particularly when the heart muscle is affected, because it can lead to heart failure. This happens because statins block the production of coenzyme Q10, an essential chemical for energy production in the body.

Statins are current number one profit-makers for the pharmaceutical industry and are rapidly becoming the most prescribed drugs in the Western world. As Dr Malcolm Kendrick has put it, "We are sleep-walking into what could become a major medical disaster, because statin drugs will soon be sold over-the-counter".

Memory loss is a very serious result of statin therapy. In fact it is possible that a considerable part of the memory loss epidemic in our ageing population is due to our ubiquitous statin prescriptions. One of the reasons for that is that acetylcholine, the chemical in the brain responsible for memory, is made from cholesterol. The brain is very cholesterol-hungry, it takes 25% of all body cholesterol and uses it for many vital jobs. Statins rob the brain of cholesterol and hence the brain cannot produce acetylcholine and accomplish many other functions.

More recently, statins have been linked to development of Parkinson's disease. Dr Xuemei Huang from North Carolina University, having researched the connection, commented "A surge in Parkinson's disease could be imminent because of the widespread use of statins."

Strong stuff, eh? I rest my case.

The problem is, what do you do if you have been a couch potato all your life, and now have heart disease? Well, you could simply reach for another pie of course. The Health Service will put you on statins and to be honest there are few other options unless you are determined to get healthy. It is difficult to change the habits of a lifetime and get out and build up to some serious exercise. Statins are an inevitable option for these people, but certainly not for those people who have an elevated cholesterol level but no chronic heart disease. Yet.

The proper thing to do is find out why your cholesterol level is elevated. I help you to do that in 'Do you have creases on your earlobe'.

The Government is committed to reducing the death rate from coronary heart disease and stroke and related diseases in people under 75 by at least 40% by 2010.

Looks like an uphill struggle. But now we know what to do don't we? No sugar, a correct fatty acid ratio, brain food and lots of strenuous exercise. Before it's too late.

Do you frequently catch colds and other respiratory infections?

If you do, you may be deficient in VITAMIN C and ZINC

Reviews of the research conducted on the use of Vitamin C over the past 20 years conclude that, in general, large doses of vitamin C have been found to decrease the duration and severity of colds, an effect that may be related to the antihistamine effects found to develop with large doses (e.g. 2 grams) of vitamin C. But large doses of vitamin C do not have a significant effect on the number of colds you catch, except for certain susceptible groups (e.g., individuals with low dietary intake, and athletes) who may be less susceptible to the common cold when taking supplemental vitamin C.

One aspect of human physiology which points towards a diet heavily reliant on fruit and vegetables, rather than meat, is our lack of ability to synthesis vitamin C.

Man, together with only one or two mammalian species cannot manufacture vitamin C, one of the most important vitamins. This suggests that we existed on a diet of fruit and vegetables, high in vitamin C, and therefore didn't need to develop the ability to manufacture it. Now, vitamin C is one of the main supplements taken in Western society. Deficiency in Vitamin C has more serious implications. Vitamin C is required for the synthesis of collagen, an important structural component of blood vessels, tendons, ligaments, and bone. Vitamin C also plays an important role in the synthesis of neurotransmitters that are critical to brain function and are known to affect mood.

Recent research also suggests that vitamin C is involved in the metabolism of cholesterol to bile acids which may have implications for blood cholesterol levels and the incidence of gallstones.

A large number of studies have also shown that increased consumption of fresh fruits and vegetables is associated with a reduced risk for most types of cancer. Such studies are the basis for dietary guidelines which recommend at least 5 servings of fruits and vegetables per day. A number of case-control studies have investigated the role of vitamin C in cancer prevention. Most have shown that higher intakes of vitamin C are associated with decreased incidence of cancers of the mouth, throat and vocal chords, oesophagus, stomach, colorectal, and lung.

But if you get a cold, don't guzzle orange juice for the vitamin C it contains. A big dose of sugar is what you'd actually be getting, making you even more ill. You'll conclude that you must not have caught the illness in time, which couldn't have been any further from the truth. The sugar simply fed your infection. If you want that much vitamin C, take a vitamin supplement, washed down with plenty of water. Sufficient zinc is also essential in maintaining immune system function. You can find plenty of information about zinc and its healing properties elsewhere in this book.

Have you experienced infertility, miscarriage or premature labour?

If you have, you may be deficient in ZINC

It has been estimated that 82% of pregnant women worldwide are likely to have inadequate zinc intakes. Poor maternal zinc nutritional status has been associated with a number of adverse outcomes of pregnancy, including low birth weight, premature delivery, and labour and delivery complications. However, the results of zinc supplements to mothers have been mixed. I have found that this is simply because these trials have not been conducted in zinc deficient populations.

ZINC AND SPERM

Semen is rich in zinc, with each ejaculation containing 5 mg which is one third of the recommended daily nutrient intake. This would imply that zinc plays an important role in sperm health. Three additional functions of zinc have been discovered apart from its important antioxidant role.

1. The genetic DNA material in the sperm nucleus is tightly wound with special proteins to form an insoluble, stable complex. This condensed structure is important for successful fertilization. Zinc is a part of this structure and protects it from breaking down.

2. The high concentration of zinc in semen damps down sperm activity, keeping them in a relatively quiescent state. This lowers their consumption of oxygen and conserves sperm energy. Once within the female reproductive tract, which contains very little zinc, zinc concentrations are rapidly diluted. This causes a sudden increase in sperm activity, speeding them up and acting like a mineral turbocharger in reverse. Galvanising them into action, you might say. (Galvanising is a process in which steel has a layer of zinc added to it to protect it from corrosion).

3. During fertilization, a sperm exposes enzymes in a sac at the sperm head to form a hole in the outer egg shell through which the sperm can pass. This is known as the acrosome reaction. In many cases of below-average fertility it seems that large numbers of sperm discharge their enzymes spontaneously before or just after ejaculation. By the time they reach the egg they are no longer capable of penetrating it. This early discharge of the acrosome reaction is believed to be linked with a zinc deficiency, and is a major cause of infertility in couples.

The Body Language of Health

High concentrations of zinc in semen help to slow down the acrosome reaction in a reversible way. Once zinc concentrations become diluted within the female tract, the acrosome reaction can occur again. It seems that zinc balance in the male is vital in maintaining the correct balance of zinc in the sperm too.

Another recent finding is that zinc deficiency changes the sequence in which seminal secretions are ejaculated. The secretions from the seminal vesicle, which are usually ejaculated last, are released along with the sperm instead. All very clever, in something that happens in a split second spurt.

There are several theories why this happens. Lack of zinc may cause swelling of the prostate gland, which will slow sperm travelling up from the testes. This swelling will also slow the release of prostatic secretions, which are usually the first fluids to be ejaculated. So perhaps zinc deficiency and prostate enlargement go hand in hand?

It is possible that this alteration in the ejaculatory sequence is a survival response to low concentrations of sperm zinc. By mixing the sperm and the relatively zinc-rich seminal vesicle secretions as early as possible, the protective effects of zinc are maximized.

This is lucky because most men do not obtain enough dietary zinc. Those that are highly sexually active may be losing more zinc per day in their semen than they can keep up with in their diet. Men ideally need a minimum of 15 mg zinc from their diet per day. That's good for three ejaculations a day, boys, so get some supplements now.

Certain individuals are more at risk of zinc deficiency than others:

Infants and children
Pregnant and lactating (breastfeeding) women, especially teenage mothers
Patients receiving total intravenous feed
Malnourished individuals, including those with protein-energy malnutrition and anorexia nervosa
Individuals with severe or persistent diarrhoea
Individuals with malabsorption syndromes, including spruce and short bowel syndrome
Individuals with inflammatory bowel disease, including Crohn's disease and ulcerative colitis
Individuals with alcoholic liver disease
Individuals with sickle cell anaemia
Older adults (65 years and older)
Sex maniacs (presumably)
Strict vegetarians

Strict vegetarian sex maniacs

The requirement for dietary zinc may be as much as fifty percent greater for strict vegetarians whose major food staples are grains and legumes because high levels of phytic acid in these foods reduce the absorption of zinc. In most cases the only answer is to use a zinc supplement. You could even say that zinc tablets should be considered an aphrodisiac.

Do you take the contraceptive pill or receive HRT treatment?

If you do, you may be deficient in ZINC, MAGNESIUM and VITAMIN B6 and have increased levels of COPPER

In 1993, the *Lancet* medical journal reported on the remains of an 18th century woman found beneath a church. Studies showed that her bones were stronger and denser than the bones of any modern women, either pre-menopausal or post-menopausal. Something in our modern lifestyle seems to be adversely affecting the density and strength of our bones, and only now are we beginning to understand what that might be.

For more than 50 years medicine has believed that lack of oestrogen was the primary cause of osteoporosis, based on the fact that osteoporosis mainly affects post-menopausal women who are short of oestrogen. Even today, medical students are taught that the treatment for osteoporosis is oestrogen replacement therapy. Oestrogen does, in fact inhibit the osteoclast cells that function to reabsorb bone and as a result can slow the rate of bone loss. But oestrogen cannot rebuild bone.

Oestrogen can be given in conjunction with another hormone, progesterone, which rebuilds bone by stimulating the osteoblast cells that re-mineralise and restore bone mass. But oestrogen has little to do with osteoporosis actually, see Page 295.

The use of oestrogen and/or progesterone are fraught with numerous side effects that have been reported: Hypertension, salt and water retention, increase in blood clotting, promotion of fat synthesis, hypothyroidism, painful breasts, fibrocysticic breast disease, increased risk of gallbladder disease and gallstones, liver dysfunction, increased risk of endometrial cancer of the uterus, pituitary prolactinoma tumour and possibly even breast cancer.

The Body Language of Health

The mineral balance in your body can easily become upset by these hormones. Deficiency of zinc and magnesium can cause elevated copper levels. Bringing more zinc and magnesium into your diet will soon redress the balance. And that's why you need zinc, magnesium, and vitamin B6 when you are on HRT or the Pill. In fact many experts recommend that you do not use HRT and look to natural remedies like Black Cohosh.

Do you or your family have a history of cancer?

If so, you may be deficient in SELENIUM

If you started at the beginning of this book you'll perhaps remember that Body Language began when my wife developed a passion for lettuce. During my investigations I found that lettuce contained chemicals called sulphorathanes which were being investigated as potential cancer treatments. Well, I wrote this section of the book a long time after that, so imagine my surprise to find that sulphorathanes appear here again in technical literature.

But let's start with selenium.

Our bodies need selenium, an antioxidant that is thought believed to control cell damage that can lead to cancer. In one study of nutrition and cancer, covering 1,300 men and women it was found that men who had taken selenium for 6½ years had approximately 60 percent fewer new cases of prostate cancer than men who were given a placebo. In 2002, this study data showed that men who took selenium for more than 7½ years had about 52 percent fewer new cases of prostate cancer than men who took the placebo.

A deficiency in the mineral selenium is associated with many types of cancer, while the presence of a chemical found in some vegetables (sulphorathane) is also known have a powerful role in cancer prevention.

Actually, there is a valuable point to make here. I think I have become pretty good at searching for information on the internet, but when I researched lettuce and sulphorathanes I failed to see any American research into these compounds. In fact America seems to pretty much be a scientific desert as far as technological breakthroughs are concerned. Can you guess why? (apart from the total scientific domination of British scientists).

Page 320

The Body Language of Health

In Britain sulphur is spelt – well..... S-U-L-P-H-U-R but in America sulphur is spelt S-U-L-F-U-R. And the internet search engines are very fickle, they will only give out what you put in. This happens a lot with scientific data, especially in chemistry. Look for the painkiller, paracetamol on the internet and all you will see is British references. That is because in America paracetamol is called Acetaminophen (or maybe it is Acetaminofen, I am not sure which), just as in America sulphur is spelt sulfur.

Of course it's not terribly important, because after all most of the world's definitive inventions and meaningful research come from Britain, but if I have missed out any American Body Language signs because of the language barrier, please check it out for yourselves using your own version of the English language.

Recently research on human cancer genes has found that foods that contain the mineral selenium and plant-based chemical sulphorathane (sulforathane) in combination may have a 13 times greater ability to protect against cancer than when these are used separately. So lettuce is great on its own, but it's even better when accompanied with a dressing of selenium.

Selenium is a mineral that is found in nuts, poultry, fish, eggs, sunflower seeds and mushrooms. Having a deficiency of selenium in the diet is known to be associated with a number of cancers, including prostate cancer. Recently we have found that game birds are rich in selenium, presumably because they and are free to roam and have a varied diet. So if you have a history of cancer, the odd pheasant or pigeon in your diet won't go amiss.

Sulphoraphane is being investigated as a potential cancer drug. It is found in foods such as broccoli, sprouts, cabbage, watercress, lettuce and salad rocket. So according to my new findings, eating a salad with nuts, game poultry, fish, eggs, sunflower seeds and mushrooms should be a cancer busting meal, because you are combining sulphorathanes and selenium together.

We know that mercury fillings leach out into the body all the time, and selenium mops up mercury, so if you have mercury fillings you'll probably be deficient in selenium. See 'Do you have mercury fillings?'

See also 'Do you have Keshan's disease?'

Vitamin E for prostate cancer prevention?

The Body Language of Health

We get vitamin E in a wide range of foods, especially vegetables, vegetable oils, nuts, and egg yolks. Vitamin E, like selenium, is an antioxidant, which might help control cell damage that can lead to cancer.

In a 1998 study of 29,100 male smokers in Finland; men who took vitamin E to prevent lung cancer had 32 percent fewer new cases of prostate cancer than men who took the placebo.

Take to the sun to beat cancer

Sunbathing has been proven to improve your chances of surviving cancer, doctors now declare. British research shows that patients diagnosed with cancer in summer and autumn live longer than those diagnosed at other times of the year.

This is undoubtedly because their vitamin D levels are topped up by sun exposure. Vitamin D can reduce the rate of cell division in tumour development and can trigger the self-destruction of cells that have been developing in the wrong way.

The study of more than one million patients suggests the season when cancer is detected and treated could make a significant difference to progress of the disease. It says that diagnosis in the summer and autumn months is 'associated with improved survival, especially in lung and breast cancer patients'.

The researchers found sunlight exposure to be a predictor of cancer survival, with results adding to a growing body of evidence that vitamin D may play an important role in cancer survival.

The study, published in the International Journal of Cancer, looked at 590,000 men and 606,000 women diagnosed between 1971 and 2002. Diagnoses made in summer and autumn - when blood levels of vitamin D are highest - had the lowest risk of death.

Women with breast cancer had a 14 per cent better chance of survival while women with bowel cancer had a 6 per cent better survival rate. There was a reduction of 6 per cent in the death rate for all cancers combined for both sexes when diagnosed in summer and autumn.

The study, which was led by Dr Henrik Moller, head of the Thames Cancer Registry based at King's College London, analysed their season of diagnosis, with summer and autumn defined as June 1 to November 30.

The researchers also obtained data on sunlight from the British Meteorological Office and calculated levels of cumulative sunlight hours for each season during the study period.

Their report says the results support the hypothesis that variation in vitamin D levels through sunlight exposure lies behind the differences in survival.

But it says data on sunlight hours probably underestimates the true effect of exposure because it does not measure the intensity of light - which is much stronger in summer and would have a more significant impact on blood levels of vitamin D.

The findings come as evidence grows that vitamin D could play a vital role in helping prevent disease, with sun exposure helping to top up natural levels more effectively than through diet.

Another study showed taking a large dose of vitamin D every day - 1,000 international units (IU) or 25mcg - could halve your chance of developing cancers such as breast, ovarian, colon, and prostate.

Oliver Gillie, who runs Health Research Forum, published a report showing that topping up levels of vitamin D could help prevent more than 25 chronic diseases.

He added: 'The research evidence shows Government advice to avoid sunbathing is misguided. Tanning should properly be seen as a sign of health, as indeed it is by most members of the public, although care should be taken to avoid burning.'

Mr Gillie said cancer patients should get advice from their doctors about whether they can safely sunbathe, as chemotherapy and radiotherapy can sensitise the skin to sunlight.

So get out there and soak up those rays.

SO DO BLONDES HAVE MORE FUN?

Have you ever wondered why Scandinavians are predominantly blonde? And do you know why men find blonde women so attractive? I have travelled quite a lot in Norway, Sweden and Finland and can confirm that there are a high proportion of Agnetha Faltskog look-alikes there. If you're not old enough to know who Agnetha Faltskog is, just look up Abba's greatest hits. Agnetha is the blonde singer with the greatest...

well you can probably guess why she's famous. Memories of her assets have endured much longer than her surname, which in contrast hardly rolls off the tip of the tongue.

Most men are highly attracted to blondes, but not many males realise why. The reason is said to be that men find their pale complexion attractive, but the answer is much more subtle, and it is all to do with fertility.

Modern men have lost the art of identifying when a woman is fertile just by looking at her complexion, but this was an essential trait for our male ancestors in the days when women would probably bear children as soon as they reached puberty, because life expectancy was poor. It was one of the survival instincts that ironically put us 'at the top of the tree' as soon as we left the forests. It was essential that the human race was replicated, so anthropologists believe that early woman would become pregnant as soon as they reached puberty. (early + woman – now there's a contradiction of terms).

When women become fertile their body temperature increases by about one degree, and this rise in temperature is one way that a couple can monitor the right time to conceive. At this point in time a woman's cheeks and neck take on a 'natural blush' for a couple of days that signals their fertility each time they ovulate. For primitive man, this would be how young virgins would become attractive to the males in the group. (Women you can get your own back here – primitive + man, yes, that sounds about right). Every month this blush would signal their fertility, making sure that each opportunity for fertilisation was satisfied. This 'natural blush' is still capitalised upon by women today who use rouge or pink blusher applied to their cheeks. And you thought 'rosy cheeks' were simply a sign of exposure to the weather!

The real reason that blondes are said to be so attractive to men seems to be that a blonde woman's pale complexion emphasises the blush that a woman radiates when she is fertile. This is a turn on to any male. It seems we have never lost that instinctive, subconscious desire for a fertile woman that we see in a blonde without realising it. Just as we have never lost the ability to crave butter for its salt, even though butter now has little salt in it, we still have this instinct for the important features that help us in the reproduction of the species. Incidentally, dyeing hair blonde is just not the same, because of a brunette's facial complexion that masks that fertile glow. It is that lack of pigmentation that is all-important to the male.

Our near neighbours also use fertility signs. Applying rouge to female cheeks is a lot more subtle than the tactics of our nearest ancestor, the chimpanzee, who has a dark, hairy face and therefore no 'fertile blush' to signal her willingness to mate. She has the indignity of having to wave her rump in the direction of a male to signal her fertility. And to be sure he gets the message her buttocks turn bright red and swell up when she becomes fertile. To us, it looks as though her bottom is inflamed and sore. Maybe that's why you rarely see chimpanzees riding a bicycle. (Sorry, it's just the imagination of a fertile mind)

You would imagine that a blonde woman's complexion would increase the likelihood of being successful, so the blonde genetic trait should dominate. But the dominant genetic pattern in humans is dark skin and brown eyes; blonde is recessive. Blonde hair and blue eyes is mainly confined to northern Caucasians such as the Scandinavians and anyone who has an element of Viking blood, such as some Britons. This means that for the Scandinavian blonde gene to predominate here, there had to be a significant biochemical advantage to having blonde hair, blue eyes and pale skin.

The answer is sunshine, which allows the skin to produces Vitamin D. In Scandinavia the sun is always shallow in the sky and in winter the sun hardly shines at all. So having a fair skin is a very distinct advantage to health, well-being and fertility because Scandinavians would be disadvantaged by the poorer sun absorption properties of dark skin. It may be no coincidence that most blonde women I know are rather active individuals, including a number of 'sporty types' clearly bursting with health and vigour.

Now that global travel is so prevalent and inter-country marriage is getting more common, it is likely that the brown eyed gene will eventually predominate, and the Scandinavians will be that bit sadder because of it.

The Scandinavians were great seafarers, and the Vikings have spread their genetic traits round much of the world, so the blonde genes have infiltrated everywhere, even though the gene is not dominant. I once became a little bit involved in genetic fingerprinting for a person's genetic history, and forensic scientists are now able to identify your forebears, including whether the family has any Viking blood in it from the past. In fact forensics has gone as far as being able to have a stab at the surname of a male murderer from a spot of blood at the scene by interrogating the genetic pattern in the DNA. Males keep their surname from one generation to the next and their family history, and hence their surname is fixed in the Y chromosome responsible for an individual being male.

'I have some news for you, Officer. Our DNA analysis from the scene of the crime has indicated the surname of the perpetrator'. 'You just need to arrest........ Mr Jones'

The Body Language of Health

So, we can infer from this that blonde women get more opportunities for sexual activity, but do they have more fun? Probably. Vitamin D can almost be thought of as the 'happy vitamin' and is responsible for many mental operations and harmonies. Blondes will have a ready supply of this vitamin, even in sun-starved (but presumably not sex-starved) Scandinavia, because they have evolved a fair complexion that maximises their sun exposure. For the rest of us, if you want to have more fun, get more sun.

SCREENING FOR CANCER

A few years ago I introduced a novel cancer test to Britain and was featured on virtually the whole of the front page of a national Daily Newspaper. Because of that I ended up having the honour of working with an eminent British laboratory that carries out a range of ground breaking screening tests for cancer specialists. Some of these are designed to diagnose cancer, others are valuable as monitoring tests to be done during treatment.

I've summarised (and tried to simplify) them and have reproduced them here to help medical professionals, but they also will be useful to sufferers as points of reference to do your own research on the internet. If you would like to have access to these medical tests, you should refer to www.mybodylanguage.co.uk for the address and details of the laboratory that performs them. However you will have to arrange for the tests through your own doctor or consultant if you are a private individual.

The body is an incredible machine, and I know of several consultants who have been able to switch on the body's own immune system to fight cancer. Once this is achieved, the body can fight defective tissue, in fact there is evidence that the body is doing this every day in all of us. Just think, your body is almost certainly fighting pre-cancerous cells right now. Cancers only get hold once the body is unable to identify and fight the defective cells so you should give them all the support you can. Mainly, you do that by eating the right food.

Cancer is not just one disease. The following section on cancer diagnosis and tracking is rather complicated, even though I have tried to make it as simple as possible. But I thought that you should be informed about the range of tests that are available to diagnose cancer, then track its progress or remission while it is being treated. These pages are just too valuable to have left them out of the book. I have found that sufferers are desperate for knowledge.

Arabinatol/Arabinose Levels
Indicates the presence of Candida Albicans.

This test is designed to distinguish between the presence of intestinal and systemic Candida infection. It has been found that Candida Albicans, which produces more than 70 toxic substances, can be a major allergen that triggers a hay fever type of reaction, resulting in asthma, irritable bowel syndrome, general malaise and other pathological conditions. So the test is very useful in determining how severe the infection is.

One of the by-products of Candida – the sugar alcohol arabinatol, is able to profoundly impair the nervous and immune systems functions, leading to other associated health problems. In the body this toxin can be transformed to the sugar, arabinose. The test uses a urine sample.

Anti - apoptotic Bcl – 2/ Pro - apoptotic Bax Genes Expression
An indicator of the ability of cancer and other abnormal cells to survive.

This test provides information related to the possibility of tumour growth without destruction, by measuring the ratio of the anti-apoptotic Bcl – 2/pro-apoptotic Bax genes expression.

Protein Bcl – 2 inhibits apoptosis, (programmed cell death), by preventing the release of apoptosis inducing factor (AIF) and cytochrome C from mitochondria. Protein Bax promotes apoptosis by triggering the release of AIF and cytochrome C from mitochondria. If the Bcl – 2 level is higher than the Bax level then apoptosis will be prevented. The ratio of Bcl – 2 to Bax in the cell can determine whether or not the cell initiates apoptosis or survives. Many cancer cells over express Bcl – 2, thus preventing apoptosis, allowing malignant growth to continue. This is a blood test.

Anti p53 Antibodies
An indicator of the ability of cancer cells to survive.

This blood assay is able to provide information relating to the presence of a wild (normal), mutated or deleted p53 gene, which is associated with the suppression of tumour development.

P53 is a tumour suppressor gene that functions as an inducer of apoptosis and is a regulator of the Bcl - 2 gene, which expresses protein inhibiting programmed cancer cell death. In cancerous cells, the p53 gene is one of the most mutated genes that express mutant forms of the p53 protein in the nucleus. This mutant p53 protein is not able to induce apoptosis of cancerous cells and they will continue to divide, thus increasing cancer growth. Also, cancerous cells with a deleted (absent, for unknown reasons p53 gene will continue to proliferate, thus increasing cancer growth.

It is not possible to convert cells with mutated or deleted p53 gene into cells with a wild (normal) gene. Thus, such cells can only be destroyed or eliminated.

Neurological Profile - Urine Based Assay

This urine based assay detects a comprehensive profile of neurotransmitters (dopamine, noradrenaline, serotonin), their precursors, metabolites, derivatives and neurotoxins.

Suppression of immune activity, adrenal insufficiency, depression and other neuropsychological problems, and many immunological and hormonal pathologies can develop if the chemical substances which make up the nervous system become imbalanced. This assay:

a) Detects and identifies abnormalities affecting the immune and hormonal systems.

b) Detect the underlying causes of various pathological conditions including cancer, chronic fatigue syndrome, multiple sclerosis, autism, depression etc.

c) Identifies possible treatment targets.

This assay provides information on the status of the nervous system by evaluating the concentration of various chemical substances, found in urine. It covers:

- The presence, and probable type, of any infection.
- The generation of damaging free radicals.
- Oxygen, vitamins and some mineral deficiencies.
- The activities of the defence system (NK cells, T cells, B cells and macrophages).
- The character of the activities of the adrenal cortex, liver, pancreas, pituitary and thyroid.
- The influence of stress.
- Fluctuations in mood and behaviour.

Hormonal Profile - Urine Based Assay

A comprehensive urine-based assay of steroid hormones such as progesterone, cortisol, corticosterone, dihyroxyepiandosterone, beta-estradiol, estriol, estrone, testosterone and some of their metabolites and toxic derivatives.

Many problems are hormone-driven, from chronic acne to breast and testicular cancer. Normal hormonal balance indicates healthy body systems. Imbalance of hormone production and utilisation, other than normal, can lead to pathological conditions, including the impairment of protein, carbohydrate and lipid metabolism, cancer (for example breast, prostate), osteoporosis and many others. This assay provides details of:

a) General male hormones.   b) General female hormones. c) Possible treatment targets.

Bactericidal Permeability Increasing (BPI) Protein Level
A marker of the response to pathogenic gram negative bacteria.

This assay is able to provide information related to the presence of pathogenic gram negative bacteria.
Bactericidal Permeability Increasing protein is a bactericidal compound that is present in leukocytes. BPI binds endotoxins, it is rapidly released by leukocytes in response to exposure to bacteria which produce endotoxic lipopolysaccharides (LPS). LPS are highly toxic components present in the cell wall of gram negative bacteria, which include many bacteria responsible for diseases. The presence of LPS in blood will lead to the development of fever, inflammation and septic shock.

Cathepsin L Level
A marker of the ability of cancer and other abnormal cells to destroy their environment, resulting in disease progression.

This assay is able to assist in the prognosis of the progression of tumour growth and also neurodegenerative and some inflammatory processes.

Cathepsin L is an enzyme, lysosomal endopeptidase, produced by certain specialised cells, such as macrophages and osteoclasts. This enzyme is also produced by many malignantly transformed cells. Since Cathepsin L has the ability to degrade the proteins of the extra-cellular matrix, it is assumed to play a crucial role in tumour progression, metastasis and numerous other disorders, where the destruction of the extra-cellular matrix is the major cause of disease. For example, rheumatoid arthritis and neurodegeneration.

Cell Viability Detection
An indicator of the presence of harmful substances and abnormal cells.

This assay is designed to reveal, indirectly, the presence of cytotoxic agents, which damage cells (drugs, preparations, natural toxins etc.) and abnormal cells (i.e. fungi and bacterial cells) in the test media. Useful to monitor the effectiveness of a treatment programme.

Cu/Zn Superoxide Dismutase (Cu/Zn SOD) Level
This is a marker of inflammation, cell destruction and organ dysfunction.

This assay is able to provide information relating to the inflammatory processes, associated dysfunctions of the liver and kidney, plus destruction of cells of the nervous system.

Radicals are generated in many physiological metabolic pathways, particularly in activated cells of the defence system – phagocytes. Radical generation is essential to kill some bacteria but liberated radicals can extend beyond the target area, which results in membrane damage, lipid and protein oxidation, followed by cell damage or destruction. Overall, free radicals have to be considered as potentially harmful and protection is provided by superoxide dismutases (SOD). Cu/Zn SOD is a soluble cytosolic enzyme and is present in the cytoplasm of virtually all eukaryotic cells. Cells, which are dying or dead cells, release Cu/Zn SOD into the media where it can be tested, thus indicating the level of apoptosis. Liver dysfunction, kidney damage and neurodegenerative pathologies could be associated with increased Cu/Zn SOD level, whilst decreased Cu/Zn SOD level means that any abnormal cells could proliferate without destruction to give clones of infected cells, cancer cells, etc.

C – Reactive Protein (CRP) Level
A marker of the response to infected or impaired cells and tissue.

This assay is able to provide information related to the presence of active inflammation or tissue destruction.

C – Reactive Protein is a protein which is not normally present in blood. However, elevated levels of CRP have been found in the blood in virtually all diseases associated with active inflammation or tissue destruction. Rheumatoid diseases, acute infectious processes, advanced and wide spread malignancy, post myocardial infarction or surgery are particularly characterised by high levels of CRP.

The Body Language of Health

Since the titre of CRP in the serum is at a maximum in the active stage of inflammation and rapidly decreases during recovery, the estimation of CRP is of considerable prognostic value.

CRP is considered to be one of the best markers for heart disease and monitoring during and after a heart attack.

E – Cadherin Level
An indicator of the ability of cancer cells to be invasive, plus a marker of inflammation and organs dysfunction.

This assay is able to assist in the prognosis of cancer invasion/metastasis and also in the estimation of systemic inflammation and associated multi-organ dysfunction. It is designed for the quantitative determination of soluble E – cadherin.

E – cadherin, also known as uvomorulin or cell – CAM120/80, is one of the sub-classes of cadherins, Ca2+ dependent cell adhesion molecules, which are responsible for the selective cell – cell adhesion.

There is evidence to suggest that the changed expression of E – cadherin is a common event in cancer progression. The level of this substance can significantly decrease in the number of solid tumours such as lung, breast and hepato-cellular carcinomas, gastric, prostatic and other tumours. Simultaneously, its level in blood could be increased.

Such distribution of E – cadherin is associated with the ability of cancer cells to be invasive, which can lead to the development of metastasis. In addition, the elevated E – cadherin level is associated with systemic inflammatory response and multi-organ dysfunction syndrome.

Endoblock Detection
An indicator of any impairment of the response to pathogenic gram negative bacteria.

The Endoblock assay is designed to detect the compounds involved in the impairment of the biological response to the toxic lipopolysaccharides (endotoxins) produced by gram negative bacteria, which are responsible for many pathological conditions.

Fas Ligand (Fas L) Gene Expression
An indicator of the ability of cancer cells to destroy cells of the immune system.

This assay is able to obtain information related to the cancer cell defence mechanism protecting against its own death.

Fas Ligand is the special protein molecule, which is able to trigger apoptosis in the Fas sensitive cells. The immune system T cells and B cells, as well as Natural Killer (NK) cells are Fas sensitive cells.

On their surface there is a special receptor molecule called Fas or CD95. When Fas Ligand interacts with the Fas receptor, the destructive mechanism of the immune system cells is triggered. Activated T cells, B cells and NK cells have an increased number of Fas receptors, which make them more Fas sensitive.

There is evidence that some cancer cells produce significant amounts of Fas Ligand. This Fas L is able to trigger destruction of the cells of the immune system, which would normally attack cancer cells. This means that cancer cells avoid destruction whilst some of the cells of the immune system could be destroyed. This phenomenon is known as the 'immune escape' of cancer cells.

Glycoprotein 90K/Mac – 2BP Level
An indicator of the presence of a viral infection.

Glycoprotein 90K/Mac – 2BP is mainly produced by the cells of the defence system: the macrophages, monocytes and to some extent by a variety of other cells. There is evidence of its involvement in immune defence mechanisms. Elevated levels of this glycoprotein are associated with viral infections and some types of cancer (probably of viral origin). In some cases, the failure to respond to treatment could be connected with increased production of this molecule.

Interferon Gamma (IFN - gamma) Gene Expression
A marker for the presence of Natural Killer (NK) and Th1 cells.

This assay is able to assist in the evaluation of the processes relating to the destruction of cancer and other abnormal cells. It has been designed to estimate the Interferon Gamma gene expression as part of the characterisation of the state of the defence system.

Production of IFN - gamma is a function of NK cells and T cells (both cytotoxic and the Th1 type). Interferon gamma is a lymphokine which has a number of properties such as anti – viral and anti – proliferative. It is able to activate the macrophages in order to destroy tumour cells by releasing reactive oxygen intermediates and Tumour Necrosis Factor – alpha. In addition, IFN - gamma is capable of down regulating (inhibiting) anti-apoptotic Bcl – 2 protein followed by the induction of cell destruction.

Interleukin 1 Beta (IL - 1beta) Gene Expression
A marker of the presence of macrophages, Th1 cells, inflammation and oxidative stress.

This assay is able to provide information related to the activation of cellular immunity. It is also designed to estimate the risk of inflammation and oxidative stress.

IL - 1beta, originally known as Lymphocyte Activating Factor (LAF), activates T lymphocytes, which then proliferate and secrete Interleukin 2. IL - 1beta is also known as endogenous pyrogen is able to mediate oxidative stress and is produced mainly by macrophages and monocytes.

Interleukin 2 (IL - 2) Gene Expression
A marker of the presence of naive T and Th1 cells.

This assay is able to assist in the estimation of specific immune response to cancer (anti-tumour immunity) and also various types of pathological conditions. It is designed to estimate the Interleukin - 2 gene expression as part of the characterisation of the Th1/Th2 immunological balance.

IL - 2 is produced by the embryo CD4+ T cells and Th1 cells and is a cytokine, which plays a central role in immune responsiveness by promoting the activation and proliferation of lymphocytes, that have been primed by antigens (antigen specific T - lymphocyte proliferation). IL - 2 also stimulates the proliferation of B cells, augments NK cell activity and inhibits granulocyte macrophage colony formation. IL - 2 displays anti-tumoural effects. Russian researchers injected IL-2 into lung tumours and in 3 months they had vanished.

Interleukin 4 (IL - 4) Gene Expression
A marker of the presence of naive T and Th2 cells

This assay is able to assist in the estimation of factors preventing the formation of the anti-tumour immunity and also to provide information related to the presence of some bacterial infections. It is designed to estimate the Interleukin 4 gene expression as part of the characterisation of the Th1/Th2 immunological balance.

IL - 4 is produced mainly by the Th2 cells, as well as Mast cells. This cytokine exerts numerous effects on various haematopoietic cell types. It can promote survival, growth and differentiation of both T and B lymphocytes, mast cells and endothelial cells. In addition, IL - 4 can inhibit the production of Tumour necrosis factor - alpha and Interleukins 1 and 6, by macrophages.

Interleukin - 5 (IL - 5) Gene Expression
A marker of the presence Th2 cells.

This assay is able to assist in the estimation of the factors preventing formation of the anti-tumour immunity and also to provide information related to the presence of parasite infections or allergens. It is designed to estimate the Interleukin - 5 gene expression as part of the characterisation of the Th1/Th2 immunological balance.

IL – 5 is a cytokine, that promotes the development and the activation of eosinophils. It is produced mainly by Th2 cells, in response to the stimulation from parasite derived antigens and allergens. In addition, various transformed B cells, Reed – Sternberg cells in Hodgkin's disease and activated eosinophils can express IL – 5. Some inflammatory processes (e.g. asthma or various allergic responses) are associated with Th2 cell activation followed by an elevated production of Interleukin 5, together with Interleukin – 6.

Interleukin 6 (IL – 6) Gene Expression
A marker of infection or trauma.

This assay is able to provide information relating to both viral and bacterial infections, trauma and cancer development.

IL – 6 is a cytokine, which is produced by a variety of cells, including macrophages and Th2 cells. Normal cells do not produce this cytokine constitutively, but its expression is induced by a variety of cytokines, bacterial or viral infections. IL – 6 has numerous properties, it acts on a wide range of tissues, exerting growth-induction, growth-inhibition or differentiation, depending on the nature of the target cells. IL – 6 is involved in other important processes, such as the proliferation of T cells, the induction of IL – 2 expression and B cell differentiation. The changed expression of IL – 6 is associated with infections, autoimmune, proliferative and neoplastic diseases and inflammatory responses to infections or trauma.

Interleukin 10 (IL – 10) Gene Expression
A marker of cellular immunosuppression and infection.

This assay is able to assist in the estimation of the level of Interleukin – 10 gene expression as part of the characterisation of the Th1/Th2 immunological balance.

IL – 10 is a cytokine, that is produced by the regulatory CD4T cells and has the ability to suppress the functions of macrophages, Th1 cells and NK cells. It is associated with the promotion of Th2 cell development and consequently with the regulation, proliferation and differentiation of B cells.

IL – 10 has immunosuppressive properties by inhibiting the production of Th1 specific cytokines and the maturation of dendritic cells and is able to exert strong anti - inflammatory activities. The expression has been shown to be elevated in parasitic infections (such as schistosoma mansoni, leishmania, toxoplasma gondii and trypanosoma), mycobacterial infections (such as mycobacterium leprae, mycobacterium tuberculosis and mycobacterium avium) and retroviral infections.

Lipid Peroxidation Products Level
An indicator of the destructive processes by free radicals.

This assay is able to provide information related to the destructive oxidative processes in the body.

Lipid peroxidation is the major indicator of oxidative stress, which is associated with the production of damaging free radicals and contributes to the formation of various pathophysiological changes in the cells and organs functioning. The lipid peroxidation of the cell membrane is very often followed by necrosis (accidental death) of such cells.

Matrix Metalloproteinase 2 (MMP – 2) Gene Expression
An indicator of the ability of cancer to be invasive and form metastasis. This assay is able to assist in the prognosis of the progression of cancer.

Matrix metalloproteinases (MMP's) are a family of zinc dependent endopeptidases, which can degrade the major components of the extra-cellular matrix. Cancer cells subvert MMP's activity to promote invasion of the surrounding tissues, as well as metastasis to distant tissues. MMP's by releasing growth factors sequestered in the extra-cellular matrix are also thought to promote the growth of these tumour cells once they are changed. The inhibition of one of the MMP enzymes can lead to the dissemination of cancer, in other words the suppression of its progression and metastasis.

Mycoplasma Detection/Gene Expression
An indicator of the presence of an infection.

This assay is able to provide information related to the presence of mycoplasma – the DNA particle of the bacterium.

Mycoplasma is able to dramatically change the properties of normal cells and to significantly impair the functions of the defence system.

Nitrotyrosine Level
An indicator of the presence of an infection and inflammation.

This assay is able to assist in the estimation of inflammatory processes triggered by pathogenic micro-organisms including gram negative bacteria.

Nitrotyrosine (modified tyrosine) is formed in the presence of peroxinitrite, which is the active metabolite of nitric oxide (NO). NO is produced by various cells in response to the inflammatory or mitogenic stimuli. The biological role of NO is defensive against non-self pathogens. However, enhanced NO production will have toxic effects. In this case, increased formation of its metabolite peroxinitrite will spontaneously lead to elevated nitrotyrosine production.

Accumulation of nitrotyrosine dramatically affects the functions of proteins, which negatively influence numerous physiological processes. Consequently, nitrotyrosine is associated with various inflammatory processes, including septic shock.

Interleukin – 12 (IL – 12) Gene Expression.
A marker of the presence of B cells, macrophages and possible stimulation of Th1 cells.

This assay is able to assist in the estimation of the formation of the anti-tumour immunity and also to provide information related to the presence of bacterial and viral infections. It is designed to estimate the Interleukin – 12 gene expression as part of the characterisation of the Th1/Th2 immunological balance.

IL – 12, which is also known as the natural killer cell stimulatory factor or the cytotoxic lymphocyte maturation factor, is a cytokine which can have multiple effects upon T cells and NK cells.

IL – 12, produced by macrophages, is associated with the promotion of Th1 cell development, followed by cell – mediated immune response. In addition, IL – 12 has been shown to be a pro – inflammatory cytokine produced by phagocytic cells, B cells and some antigen – presenting cells that modulate adaptive immune responses.

The critical role of Interleukin 12 in several pathologies has been demonstrated. Significant elevations were measured in autistic patients and sufferers of multiple sclerosis. Auto-immune diseases, cancer and chronic inflammatory reactions can all be accompanied by an increase in the level of IL – 12. Additionally, a large number of bacterial & viral infections are capable of changing the expressed levels of Interleukin 12.

Non – Genomic DNA Level
An indicator of the presence of a viral infection or mycoplasma.

This assay is designed to measure the concentration of extra cellular (non genomic) DNA.

This type of DNA could be of viral origin or even originated from mycoplasma. In some cases, patients who relapse have an increased level of DNA in the blood. In addition, there is some evidence that non – genomic DNA could be an indicator of the presence of oncoviruses.

Non – Genomic RNA Level
An indicator of the presence of a viral infection.

This assay is designed to measure the concentration of extra cellular (non genomic) RNA.

This type of RNA could be of viral origin and, as an antigen, can negatively affect the functioning of the immune system. This can be of particular significance if there are problems with the enzyme ribonuclease which is responsible for degradation of RNA. There is evidence that CFS is associated with abnormal ribonuclease. In addition, there is some evidence that non – genomic RNA could be an indicator of the presence of oncoviruses.

Soluble p185 Her – 2 Protein Level
An indicator of the ability of cancer cells to metastasize.
This assay is able to provide information related to very early oncogenic changes and is able to assist in the monitoring of tumour spread, post-operative relapse and metastatic risk.

P185 protein is a transmembrane growth factor receptor, which belongs to a class of oncogenes related to tyrosine protein kinase, which possess tumorigenic or transformation activity. It is involved in all cell growth and cell transformation. It is possible to detect increased levels of p185 in the blood of individuals who will subsequently develop cancer up to 60 months before clinical diagnosis.

Superoxide Dismutase (SOD) Activity
An indicator of the ability of the defence system to scavenge and neutralise the damaging effects of the reactive oxygen species.

This assay is able to provide information related to the destructive oxidative processes in the body.

Reactive oxygen species, such as free radicals and the superoxide anion are generated during a number of chemical reactions within the cell. These species may cause severe damage within the cell, however several enzymes have evolved which scavenge and neutralise the effects of the reactive oxygen species. Superoxide Dismutase, a metallo enzyme, is one key enzyme involved in the protection of cells from damaging free radicals. Any one of three metals will work together with SOD by catalysing the dismutation of superoxide anion into oxygen and hydrogen peroxide, these are manganese, iron and copper. There is evidence to suggest that many disease processes could be associated with extremely low superoxide dismutase activity.

Survivin Level
A marker of the ability of cancer cells to inhibit their own death.
This assay is able to assist in the estimation of cancer cells to survive the normal destructive process and to continue the growth process.
Survivin is a protein, which is produced in many fetal tissues, such as the kidneys, liver, lungs and brain in addition to transformed cell lines and most cancers. Survivin is not found in terminally differentiated adult tissues. Whilst a critical role for Survivin in tumour growth has been established, overproduction of Survivin in rapidly growing cells may explain its abundance in tumours.

Transforming Growth Factor – Beta (TGF - beta) Gene Expression
A marker of the presence of cells with immunosuppressive properties.

This assay is able to assist in the estimation of the level of TGF - b gene expression as part of the characterization of the state of the defence system.

TGF - beta is a multi-functional protein, which is produced mainly by mammalian cells. TGF - beta is capable of influencing differentiation, proliferation and a variety of cellular functions. This protein generally slows immunosuppressive and anti-inflammatory activities but is able to stimulate the macrophages and monocytes. TGF - beta overproduction is linked to tumour growth, perhaps as an indirect result of its other actions.

Tumour M2 – Pyruvate Kinase (TM2 – PK)
A marker of active tumour cells.

Pyruvate Kinase (PK) or pyruvic acid kinase is an enzyme which catalyses the transfer of a phosphate group from phosphoenolpyruvic acid to adenosine diphosphate (ADP) with the formation of an 'energy' molecule – adenosine triphosphate (ATP). This reaction is very important in the glycolytic pathway. This enzyme has an absolute requirement for magnesium and is inhibited by calcium. Whilst the conventional form of pyruvate kinase is a tetrameric molecule, a dimeric isoform of PK is over produced by a wide range of different tumours. This appears to be linked to the different metabolic requirements shown by tumour cells, which leads to these cells using a metabolic shortcut to 'save energy' for cell multiplication. In this process the proportion of pyruvate kinase present as the dimer form is increased. Therefore the level of the dimer, namely Tumour M2 – PK, is significantly increased in tumour cells.

In rare cases however, a somewhat increased TM2 – PK level could be associated with the presence of impaired glucose utilization which may not be cancer cells, eg. chronic inflammatory processes such as diabetic nephritis.

Tumour Necrosis Factor – Alpha (TNF - alpha) Gene Expression
A marker of the presence of macrophages, Th1 cells and neurotoxicity.

This assay is able to assist in the estimation of the formation of anti-tumour immunity and also to provide information related to the presence of pathogenic micro-organisms and inflammatory processes. It is designed to measure the tumour necrosis factor – alpha gene expression as part of the characterisation of the state of the defence system.

TNF - alpha, also known as cachetin, is a cytokine which is produced mainly by monocytes and macrophages. Endotoxins and Interferon – gamma promote the production of TNF - alpha and it functions as a modulator of the immune response by activating dendritic and Th1 cells. It may play a role in the pathogenesis of many disease states and, in particular, inflammatory diseases. In high quantities, this cytokine acts as a pyrogen and neurotoxin by increasing the permeability of the blood/brain barrier and destroying the serotonin containing cells of the nervous system.

TNF-alpha is responsible for the inflammatory response in rheumatoid arthritis and Crohn's disease.

Telomerase - Number of Cells with Active Telomerase
An indicator of the presence of cancer cells or their precursors

This assay is able to provide information related to the very early oncogenic changes prior to the definitive formation of any tumour and clinical diagnosis. When the tumour is formed, this assay is able to assist in the prognosis of cancer regression or progression.

Specific structures found at the ends of chromosomes in eukaryotes are known as telomeres. These telomeres protect chromosome ends from undergoing fusion, rearrangement and translocation. In somatic cells the telomere length is progressively shortened with each division due to the inability of the DNA polymerase complex to replicate the 5' end of the lagging strand.

Telomerase is a unique enzyme, which is a ribonucleoprotein that synthesises and directs the telomeric repeats on to the 3' end of existing telomeres using its RNA component. Telomerase activity becomes suppressed through the ageing process but activation of telomerase is regarded as essential to most cancer.

Telomerase activity has been shown to be specifically expressed in immortal cells, cancer and germ cells where it compensates for telomere shortening during its DNA replication and this stabilises telomere length. The expression of telomerase activity in cancer cells is a necessary step for tumour development and growth. This means that there is a specific association of human telomerase activity with cancer and it is usually high in cancer patients. It is considered that the regression of telomerase activity could be one of the mechanisms for cancer regression.

Low telomerase activity in the blood of cancer patients can be associated with:-

- The tumour being in an encapsulated form.
- Remission of cancer.
- The inability to create tumour immunogenicity, eg. recognition of cancer cells by the immune cells.

High telomerase activity in the blood of cancer patients can be associated with:-

- A risk of further tumour development.
- The destruction of the tumour during effective treatment and two to four weeks after such a treatment.

To correlate the level of telomerase activity with one of these indicators, additional information is necessary. The special packages for cancer (p 4) are able to provide this information.

Parasites and Smears Detection
An indicator of the presence of an infection.

This assay is able to provide information related to the presence of blood parasites or smears. Parasites and their by-products are able to significantly impair the functions of the nervous and immune systems, which can lead to the development of various pathological conditions.

Perforin Level
A marker of the presence of active NK cells and cytotoxic T cells.

This assay is able to provide information related to the presence of the necrotic process.

The Body Language of Health

Human perforin (cytolysin) is one of the major effector molecules used by NK cells and cytotoxic T cells to mediate targeted cell lysis or necrosis (accidental cell death). Perforin expression is constitutive on NK cells, but increases in resting CD8+ cytotoxic cells upon activation.

Many cancer cells are resistant to destruction through apoptosis. Stimulated by perforin, necrosis is the only mechanism of destruction of such cells.

Protein Fractions Level
An indicator of organ dysfunction.

It is possible to obtain three specific pieces of information from this assay, namely:-

a. The concentration of total high molecular protein.
b. The concentration of 'bonded' protein which could be part of the antibody – antigen complexes, which result from immunostimulation or could be associated with adhesion molecules involved in the cells aggregation.
c. The concentration of total small peptides in blood.

The latter is of particular importance as some of these peptides can have a negative affect upon the nervous and immune systems. Total peptides can serve as an indicator of gut problems.

Tumour Necrosis Factor – Beta (TNF - beta) Gene Expression
A marker of the presence of Th1 cells.

This assay is able to assist in the estimation of the formation of cell-mediated immunity. The tumour necrosis factor - beta (TNF - beta), also known as lymphotoxin alpha, and the tumour necrosis factor - alpha are two closely related proteins that bind to the same cell surface receptor and show many common biological functions. TNF - beta plays a central role in lymphoid development and in normal host resistance to infection and to the growth of malignant tumours, serving as an immunostimulant and as a mediator of the inflammatory response. It is produced by activated T , B and NK cells, astrocytes and human myeloma cells. Excessive production has been found to play a very significant role in a number of autoimmune disorders including multiple sclerosis, insulin dependent diabetes and rheumatoid arthritis.

The Body Language of Health

Vascular Endothelial Growth Factor (VEGF) Gene Expression
A marker of the angiogenic process which stimulates the growth of tumours.

This assay is able to assist in the estimation of the risk factor which is able to suppress the host anti-tumour immune response and stimulate tumour growth.

Vascular Endothelial Growth Factor is a family of closely related growth factors which are polypeptides. VEGF is a potent growth factor for blood vessel endothelial cells, showing pleiotropic responses that facilitate cell migration, proliferation, tube formation and survival. It is also one of the most potent permeability factors, so VEGF is a common link of inflammation permeability and angiogenesis.

Local hypoxia is a potent inducer of VEGF production from adjacent cells but it is not synthesized in endothelial cells. Expression of VEGF can be induced in macrophages, T cells, astrocytes, osteoblasts, smooth muscle cells, fibroblasts, endothelial cells, cardiomyocytes, skeletal muscle cells and keratinocytes.

It is also expressed in a variety of human tumours. In fact, the VEGF, which is the most active angiogenic factor, appears to inhibit the maturation of the dendritic cells, whose fundamental role in the activation of an effective anti-cancer immunity has been well documented. In addition, the evidence of abnormally high pre-treatment levels of VEGF has appeared to be associated with reduced efficacy of IL – 2 cancer immunotherapy.

In this case, the concomitant administration of anti-angiogenic drugs could enhance the anti-cancer immunotherapy. Therefore information related to the VEGF expression could be used to control the angiogenic processes, which have been proven to stimulate cancer growth not only through stimulation of cancer related neo-angiogenesis, but also by inducing a suppression of host anti-cancer immune response.

Yeast Gene Expression
An indicator of the factors which are negatively influencing the nervous and immune systems. This assay is able to provide information related to the presence of yeast. Yeast and its by-products are able to significantly impair the functions of the nervous and immune systems, which can lead to the development of various pathological conditions.

Cytokine Assays
Interleukins, TNF's, etc. assayed by special request
Previously ignored by everyone, the laboratory I have described was probably the first laboratory to take cytokine analysis seriously. I actually attended the First Symposium on Cytokine Medicine, held in Manchester, February 2003, several years

The Body Language of Health

after they were offering cytokine assays as a way of identifying illness and looking at the inflammatory response.

Cytokine mapping gives clues to many ailments and maladies including Crohn's disease, rheumatoid arthritis, asthma, inflammatory bowel disease, and many others. Ideal if you're considering using one of the anti-TNF antibody treatments like Infliximab.

Oxidative Stress, (ROS), Inflammation Assessment Profile
Comprehensive profile of products from lipid peroxidation and cell destruction.

Provides information on the following:
a)   The level of damaging or destructive processes within the body.
b)   The ability of the body to normalise the level of oxidative stress.
c)   Possible causes for the abnormal level of oxidative stress.
d)   Possible treatment targets.

The process of damage and destruction of the bodily cells by the action of reactive oxygen species (R.O.S.), including free radicals, is called oxidative stress. Under normal circumstances, this process is involved in the destruction of abnormal cells, particles and substances from bacterial, viral, fungal and parasitic origin. If the level of oxidative stress is below the normal range, then an accumulation of harmful agents will result.

Conversely, if the level of oxidative stress is above the normal range, then it will result in the destruction of normal, healthy cells. In both cases pathological conditions, including; liver dysfunction, kidney failure, arteriosclerosis, neurological disorders and cancer, may develop.

Glucose – 6 – Phosphate Dehydrogenase (G – 6 – PDH) Deficiency Detection
An indicator of the suitability of Vitamin C therapy, vitamin B17 therapy or drug therapy.

This test is able to provide information related to the risk of developing drug induced haemolytic anaemia.

G- 6 – Phosphate Dehydrogenase is an enzyme which catalyses the oxidation of glucose – 6 phosphate in the phosphogluconate oxidative pathway of glucose metabolism. During this reaction reduced triphosphopyridine nucleotide (TPNH) is formed. TPNH particles in maintaining glutathione in a reduced state in normal erythrocytes which protect them from haemolysis by peroxides generated during drug-related destruction of abnormal (cancer, infected) cells. Therefore G – 6 – PDH deficiency will lead to TPNH deficiency and the development of over sensitivity of erythrocytes to the peroxides generated by some treatment strategies. G – 6 – PDH deficiency can occur as a result of the inhibition of this enzyme by fatty acids.

There is also quite a lot of information on the web about the detrimental effect of hormones in dairy produce that may adversely affect many cancers, notably breast cancer. These sites do not recommend diary products as a diet source.

Do you have Cardiomyopathies (Keshan's disease)?

If you do, you may be deficient in SELENIUM

Keshan's disease is a type of heart disease called cardiomyopathy (which simply means 'heart muscle disease') that particularly affects young women and children in a selenium deficient region of China. Keshan's disease is closely associated with very low dietary intakes of selenium, and selenium supplements has been found to protect people from developing Keshan disease although it cannot reverse heart muscle damage once it has occurred.

Despite the strong evidence that selenium deficiency is a fundamental factor in Keshan's disease, it is seasonal and the cause appears to be a virus that produces inflammation of the heart. The same happens to selenium-deficient mice.

HIV patients and hepatitis sufferers are also usually deficient in selenium, so it appears that low selenium causes a risk of viral infections. Maybe this suggests the route to a prevention and cure for the common cold.

Some researchers claim that instead of the billions spent on viral drugs, a few pennies would be better spent on providing selenium in the diet of viral infection sufferers such as HIV victims.

Bird Flu from China

It may be no coincidence that the regular new flu viruses come from China/Hong Kong as there is a well-known vast area in China that is selenium deficient. The same area produced Keshan's cardiomyopathy and pandemics of oesophageal and gastric cancer until the villagers were instructed to take extra selenium, after which both illnesses abated. It appears to be an established fact that viruses readily mutate in selenium deficient hosts as well as being more virulent, as shown in selenium-deficient mice where respiratory viruses caused greater morbidity and mortality.

I doubt that man is any different. Two more areas of study also comes to mind, namely, the Congo with its Ebola outbreak, and the rest of Africa with its pandemic of HIV and AIDS, currently running at over 30-40% of the various indigent populations. These populations are also selenium deficient. However, Senegal, a country on the West African coast, apparently has an HIV incidence of only about 1% even though the population has the same sexual habits as its neighbours. The only difference is that Senegal lies on top of an old seabed and the soil has a very high mineral content that includes selenium. I understand that the Senegalese have some of the highest blood selenium levels in the world. Maybe it could be worthwhile if everyone took some extra selenium. Extracts from garlic are very good anti-viral treatments too.

SELENIUM AND CHRONIC INFECTIONS

In New Zealand, where selenium daily intake is less than 40mcg, and where both cancer, heart disease and virus infections are rampant, it would seem appropriate to increase the intake to over 200mcg/day. New Zealand farmers and horse breeders make sure that their animals get selenium but then their animals have to be healthy to be commercially valuable.

Bird flu could be the next viral epidemic to strike, and millions have already been spent on Tamiflu. Personally, I know what I will be taking to help ward off the virus.

Incidentally I have been experimenting with garlic patches recently. Garlic is so good at getting through the skin, that you can do a little experiment to prove to yourself just how porous your feet really are. Take a clove of garlic, crush it, and rub it on your feet. Within an hour your breath will smell of garlic. The allicin in the garlic has diffused through your skin and into the bloodstream, and has come out into the breath in your lungs.

Garlic is an excellent anti-viral product. And guess what? Garlic is rich in selenium. That is quite possibly why garlic is well known to have powerful anti-cancer properties.

Good sources of selenium

- rice, wheat
- seafood, fish, meat, poultry
- nuts, especially Brazil nuts
- eggs
- sunflower seeds
- mushrooms, garlic

Good sources of sulphoraphane which should also be taken with selenium

- fish
- eggs
- sunflower seeds
- broccoli, sprouts
- cabbage
- watercress, lettuce, salad rocket

Have you had, or are you prone to heart attacks?

You may be deficient in VITAMIN E

Preliminary research has led to a widely held belief that vitamin E may help prevent or delay coronary heart disease by limiting the oxidation of LDL-cholesterol. Vitamin E also may help prevent the formation of blood clots which could cause a stroke. Observational studies have associated lower rates of heart disease with higher vitamin E intake. A study of approximately 90,000 nurses suggested that the incidence of heart disease was 30% to 40% lower among nurses with the highest intake of vitamin E from diet and supplements.

A 1994 review of 5,133 Finnish men and women aged 30-69 years also suggested that increased dietary intake of vitamin E was associated with decreased mortality (that's a medical term for more deaths) from heart disease.

Even though these observations are promising, randomised clinical trials raise questions about the efficacy of vitamin E supplements in the prevention of heart disease, but again these people were probably not deficient to start with.

Previous studies have suggested that vitamin E reduces the risk of prostate cancer in male smokers, decreases the risk of Alzheimer's disease when taken with vitamin C and protects against Parkinson's disease. Several other sections in this book refer to heart disease, take a look in the index and review other sections for a more complete picture, so as to keep your finger on the pulse.

Do you experience Carpal tunnel syndrome?

If you do you may be deficient in VITAMIN B6

Studies have found vitamin B6 deficiency to be common in people with carpal tunnel syndrome (CTS). Supplementation with vitamin B6 has reportedly relieved the symptoms of CTS in many cases. Various clinical biochemistry tests tend to show that carpal tunnel patients have distinct and often severe deficiency of vitamin B6. Numerous studies debate the point whether vitamin B6 deficiency causes CTS. Regardless, the volume of studies weighs heavily in favour of its use in treatment and rehabilitation of carpal tunnel patients whether surgery or steroid injection treatment is to be used or not.

Symptoms of CTS include recurrent numbness, tingling, weakness, or pain in one or both hands in a characteristic location defined by the median nerve, which is compressed as it passes through the carpal tunnel in the wrist. Symptoms are usually worse at night and after prolonged use of the hands. Some people may experience clumsiness in handling objects, with a tendency to drop things, and may also have a decreased ability to feel hot and cold.

CTS is typically treated with nonsteroidal anti-inflammatory drugs such as aspirin and ibuprofen, oral diuretic medications, and injections of corticosteroids into the wrist in order to reduce swelling. Splints are often recommended to immobilize the wrist, theoretically protecting it from repetitive motion injury. Sometimes a physical therapy program of hand- and wrist-strengthening exercises and the use of a wrist brace is recommended. In more advanced cases, a surgical procedure called a "release" may be used to separate the ligaments covering the carpal tunnel in the wrist in order to relieve the pressure on the median nerve.

Indiscriminate use of supplements can lead to high levels of Vitamin B6 which have been reported as harmful, so again the message from this website is that you should concentrate your efforts on finding the right food that is wholesome and fresh.

Have you had a Gastrectomy?

You may be deficient in VITAMIN B12 and HYDROCHLORIC ACID

One of the issues arising out of alimentary canal surgery is something called post-gastrectomy syndrome. It shows as anaemia due to low levels of vitamin B12 ,iron and higher risk of osteoporosis. These problems generally occur months or even years after gastric surgery.

Vitamin B12 malabsorption occurs when a protein known as intrinsic factor is either not produced by the stomach (a condition called pernicious anaemia) or when the portion of the stomach producing intrinsic factor has been removed. Under normal circumstances intrinsic factor binds to vitamin B12 and assists with the absorption of this vitamin in the lower portion of the small bowel. When vitamin B12 is poorly absorbed, anaemia and, in some cases, poor nerve function can occur. This generally does not happen for several years because vitamin B12 is stored in large amounts in the liver and has to become exhausted first. This makes the link hard to track down

Iron deficiency anaemia develops because removal of the stomach often leads to a marked decrease in the production of gastric acid. This acid is necessary to convert dietary iron to a form that is more readily absorbed in the duodenum. Anaemia usually does not occur for a few years after gastric surgery because iron is stored in moderately large amounts in the bone marrow, where red blood cells are produced.

Osteoporosis develops as a result of poor calcium absorption, another problem that occurs after gastric surgery. Under normal circumstances, calcium absorption, which occurs in the duodenum and proximal small bowel, is modest at best, with large amounts being lost in the bowel movement. Following gastric surgery, calcium absorption is even less efficient as a result of rapid emptying of the stomach. Calcium also binds tightly to unabsorbed dietary fat which further interferes with its absorption. Symptoms of osteoporosis may develop ten or more years after gastric surgery because of the large amount of calcium that is normally stored in bone.

So it is important to adjust your diet to allow for these factors, and eat the best quality food you can buy, preferably organic and grown in fertile, manured soil.

Have you had an intestinal problem or Irritable Bowel Syndrome (IBS)?

Thanks to our modern diet, one in four surgical operations in the UK are now on some part of the digestive tract. Maybe this is because the average person in the West eats 65 tons of food and drink in their life, and much of it is unnatural.

We've cured the old diseases like diphtheria, polio and smallpox, and replaced them with modern killers like cancer and heart disease, due to our unsuitable diets. About one in five UK adults suffer from Irritable Bowel Syndrome (IBS). Some think IBS is now 'usual' - the legacy of combining fast-paced lifestyles with rich food and reduced exercise.

So, we each eat about half a ton of food per year. Current research shows that the prevalence of food hypersensitivities in the general population is estimated at about 5 per cent, and up to 65 per cent of IBS patients attribute their symptoms to food allergies.

Many irritable bowels are caused by smoking, one of the commonest causes of Crohn's disease as well.

Look after your gut, it is your powerhouse

- Eat plenty of fibre (for more details see haemorrhoids)
- Don't smoke
- Eat a varied diet (Japanese eat 40 different foods a day)
- Eat plenty of coloured vegetables
- Eat fresh food that is in season from a proper greengrocer selling fresh food
- Avoid convenience foods, confectionery and sweets.
- Don't microwave food

If you fancy a snack, first try something from this list:

nuts and raisins, dried fruit, fresh fruit, carrots, vegetable sticks dipped in hummus, dry muesli, seeds, vegetable crisps, rice crackers, sesame seed sticks, and porridge, are all ideal. I am sure you could add a few favourites of your own.

IRRITABLE BOWEL SYNDROME

Researchers have found that IBS patients have elevated antibodies to common foods such as wheat, beef, pork, lamb, and Soya bean. These findings, published in the *American Journal of Gastroenterology*, suggest that food hypersensitivities play a role in IBS and the observations made are consistent for three subgroups of IBS tested - diarrhoea, constipation and both. "With this simple test, we have scientifically shown that these symptoms may be due to the body's response to what we eat in our daily diet. It opens up a new avenue for the management for this large and complex group of patients," said Dr. Devinder Kumar of St. George's Hospital in London. Since this study has been conducted, the researchers have now performed a diet exclusion study based on the findings of the food hypersensitivity test and "preliminary results are very encouraging."

Whether simply digestive discomfort caused by holiday tummy, constipation, diarrhoea or indigestion, or more serious digestive problems such as irritable bowel syndrome, we have all suffered at some point. What is less commonly acknowledged, however, is that poor digestive health is also the root cause of many of our most frequently suffered allergies, which is just another of the many reasons reason why taking a little time to care for our gut will boost general health and well-being.

- Deaths from digestive illness - including colon cancer, liver disease, pancreatitis and diverticular disease - now account for 12 per cent of all UK deaths and one in eight of all admissions to general hospitals in the UK are connected with the digestive tract.
- Most problems can be linked to over-milled flour. When we have to break down the wheat cells in our gut, gluten release is slow and controlled, but milled flour in which cells have ruptured gives us a massive slug of gluten our digestive system can't handle. Commercial bread is not a product we have evolved to eat.

Are you over 60 years of age?

You may be deficient in VITAMINS and MINERALS, especially the B VITAMINS.

Most elderly people are deficient in their diet. Researchers have found that seemingly healthy, elderly subjects can still exhibit low vitamin levels which reduce their ability to fight disease. There are several reasons for this. As we get older we tend to rely more on processed foods which are a poor substitute for a proper diet. We may not be able to chew food as well as we used to, so we tend to leave out certain foods from our diet. We may even find that shopping for food is more difficult because of changing shopping patterns and less mobility.

I have been saying that there is no substitute for a fresh and varied diet, but for the over 60's the answer seems to be to rely on additional supplements of minerals and vitamins. There are some excellent vitamin and mineral combinations around that will cater for most of your daily needs.

It is also worth pointing out that there are a number of myths about old age that are just not true. I have included them here to give us all hope for our old age.

Myth No 1. Many of us view the elderly as doddering old fogies. In reality, true senility only strikes a very small proportion of elderly people, and even then, some age-related reduction in mental functioning can be prevented or even reversed.

Scientists have discovered that vitamin deficiencies account for many of the symptoms of senility. For example, low folate levels in the elderly can cause forgetfulness, irritability and possibly depression. Vitamin B6, a nutrient required to make many neurotransmitters, may lead to peripheral neuropathy (a disorder of the nervous system where the limbs feel numb or tingle) if deficient. The nutrient that ensures nerves are protected with a myelin sheath, vitamin B12, can be responsible for delusions and mood disturbances when levels fall below normal.

Statins also rob you of your mental powers and there is no evidence they protect you against heart disease. You should stop taking them unless you already have heart problems. Even then, it is worth discussing your medication with your doctor.

Myth No2: Old age means losing all my teeth.

The Body Language of Health

Even if you're not worried about losing your mind when you're old, you might fret about losing your teeth. Part of the problem, said investigators, was that education and dental care for the elderly are overlooked by both dentists and the patients themselves.

Proper dental hygiene and regular cleanings by the dentist are usually enough to stave off infection. Another simple and inexpensive way of preventing or at least halting the progression of periodontal disease is to store and replace your toothbrush properly. Although most of us are in the habit of keeping our toothbrush in the bathroom, this is not recommended. Bathrooms are the most contaminated room in the house. It is not a bad idea to change your toothbrush when you have recovered from an illness too.

Finally, an important aspect of both dental and general health is immunity. Cigarette smoking is the worst thing you can do. Other lifestyle behaviours that theoretically could do the same include poor eating habits, stress and other immune depressors.

Myth No 3: The older I get, the sicker I'll get.

Old age doesn't have to mean being sick and tired of feeling sick and tired. An important part of staying well into the older years is keeping your immune system operating at its peak.

By taking the right nutrients, exercise and other measures, you can prevent many age-related diseases. For example, there is evidence that smoking and low plasma levels of vitamins C and E, and beta-carotene contribute to cataracts. Experts have shown that a one year program of stress management, moderate exercise, no smoking and a good vegetarian diet may reverse the development of heart disease. Left untreated, those fatty plaques usually continue to grow.

Why not get a pet? Cats are well known to give health benefits (unless you are allergic to cats of course) and take little looking after. Dogs are also great companions and taking it for walks will keep you fit. Even a soft toy to pet and cuddle has been shown to have health benefits. I hesitate here to suggest a pet goat – originally I thought that Sally would feast on our abundant grass not realising she would much prefer the roses, rhododendrons, camellias…. etc.

Many other chronic diseases can also be prevented or treated with lifestyle changes. Zinc and magnesium supplementation helps some individuals with hypertension. Most are helped by high potassium foods (fruits and vegetables), and weight maintenance. Keeping blood pressure under control can also decrease the risk of a stroke.

The Body Language of Health

Adult-onset diabetes is usually treated best with dietary measures such as removing simple sugars, consuming a lot of fibre and taking chromium supplements. It is estimated that at least half of all types of cancer are linked to diet. This explains why less fat, lots of fruits, vegetables and fibre, vitamins A, B6, C and E and zinc and selenium all appear to play a role in cancer prevention.

You will find plenty of health advice about these issues elsewhere in this book

Myth No 4: Lifestyle changes won't help me when I get old.

It's a mistaken notion that at a certain age, you reach the lifestyle modification point of no return. If you've used this as an excuse to cling to old, comfortable, unhealthy habits, it's time to let go. Of course, it's always best to live as healthy as possible as young as possible. But for those of us in our golden years, there is still plenty of hope.

Two of the most difficult habits to break, smoking and a sedentary lifestyle, can change our life for the better if we can break the habits of a lifetime.

Frailty in the older person can't be totally blamed on aging. At least some weakness occurs because of physical inactivity. A regular exercise program not only decreases the risk of chronic illness, but also can help prevent early death. Those who begin exercising later in life can slow or even reverse organ deterioration.

Exercising, at any age, helps fight chronic diseases, increases heart strength, muscles are more fit and flexible, mood is enhanced, and falls and fractures are less frequent. While exercise alone probably doesn't significantly extend life beyond 80 years old, it can improve your quality of life. Some of our friends say dance classes are brilliant.

Sex can still be invigorating and enjoyable at any age, you just have to take your time. And if you find yourself on your own, many elderly people find fulfilment and companionship in their retirement and discover a new lease of life with a fresh partner. Find a new one at your local dancing classes, perhaps.

Myth No 5: As long as I maintain the eating habits I had when I was younger, I'll stay healthy.

Perhaps one of the biggest fallacies of good health is that nutritional needs don't change with age. Just as children and teens have different dietary requirements than adults, so do the elderly differ in their needs from youngsters.

The Body Language of Health

A number of factors cause poor dietary intake. Chronic diseases, both physical and mental, can cause nutritional problems. Various medications can impair nutrient availability or discourage eating due to loss of appetite. If you wear ill-fitting dentures, pain can prevent you from eating. Elderly who live alone may feel isolated and uninterested in eating. Even the diet in a nursing home can be lacking in nutrition, and some food provided in hospital is scandalously poor, just when you need it most to promote healing.

But even if you are older and healthy, the very process of ageing alters your metabolism and physiology. Stomach acid declines, thus affecting some nutrient absorption. Many older people feel full quicker because of an increased sensitivity to the 'I'm full' system. Ageing also dampens the body's appetite centre, and consequently you lose your appetite. Finally, it's suspected that an older palate is less sensitive to those senses that drive us to the dinner table.

The answer is to make dining an event to be enjoyed. How about eating with friends now and again? Or setting up a circle of friends or relatives who try out restaurants, or even club together to make a meal at home and share a bottle of wine?

If you dine out, try to be discriminating because chefs tell me that quite a lot of 'pub meals' are made from microwaved cheap produce and they wouldn't eat it themselves. You do need to choose good quality food. At the time of going to print, these chefs suggested that anything below £6 for a main course is probably not going to be very nutritious. You're better to buy one decent meal that is a bit more expensive than buy three that are cheap. Money spent on nutritious food is an excellent investment.

Ageing is inevitable. Poor health is not. Regular exercise, nutritious eating (appropriate for your age) and a lucky roll of the genetic dice can help you to age with grace and good health.

Take a browse through other sections of the book, or view our website on www.mybodylanguage.com , and get up to speed on diet and nutritional requirements.

CONCLUSIONS

Looking back, I suppose I became interested in the link between health, environment and diet many years before the trigger for this book when my wife took up an association with lettuce.

Some years previous I had developed an interest in water. It started when I met an eminent Russian scientist who seemed to know a lot more about water than I did, and I was fascinated by the Russian technology that had evolved along a totally different thought path to the way we think in the West, because of the isolation of scientific learning that the iron curtain had caused. To a scientist, this was like the excitement that Darwin must have felt when he visited the Galapagos Islands and discovered the fascinating flora and fauna that had developed because the islands were isolated from creatures on the mainland.

Remember, this was at a time when Russians were very restricted in their travel, and this eminent Russian professor had to have all the necessary invitations from me to make the journey to Britain to see me at all. I was very honoured to see him, since his status in Moscow was equivalent to an Ambassador. Imagine then, to find that he had only once been out of Russia, for a similar meeting in Moldova the year before. When he arrived in Moldova, there was no-one waiting for him at the airport, and he was unable to contact his host. All he had was a change of clothes and his ticket back home. Not even any spare money and certainly no credit cards. So he had to sleep rough in the Airport until it was time to get on his plane and go back home.

So I found out some months later that when he came to visit me he had come prepared, fearing that he would suffer the same fate in Britain as he had in Moldova. As a safeguard he had brought a giant Russian Polony sausage in his suitcase, so that he would at least have something to eat if I failed to meet him. Fortunately this unusual parcel was not picked up by our Customs, or else he would have had some difficult explaining to do.

In particular, as a result of my interest I started to investigate the irrefutable stories behind 'healing wells'. Why is the water in so many of these wells capable of miraculous healing? Is it to do with the minerals in the water?

I managed to get hold of several water samples from healing wells round the world, as well as water from the Jordan and the Ganges, and at the time we had an instrument at work called an ion chromatograph. You could inject the sample into the machine and out came a series of peaks representing the metal ions in the water. A printer then gave me a list of the elements and their concentration in the water.

The Body Language of Health

I found that these wells and springs had one thing in common. They were loaded with the elements we all associate with their horrible taste; sulphur, carbonate, iron. And there was a powerful supply of boron, manganese, magnesium, zinc and a host of other trace elements that are usually missing from our tap water. This is not surprising because our water comes from reservoirs, and in order to have water run off the hillside and keep the water in a lake you need to have a rock system that is non-porous. This generally means that the reservoir is in a part of the country where the rock is granite or dense sandstone. It is no good making a reservoir in a part of the country where the ground consists of chalk or limestone, because these rocks are porous and the water won't stay there for five minutes. But because granite and sandstone are non porous and non-soluble, the water running straight off into the reservoir is generally inert and free from hardly any significant levels of any minerals at all. It's actually a rather unnatural source of water for humans.

In contrast, many healing wells tend to be at junctions where sandstone or granite meets limestone or chalk. The run-off from the non-porous rock meets soluble rock, and here we usually find caves, swallow-holes and steep valleys and dales. The very places where mankind would have developed. Here the water slowly dissolves the rock so the water contains all the elements that are in the rock. These places have special benefits and have become known as spa towns, mostly made famous by the Romans. In Britain, Harrogate, Buxton, and Bath are typical examples. These towns became highly prized again in Victorian times, and it was popular to visit and 'take the water' but they have fallen out of favour recently. The water is so loaded with minerals that it forms stalactites and stalagmites in the caves as it evaporates, and dissolved elements give the water a strong mineral or sulphurous flavour which takes some getting used to. But as a mineral tonic it takes some beating.

The Russians had experimented with the structure of water to the extent that their belief in its beneficial properties bordered on the religious. I was never able to get to grips with the science behind their philosophy and got diverted, but scientists with a different line of research should be encouraged rather than scorned.

You will remember the particular doctor who went into practice having been taught that everything to be discovered about medicine had already been discovered? Well, most scientists seem to be like that too these days. I have realised a long time ago that scientists usually end up researching the wrong things nowadays because of the commercial pressure from their funding providers. No longer are these people their benefactors, as they were in Victorian times. Nowadays it is the financial reward that is most interesting to these people. So the scientist's career path is dictated by how many papers they publish, and that in turn is fuelled by how complex their research is. No-one wants to do the basics, so the profession is top heavy with boffins researching the unfathomable.

The Body Language of Health

So more and more researchers do more and more obscure research. There is now more scope for career enhancement by working in obscure cancer genetics that will be of little benefit to anyone, than in proving that the appropriate amount of sunshine cures cancer, or that the selenium in garlic wards off cancer as well as pesky vampires.

A researcher will get more recognition creating one-off babies in a test tube, than by demonstrating that our epidemic of infertility is due to zinc deficiency.

A doctor will be paid much more handsomely for prescribing cholesterol reducing drugs than he will in teaching the nation to eat a healthy diet, which has the same ultimate end, better in fact if you have read the section on cholesterol.

And even at the time of going to press 10% of hospital deaths in Britain were being caused by hospitals failing to follow official guidelines on the prevention of blood clots in patients. Researchers at the University of Birmingham say this causes ten times more deaths than MRSA and five times more deaths than breast cancer, AIDS and road accidents combined. Yet the government has just one obsession and that is to cut the miniscule number of road deaths even further. Why is there this discrepancy in priorities? Well, on the one hand a death in hospital is one patient less to have to treat, and on the other hand motorists are an easy target as a financial resource with no opportunity to stand up for their individual rights.

But politicians should beware, because the British can only be pushed so far. Not long ago in Canada a political party had just one agenda in their manifesto - scrap speed cameras. And they won the national election by a landslide victory. I am surprised this has not been a manifesto choice in Britain yet, because it is sure to be a winner for whichever party embraces it.

Unfortunately while researchers bury their heads in obscure work, no-one is doing the basics. But Body Language shows that many of today's health problems can be solved quite easily. All we need is to focus on the real facts, eat a properly nutritious diet and get more exercise. And we can do that if we fertilise the soil properly so that we can once again grow nutritious food, and legislate against junk food and unnatural products, but only if the authorities stop feeding us their rubbish ideas.

Britain has always been a fountain of knowledge. In the days of Newton and Hooke, the philosophers would meet in their offices round Bloomsbury Square, in London, and they inspired the world with their great discoveries. It is said that since the last war, a staggering 80 percent of all the world's inventions have originated from Britain. They include some pretty influential products; the computer, the CAT scanner, immunoassay technology and the discovery of DNA which has led to innovation in genetics. Throughout this book I have been amazed that virtually all the scientific breakthroughs have been from British scientists or from foreign scientists like Casimir Funk working in Britain.

But recently, our focus on the complex has pushed us down a scientific blind alley. The benefits of antibiotics, great though they are, are still dwarfed by the even greater benefits that better hygiene has given us. Artificial joints are an expensive and complicated answer to a balanced diet containing boron.

Perhaps I have been able to show you that the basics of Body Language can be sexy after all (well, in parts perhaps). Maybe it is time for Britain to start afresh with our perceptive powers. There is still plenty to be discovered if we go back to the simple basics.

Take energy saving as an example. We started the world's clock manufacturing industry in London and astronomers unified the world's time by implementing Greenwich Mean Time, GMT (primarily so that all Britain's trains would run to the same timetable). Now all the world sets its timepieces to the median that goes through Greenwich, London.

Recently, Parliament broke off their constant bickering about global warming to debate whether Britain should continue with British Summertime. They were contemplating whether to scrap British Summertime and stay with GMT all year, since the extra light that an added hour gave to farmers was not needed now we are no longer at war (everyone conveniently ignores Iraq, Afghanistan, the Congo etc.) and we fly in all our food in from the other side of the world.

They decided to leave the British summer time arrangement in place and leave the clocks as they were.

In the days of Newton we would have the ability to think laterally. But no longer, it seems. Sometimes I wonder if politicians are capable of lateral thought at all.

In Britain in Spring, Summer and Autumn we all typically get up four hours after it gets light and go to bed four hour hours after it gets dark. In those last four hours we all turn on the lights and turn up the central heating once the sun goes down.

Even in winter, most of us get up when it is broad daylight, and get back home long after it has got dark. OK, in December, the darkest month, maybe most of us will get up around dawn, but our morning use of electricity is limited to a kettle, toaster and maybe a couple of lights, whereas at night in the dark we become major consumers of energy. Certainly it has been light many hours before we get to work and we are already turning on the lights around 4pm.

So let's put the clocks BACK four hours so that we make the most of the sunshine throughout the whole year. We will then be more attuned to getting up at dawn and going to bed at dusk. That would save billions of tons of CO_2 from belching into the atmosphere from our power stations. (Blyth Power Station alone emits as much CO_2 as one quarter of all the cars in Britain), and save us making new power stations. And if Britain did it, the whole world would do it. We'd all be healthier too, because sunshine is vital for health and happiness, as you are now well aware.

Several countries have messed around with the odd hour here or there and argued that children have to walk to school in the dark, which is not really true any more. But changing the times by four hours will put us into another time scale (literally) and we would soon get used to a day based around sunshine again like our ancestors did. Considering the vast amount of energy we would save, it would be a major message to the whole world.

THAT'S the sort of fundamental thinking that made Britain great. But politicians were a lot smarter then in those days and less full of their own importance and hot air. Hey, maybe I have just discovered another major factor in global warming.

Britain often starts a new way of thinking, that's why the industrial revolution, the democratic system, the monetary system and the health service; all these and more have been copied round the world from the British model. Will we now start a new angle on how we look at our health, reducing our dependence on drugs and increasing the balance back to appropriate food? I sincerely hope so.

So that's Body Language, and as they say in politics, I commend it to the House. I hope you have found it entertaining and enlightening. Body Language is an ever expanding and changing field, so if you have any comments, observations, case studies or criticisms, please email them to me on info@mybodylanguage.co.uk

I cannot guarantee to respond individually but I can assure you every one will be carefully considered. And wherever possible I will add information supplied to the mybodylanguage website so that it remains a powerful resource and reference point for everyone the world over. Your comments will be valued whether favourable or not, and I would like to thank you now for taking the time to correspond and for sticking with me to the end.

The end.
Hamish MacGregor

ACKNOWLEDGEMENTS

I was lucky enough to start my career with some of the best forensic scientists. As I worked my way up, I came to realise that these people had the integrity, sharpness of mind, and unerring logic that had shaped my way of thinking too. I owe a lot to them.

During my later career I have been very fortunate to come into contact with a number of eminent people who stood out as being at the forefront of their chosen branch of science. These people are not household names, and you're unlikely to see them on television. I would love to acknowledge them by name here, but I think they would be embarrassed by fame and would prefer to remain anonymous.

No, these dedicated people have come to my attention because they are refreshingly different, and it has been an honour to know them. In their profession, one might even go as far as to call them mavericks. Instead of going with the flow they have been prepared to question the way things are done now, and work out how they could do things better. And I think that is the crux of what science is all about. If we didn't question how things are, we wouldn't progress.

These people assume everyone thinks like them, and they probably didn't even realise they were influencing me. But they showed me that you could look at things including health differently. If you are an acquaintance of mine and cannot find your name quoted anywhere, I apologise, but you can be sure that our associations together have been an influencing factor.

I would like to thank Elsie my wife for inspiration in the first place, and for her constructive comments throughout. Her advice has kept the number of Body Language references to genitalia and excrement to a respectable minimum - you wouldn't believe how many Body Language signs there are in this category. (Her first comments were 'there's too much sex and shit in here'). So I am sure she also receives your eternal thanks too. Ah well, there's always the Second Edition to look forward to.

Thanks also go to my three sons for advice and help in preparing the final draft and print setup to make the whole process of publishing a painless experience, and for the herculanean task of compiling the Body Language Medical Questionnaire website with its associated expert system that you can use on www.mybodylanguage.co.uk

And I would like to thank you, the reader, for persevering this far. I hope you find yourself able to take advantage of your new knowledge about your body, and have been satisfied with my coverage of your favourite bits.

INDEX

Note: Subject headings are not included in this index; if what you are seeking is not here, review the Contents list at the start of the book.

The Body Language of Health

Osteoporosis	31-3, 63, 74, 90, 135, 154, 163, 182, 206, 272, 283, 295-8, 319, 328, 348
Osteoporosis home test	298
Oysters	91-2, 203, 278
PABA (see para amino benzoic acid)	
Pantothenic acid (see Vitamin B5)	
Para amino benzoic acid	233-4
Pellagra	74, 184, 235, 270
Penis	95-8
Pernicious anaemia	148, 261=3, 348
Phenylethylamine	41, 72-3
Photosynthesis	68
Pica	8-11, 19, 27
Pickled onions	19-20
Pirates	193
Plants	42, 54, 61, 69-70, 80, 103, 159,209
Post-prandial drowsiness	43
Potassium	18, 19, 30, 62, 95, 161, 165-167, 288-292
Prehistoric beginnings	55
Prostaglandin	48, 120, 122, 218, 311-2
Prostate	237
Ptyalin	57
Pyridoxine (see Vitamin B6)	
Pyrroluria	136-7
Retinol (see Vitamin A)	
Riboflavin (see Vitamin B2)	
Sally the Goat	17, 20, 252
Salt	15-25, 31, 37, 52, 67, 78, 94, 103, 167, 214, 223, 243, 273, 292
Salicylates	197, 209-11
Schizophrenia	42, 136, 182, 193, 228, 234
Selenium	101, 186-8, 215, 261, 281, 296, 320-2, 344-5,
Semen	92, 119, 143-4, 317
Serotonin	37, 41, 72, 78-9, 124, 135, 229, 328
Sewage	60, 64-7, 208
Sex	42, 47, 73, 89, 91, 97, 119, 143, 157, 241, 258, 299, 309, 352
Sleep	43-4, 77-8, 80-3, 110, 143, 160, 180, 193, 204, 290
Sodium	15-24, 67, 167, 214, 292
Statins	215-7, 305-7, 314-5
Steroids	40, 114, 139, 309, 311

Stomach acid	27, 57, 99, 119, 136, 250, 353
Stools	14, 27, 106, 147, 170, 226-7, 253, 293
Sugar	33-40, 43-4, 50, 54, 59, 63, 68-9, 78, 94, 111, 123, 127, 152, 154-5, 160, 173, 197, 205, 222, 224, 229, 239, 243, 254-8, 265, 268, 274, 284, 297, 302, 310, 313, 316, 327, 352
Sulphites	28-9, 177, 211-2
Sulphorathanes	6, 9, 320-1
Sulphur	28, 115, 172, 182, 211, 228, 282, 297, 320, 356
Sun (sunshine)	6, 68, 105, 137, 194, 205, 217, 228-9, 235, 297-8, 309, 322-5, 357
Tamoxifen	128, 191
Tea	9, 27, 83, 197, 244-5
Testosterone	98-100, 236, 309, 328
Thiamine (see Vitamin B1)	
Thrush	172-4
Thyroid	217, 233, 251, 273, 293, 310, 319, 328
Tinnitus	149, 220-2
Trans-fats	124, 219
Triffids	264-7
Triumph Spitfire	118
Tryptophan	37, 41, 43, 78-80, 229, 235
Ulcer	13, 84, 147, 170, 175, 180, 189, 210, 249-52, 318
Urine	22, 30, 74, 119, 136, 147, 150, 173, 211, 222-4, 255, 263, 288, 290, 293, 327
Vagina	97-8, 154, 173, 272, 279
Vanadium	34, 44, 102, 217-8, 257
Vegan	53, 149, 177, 230, 262
Vegetarian	13, 53, 132, 150, 177, 190, 235, 262, 318, 352
Vitamin A	75, 92, 105, 198-202, 206, 220, 230, 243, 247, 257, 280, 286-8
Vitamin B1	74, 75, 86-8, 182, 229-31
Vitamin B2	75, 134, 175, 177, 183, 191, 272
Vitamin B3	74, 75, 217, 234
Vitamin B4	76
Vitamin B5	75, 78, 159, 233
Vitamin B6	72, 75, 78, 135-7, 196, 272, 319, 347, 351
Vitamin B7	75, 151
Vitamin B12	53, 74, 78, 99, 135, 147-51, 189, 220-1, 229, 261-3, 348
Vitamin C	58, 75, 184

About the Author

Hamish MacGregor trained as a forensic scientist and began in pathology and drug analysis in 1968. He transferred to criminalistics and gained an honours degree in Metallurgy and Materials at Owen's College, Victoria University of Manchester, England. Later he ran other laboratories and then started his own independent forensic laboratory.

He has always felt that a forensic scientist has to have a working knowledge about many things, because when giving evidence they are asked about lots of scientific aspects of the career, not just their core skill. And the courts don't really want a true expert – someone who is at the peak of his or her career in some specialist subject – they want an objective, rounded overview. He will tell you that a good forensic scientist is proficient at many things, but their core skill is identifying the truth and explaining it in a way that the jury and the judge can understand. Of course, many forensic scientists do have a core skill – whether it is chemistry, mechanics, biology etc. or whatever; but the best experts have that rare ability to cut through the waffle and explain the complex in simple terms. The British system of justice demands it, because it is based on twelve 'lay persons' that form the jury in a court of criminal law, and these people are drafted from all walks of life so most of them have some difficulty with the principles on which forensic science is based. Even the judge sometimes has difficulty in understanding the mechanics behind the science, and has to be guided through it accurately and painstakingly.

Hamish admits it is probably that ability to explain the complex in understandable terms that has led him to look at health in a different way. In forensic science if the answer is blindingly obvious, it is usually right. The obscure does come along, and has to be investigated, indeed that is why a forensic scientist can rarely say that an event was 'irrefutable'. But if it seems right, well, you can jolly well bet that it usually is. It seems pretty obvious to a forensic scientist that if cystic fibrosis sufferers have a problem with salt retention, and the mucous in the lungs is affected by an absence of salt in the lining of the lungs, then a salt spray inhaler will help them. So we should not be surprised to find that cystic fibrosis sufferers benefit from going surfing. If too much Omega 6 and not enough Omega 3 affects mood and behaviour, you can bet that feeding Omega 3 to prisoners will improve their chances of integrating with society. And it does. Body Language is peppered with these examples. It is just a shame no-one has taken any notice until now.

Forensic science has recently been popularised by a number of television programmes and most universities offer forensic science courses, but there are very few jobs for graduates. Hamish is often asked by forensic science students where they can look for jobs, and he has opened their eyes to many areas of industry and commerce where

The Body Language of Health

their skills are invaluable. Forensic skills are not just confined to bodies under floorboards, after all. A degree in forensic science is a degree in common sense and logical, rational thinking; skills which many industries need. It is all a matter of application. Forensic science deserves to be more widely appreciated as an organised way of looking objectively at things.

So we should not be surprised to find that a forensic scientist's view of health has focussed on the obvious. Healthcare should be about prevention, not cure. Health should be about giving our body what it needs, and about observing those telltale clues.

Hamish MacGregor still practices forensic science and often attends courts giving evidence in his main areas of expertise of physical damage, tool marks, failure analysis and accident reconstruction, but he also finds time for his extra-curricular activities which include tinkering with old cars and various restoration projects.

Hamish MacGregor, of course, doesn't actually exist, it is a pseudonym, but all other references to Hamish's profession, contacts and events are absolutely real. It is bad enough in the medical world to be seen as a maverick, and even worse to spill the beans about the secret Body Language code that doctors use when they are in consultation with a patient. But there are powerful forces in the medical and pharmaceutical world that require a professional to assume a pseudonym to avoid adverse publicity; notoriety even.

However, although you don't actually know the true identity of the author you can be sure of one thing. The content of this book is sincere, carefully researched and has been written with the best of intentions by a real life forensic scientist of some standing. And like all good forensic reports, it comes with the following final reservations from the author.

'I can only write about the facts as I see them. I have tried to authenticate each section by referring to multiple works by others, but cannot vouch for its accuracy. In fact some of the more radical thoughts out there have gathered a wave of enthusiasm that adds authenticity, but then this is no more than some of the carefully chosen trials and reports that make a few of the latest developments in medicine appear to be the answer to all the health problems of humanity'.

'So take what I have said at face value, try it, but don't rely on it as my answer to humanity either. Body Language is meant to be a bit of fun, not life or death. What I have tried to do is give you a balanced, considered view and possibly open your eyes to some research you could do yourself about your particular condition. If at any time you have any doubts about your health, you should see your doctor. Do not attempt to make a diagnosis solely on the contents of this book'.

'If you have any reason to suggest that I have not represented the facts correctly, or that I should be aware of other factors that have not yet been disclosed to me, I would be happy to consider them and amplify or amend the content of the book accordingly for the future. Please send any communications to me at www.mybodylanguage.co.uk' I cannot reply personally but you can be certain that every communications will be read, considered and acted upon'.

I wrote this book because I was concerned that the EU were eroding the opportunities of the public to buy supplements. Did you know that most of our common herbs, and many of the essential ingredients to herbal and mineral remedies will no longer be available once the legislation kicks in? All because the greedy pharmaceutiucal giants want all the business for themselves. Time to kick them out, I say.

Please do your best to support the supply of natural herbs and minerals. NOW you can see how essential they are to your health. Please look at http://www.alliance-natural-health.org/ now and write to your MP telling them you want to have access to nature's healing products. Before it is too late.

I wish you the best of health with your new-found knowledge.

FURTHER READING

As I have said already, be careful what you read on the internet. But to be honest, the internet does present itself as an incredible source of information and stimulating debate. I will only recommend a few references here, because there is nothing worse than information overload. But these references are tried and tested and in my opinion represent a reasonably balanced view.

1. The McCarrison Society. http://mccarrisonsociety.org.uk The purpose of the Society is to assemble scientific knowledge on nutrition and health that is free from economic and political pressures with the object of securing the physical and mental health of future generations.
2. British Society of Integrated Medicine. http://www.bsim.org.uk Its mission is to form an open-minded forum of integrated medicine doctors, dentists, vets, complementary therapists and also to incorporate a patient 'voice'.
3. Newstarget Health. http://www.newstarget.com Ongoing review of health and environmental issues.
4. Prince Charles' Foundation for Integrated Health http://www.fih.org.uk The Foundation works towards a culture of health and wellbeing with people and communities taking more responsibility for their own health, and where health professionals collaborate and share learning in the best interests of their patients.
5. Dr Harry Morrow Brown's allergies website www.allergiesexplained.com recording his own extensive experience in asthma, allergies and eczema over a career spanning seventy years, with numerous illustrations.
6. www.mybodylanguage.co.uk of course, where you can also contribute your own views or favourite Body language signs.

We are currently working on a mammoth Body Language diagnostic tool incorporating those staggering 1400 Body language questions from which this book was compiled. I can say this because it will be true whenever you are reading this – it will be a developing, progressing website. Whenever you visit…… well, we will be working on it. So be sure to review what's new as often as you like, and contribute to the text yourself if you feel able.

The Body Language of Health

©First Edition 2008
Printed in Comic Sans
Published & distributed by

Eclipse Naturalcare Ltd
1 Prime Parkway
Derby
DE1 3QB
United Kingdom
Tel: 0044 (0)1332 365318
Fax 0044 (0)1332 292230
Email: info@eclipsenaturalcare.com
Web: www.eclipsenaturalcare.com

Printed by Biddles Limited
24 Rollesby Road
Hardwick Industrial Estate
King's Lynn
Norfolk
PE30 4LS
t: 00 44 1553 764728 f: 00 44 1553 764633
e: enquiries@biddles.co.uk w: www.biddles.co.uk

ISBN 978-0-9557909-0-4
PRICED £11.95 IN THE UK